RNA VIRUSES AND HOST GENOME IN ONCOGENESIS

RNA VIRUSES AND HOST GENOME IN ONCOGENESIS

Proceedings of a Conference,
held in Amsterdam, May 12-15, 1971

Editors

P. EMMELOT
Antoni van Leeuwenhoekhuis, Amsterdam

P. BENTVELZEN
Radiobiologisch Instituut, TNO, Rijswijk

1972

NORTH-HOLLAND PUBLISHING COMPANY – AMSTERDAM·LONDON
AMERICAN ELSEVIER PUBLISHING CO., INC. – NEW YORK

Library of Congress Catalog Number 70-183611

ISBN North-Holland 0 7204 4105 6
ISBN American Elsevier 0 444 10367 8
100 tables, 65 illustrations

Publishers:
NORTH-HOLLAND PUBLISHING COMPANY – AMSTERDAM
NORTH-HOLLAND PUBLISHING COMPANY, Ltd. – LONDON

Sole distributors for the U.S.A. and Canada:
AMERICAN ELSEVIER PUBLISHING COMPANY, INC.
52 Vanderbilt Avenue, New York, N.Y. 10017

PRINTED IN THE NETHERLANDS

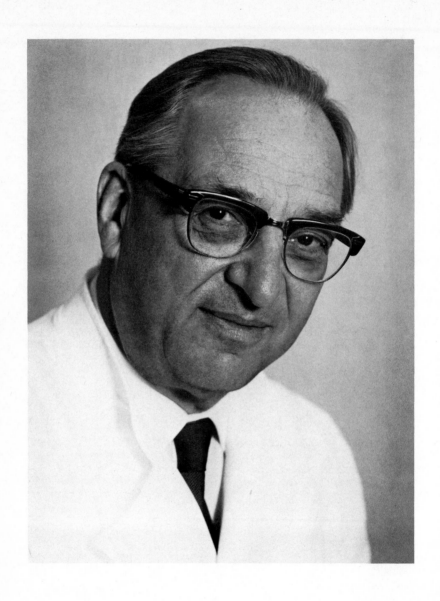

Professor Otto Mühlbock

This Conference was held on the occasion of the 65th birthday of Professor O. Mühlbock, retiring head of the Department of Biology, Antoni van Leeuwenhoekhuis, the Netherlands Cancer Institute.

It was organized by the Netherlands Cancer Institute and the Netherlands Organization for the Fight against Cancer (Koningin Wilhelmina Fonds). It was supported by the International Union against Cancer (U.I.C.C.); the Special Virus Cancer Program of the National Cancer Institute, Department of Health, Education, and Welfare, U.S.A. (Contract no. NIH-71-678); and the United Nations Educational, Scientific and Cultural Organization by way of the International Cell Research Organization.

PREFACE

Cancer is a pressing medical as well as a fundamental biological problem. It challenges the investigator because of its complex nature, which is not only reflected by the great variation in morphological, biological and biochemical characteristics found among separate tumors or displayed by individual tumors during their natural history (progression), but also by the multitude of etiological factors involved. The interaction between the various inducing agents or conditions is an intricate problem of cancer research, and is of paramount importance since human cancers may be of multifactorial origin. Also, endogenous factors or systems, such as immunity and genetic make-up, are decisive for the outcome of the cancerous process. Thus, cancer appears to arise by an interplay of exogenous and endogenous factors with inducing and permissive capacities.

We thought it a worthy tribute to Professor Otto Mühlbock, on occasion of his 65th birthday and retirement as head of the Biological Department of The Netherlands Cancer Institute, to organize a conference dealing with the interaction between various factors involved in the genesis of cancer. Professor Mühlbock has devoted the last 25 years to the study of the genesis of mammary cancer in mice. He and his collaborators paid much attention to the analysis and investigation of the various factors concerned, *viz.* viruses, hormones, genes and environmental conditions. A very important aspect of their work is the emphasis on the interrelation between these factors in the cancerous process.

It appeared to us to be the most promising to organize a conference with a limited scope rather than to cover the whole field of carcinogenesis. We decided upon "RNA viruses and host genome in oncogenesis" for several reasons. First, the mouse mammary tumor viruses belong to the group of RNA tumor viruses. Secondly, significant progress has been made in recent years in the field of the RNA tumor viruses which also had some impact on molecular biology in general. Thirdly, if some human cancers have a viral etiology, RNA tumor viruses are among the likely candidates. In several recent conferences these developments have been discussed. We are confident, however, that the present conference is not a mere replica of previous ones since here virologists and geneticists were discussing a common theme.

It cannot be ignored that work with the mouse mammary tumor viruses has not yet reached that stage of sophistication obtained with some other RNA oncogenic viruses, mainly because of the failure to develop an assay system for the virus *in vitro*. By bringing mammary-tumor virologists and investigators of other RNA tumor viruses together, it was hoped to provide the former with some new ideas whereas the latter might contemplate some aspects hitherto unique for the mammary tumor system. For instance, what is the significance of molecular models, such as the Temin provirus hypothesis, for the mammary tumor system? On the other hand, the discovery of very avirulent mammary tumor virus strains, which induce tumors in mice at a very late age, might imply that late appearing leukoses in chicken are induced by such slow viruses, and may lead investigators working with "explosive viruses" not to label a virus too soon as nontransforming. Evidently slow viruses could also be of prime importance in the etiology of various human cancers. In this connection it seems to make sense to distinguish both as to agents and mode of action, between the "natural disease" with a long latency and those experimentally-induced cancers which develop rapidly.

The classical relationship between viruses and host genetic factors is the genetically controlled susceptibility to a given virus. Although this relationship may seem not to be as complex in genetic terms as has been thought a decade ago, as yet relatively little is known as to how genes cause this susceptibility. One may theorize that gene products act at the level of virus penetration into the cell (*e.g.* "recognition"), the rate of virus replication, or control of the effects of the virus, *i.e.* neoplastic transformation. Highly interesting are the data which suggest that histocompatibility genes may play an important role in susceptibility to RNA tumor viruses. Although nothing definite is known yet about a viral etiology of human tumors – but circumstantial evidence is now accumulating that such tumors may indeed exist –, the observed correlation between certain histocompatibility genes in man and susceptibility to some forms of cancer, was reason enough to include this topic into the program.

Viral transformation is also governed by target-cell genome expression. Although RNA tumor viruses may replicate in many different tissues of a susceptible animal, neoplastic transformation seems to be restricted to mostly one cell type. Histocompatibility antigens being similar in these cases, it means that for transformation to occur the virus (products) should fit into a cell-specific program of gene activities.

Other aspects of the role of the host genome in the replication of RNA tumor viruses were also covered by the program of the conference. With regard to the molecular mechanism of replication, Temin once supposed that a DNA copy of the viral RNA would be made and, after integration into the host genome, serve as a template for the synthesis of viral RNA. The recent finding of the reverse transcriptase in the virions of many RNA tumor viruses seems to substantiate this originally heretic idea. In view of related activities in many growing tissues including tumors, it appears that the enzyme should be defined according to the chemical structure of its template, *i.e.* single-stranded RNA in the case of the tumor viruses, and the formation of RNA–DNA hybrids.

Finally, experimental support for the view that several RNA tumor viruses are genetically transmitted and much speculation as to its significance, has also been presented in recent years. Relevant data concerning both B particle-type (mammary tumor) and C particle-type (leukemia, sarcoma) viruses, were discussed in the present conference.

As well as by viruses, tumors can be induced by irradiation and chemical carcinogens. These agents have not been explicitly dealt with but were discussed in the restricted sense of "inducers" or potentiators of latent RNA tumor viruses, which might have been genetically transmitted. It is not our intention to suggest that all cancers can be explained on a viral basis. It may even be questioned whether in some cases a carcinogenic agent in the classical sense is needed altogether. Mere isolation of tissue cells from host regulatory factors, such as seems to be exemplified by cell culture and solid state carcinogenesis, would be enough. However, it is clear that studies on RNA viral oncogenesis and tumors in animals will be fruitful for our detecting, understanding, and hopefully curing such human cancers of this viral origin as might exist. In this respect the conference has tried to contribute a little to the medical problem.

We deeply appreciate the cooperation of all those institutions and individuals who have made the organization of this conference possible. We are most grateful to the International Union for the Fight against Cancer (U.I.C.C.), the special Cancer Virus Program of the National Cancer Institute of the U.S.A., and the United Nations Educational, Scientific and Cultural Organization via the International Cell Research Organization for financial support.

Finally we want to thank our colleagues of the Organizing Committee, in particular Drs. L.M. Boot and G. Röpcke who have been indefatigable in getting this meeting organized and going.

P. EMMELOT
P. BENTVELZEN

LIST OF CONTRIBUTORS

CONTENTS

Part 6. *Mammary tumorigenesis in mice*

Part 7. *The fourth Wassink Lecture*

Part 8. *DNA, RNA and viral carcinogenesis*

Part 1

INTRODUCTION

André LWOFF

Institut de Recherches Scientifiques
sur le Cancer, B.P. 8, 94-Villejuif, France

A number of distinguished workers, interested in the problem of RNA oncogenic viruses, are assembled in Amsterdam in order to pay tribute to Professor Otto Mühlbock on the occasion of his 65th birthday.

When I was invited to deliver the introductory lecture, I accepted gratefully and I selected an uncompromising title because I had no idea of what I was going to say. As a matter of fact, I find myself in a rather difficult position for I have never worked with an oncogenic virus. The late Francisco Duran-Reynals [1], in a review on "Neoplastic infection and cancer" which appeared in the *American Journal of Medicine,* wrote the following in 1950: "Evidently, the specialized worker suffers from some professional deformity with a touch of professional vanity, that makes him look at the agents and phenomena with which he is so familiar as capable of accomplishing what is inconceivable to another specialist equally deformed by his knowledge."

So far as oncogenic viruses are concerned, I feel unprejudiced and might thus be in a privileged position, but this did not solve my problem.

Since a few months, oncogenic RNA viruses have been discussed in a dozen meetings. So, everyone here knows everything about these viruses. Moreover, within a few days, everyone will have learned the present status of the subject. Yet, the present is essentially a transient, metastable state squeezed between a threatening past and unpredictable future veiled in the hazes of uncertainty.

In view of all these difficulties, I decided to act as a historian. My aim is to show some of the difficulties encountered with oncogenic viruses.

Oncogenic viruses

Up to 1934, the history of oncogenic viruses is relatively simple. In 1903, Amédé Borel [2] put forward the hypothesis according to which cancer is caused by viruses. Within the next thirty-five years, six cancers were shown to be transmitted by extracts or filtrates of tumors.

1908: Ellermann and Bang, Erythromyeloblastic form of chicken leukemia,
1911: Rous, Chicken sarcoma,
1932: Shope, Rabbit fibroma,
1933: Shope, Rabbit papilloma,
1936: Bittner, Mouse mammary carcinoma,
1938: Lucké, Frog kidney carcinoma.

At that time, cancer research was dominated by pathologists who often expressed their distrust of the so-called viral theory. The situation was analyzed by Duran-Reynals [1] who wrote the following: "It is not easy to know what is the reaction of people to the so-called "virus theory of cancer". . . Judging by what is written it is far from popular, but the opinion of people who think and do not write is just as good as the opinion of people who think and do write."

Yet, in 1943, Cornell University Press had published a book on "Virus diseases". Rous [3] contributed an article entitled "Viruses and cancer". It is an excellent review of oncogenic viruses. Here are his conclusions: "You may recall that the stated task of this lecture was a discussion of whether the relationship of viruses to tumors is casual or significant. Significant it assuredly is as making for enlarged thought and effort upon the tumor problem. Yet so little is known concerning tumors that it is still possible to conjure up a legion of causes for them as large as the imagination. But save for the viruses this legion is shadowy. The viruses are actual workmen in the cellular world."

Cancerologists should have been convinced but they were not. In 1952, the New York Academy of Sciences organized a symposium on "Viruses as causative agents in cancer". Rhoads [14], at the time director of the Sloan Kettering Institute, gave the introduction and wrote: "It may not be enough to invoke virus origin if a new neoplasm is caused by the injection of a cell-free extract of an old one. This does establish, of course, the importance of cellular components of less than cellular size. It does not, however, necessarily indicate that the sole cause of the neoplasm is a ubiquitous, foreign, semi-autonomous organism capable of evoking immune response. There is, in short, an important distinction to be drawn between cancer as the response to a contagious, infecting agent of conventional type, and cancer as a process of aggressive cellular growth due to the inheritance of new characteristics, consequent to the modification, by mutation, of components small and filterable, or large and non-filterable, which are responsible for old characteristics."

If we assume that these statements represent the view of conventional oncologists it appears that the situation was rather confused. Here is another example of scepticism against the virus. In 1952, again in New York, Gross [5] discusses his experiments on mouse leukemia and concludes: "These experiments suggest that the centrifugated leukemic extracts contain a transmissible pathogenic agent, which apparently exists in such extracts in an inactive form. When inoculated into a susceptible host, the agent remains dormant, or harmless for its host, until the host reaches middle age. At that time, for obscure reasons, the hitherto latent agent becomes activated, causing rapid multiplication of cells harboring it. This results in the development of leukemia and death of the host.

Since the leukemic agent apparently passes from the inoculated parents to their offspring, causing the development of leukemia in both these generations of mice, it is possible to assume that a similar phenomenon may take place, later on, in subsequent generations of mice. If this assumption is correct, it would then logically follow that the leukemic agent would continue the "vertical" trend of transmission, passing through the embryos from one generation to another, in this particular line of mice."

In 1957, the New York Academy of Sciences held another symposium on: "Subcellular particles in the neoplastic process". Law [6] discusses oncogenic viruses: "The recent flood of literature relating specifically to the role of cell-free agents in the etiology of "leukemia", principally in the mouse, has led to speculation and interpretations not wholly in accord with the basic knowledge gained through long, tedious, and well-controlled studies of many investigators.

The role of cell-free materials in the spontaneous occurrence of leukemia in mice and in the X-ray-, estrogen-, and carcinogen-induced diseases is by no means clear. It has been stated that filtrates from tissues of high-leukemic mice induce leukemia in a non-leukemic C3H/Bi strain. It appears that such materials may merely enhance the appearance of these neoplasms in a manner similar to that observed in (C3H x AKR)F_1 mice and in the AKR strain.

Although several investigators accept the viral nature of the filterable agent(s) in mouse leukemia, it is clear that no one had described properties specific to this agent that would set it apart from other possible biochemical complexes that possess leukemogenic activity.

The relationship of certain acellular materials to the spontaneous disease, or to its induction or enhancement by X-rays, estrogens, and carcinogenic hydrocarbons, has not been established as yet. It would indeed be premature, on the basis of present evidence, to state that "mouse leukemia was demonstrably caused by a filterable virus", that the disease is an "egg-borne virus disease", or that "the mouse leukemia virus is a spherical particle less than

70 mμ in diameter". The burden of proof rests with investigators who make these claims."

Yet, in the very same 1957 symposium, Andervont [7] expressed his faith in the viral theory: "In conclusion, no one can dispute the fact that viruses are involved in the cancer process. The virus theory no longer elicits violent reactions from its opponents, and its proponents in this publication have conceded that viruses may not be involved in all forms of cancer. The theory has attained a high level of respect in cancer research, for it enables the investigator to design an intelligent approach to the many problems to be confronted. Those who pursue this course objectively are certain to contribute to the control of the disease; for it is no longer a question of whether viruses induce tumors, but in how many neoplastic processes of different species they are involved."

Difficulties of the viral theory

In 1933, an eminent geneticist, Haldane [8], expressed his viewpoint about the viral theory: "Cancer cells do not reproduce sexually and it is only by sexual reproduction that the geneticists can distinguish nuclear changes from plasmatic changes or virus infections." I am afraid that nobody paid any attention to this pessimistic statement.

The difficulties encountered by the viral theory of cancer up to around 1950 were manifold and, among them, cytoplasmic particles. For the 1940-1955 period was obscured by plasmagenes. Here is a quotation of a review by Haddow [9], which appeared in 1944 in *Nature*: "Woods and DuBuy have recently brought evidence that the characteristics of plastid-controlled variegations are intermediate between those of normal plants and virus-diseased plants, and have endeavored to connect virus proteins phylogenetically over the variegation-inducing agents (abnormal plastids) with proteins of the normal plastids. There is little reason to doubt that variegation-inducing plastids frequently behave like viruses, just as the plant viruses have properties often shown by plasmagenes in interspecific crosses.

But, in certain cases similarity of behavior becomes identity, and, for the Rous agent at least, no real distinction can be drawn between its typical activity and that of a mutant plastogene." So, plasmagenes and plastogenes were in part responsible for the suspicion in which oncogenic viruses were held. More serious reasons existed.

Virology was slowly developing from its medical into its molecular phase. The development had been long and difficult. Twort had discovered bacteriophagy in 1915 but, around 1921, the very existence of bacteriophagy was questioned by most bacteriologists. When bacteriophagy was finally accepted, fierce polemics developed about the nature of bacteriophage. They raged until around 1935. Twort considered that bacteriophagy could be due to a virus. From the very beginning d'Hérelle was convinced that the bacteriophage was a virus. But, as late as 1931, a very eminent microbiologist claimed: "The invisible virus of d'Hérelle does not exist. The intense lytic action to which the name of bacteriophagy is given represents the pathological exaggeration of a function belonging to the physiology of bacteria."

Although the genetic material had been identified in 1944 as nucleic acid, as late as 1955, Burnet [10], in his "Principles of virology", still claimed that the protein of the papilloma virus is the infectious material and represents the virus.
      For many animal and plant virologists, the term "virus" designated the infectious particle. When no infectious particles were detectable, it was often concluded that no virus was present. Yet, plants or animals devoid of detectable virus sometimes start producing infectious particles. Consequently, it was admitted that viruses can arise *de novo*. At a time when plant virology was ahead of animal virology, the King Edward Potato had become fashionable. This potato was supposed by Salaman [11] "to create its own virus" and that this virus might be "a plastogene or a gene displaced from the chromosome". To allow myself a short digression: Modern sociologists think that society is shaped by capitalism, communism, or by some other "ism". They could perhaps read with profit the book published by Salaman in 1952 entitled: "The potato's influence in shaping society".
      The appearance of infectious particles had also been observed in animals where no virus could be detected beforehand. This was the case for mice and mammary tumor agent and Bittner [12] in 1952, had concluded that "the active milk influence" can arise *de novo*. Yet, some virologists did not accept the *de novo* hypothesis and admitted that virus, although not detectable, could nevertheless be present. It could be present in a masked state. What masking meant was not clear.
      Up to 1950, the modern students of bacteriophages in America did not believe in the existence of lysogenic bacteria. It is therefore not too surprising that viral oncologists did not pay any attention to lysogeny which could have provided them with useful models. It would have been beneficial for them to be aware of the fact discovered by Burnet and McKie [13], in 1929, that lysogenic bacteria do *not* contain phage particles. It would have helped them to be aware of the fact disclosed by Eugène Wollman [14] in 1937 that after infection of a bacterium by a bacteriophage there is a *non-infectious* phase.

It was only in 1953 that a cancer worker, namely Duran-Reynals [15], took advantage of the work on bacteriophagy. It had been shown that the genetic material of the bacteriophage can be integrated as prophage. Duran-Reynals realized that masking, that is absence of infectious particles, could be due to the fact that the virus either was in its vegetative phase or be present as a provirus. Masking, added Duran-Reynals, did not exist in bacterial infections. It was a specific feature of viruses. A clear-cut difference between viral and bacterial infections was established. In fact, it is only in 1953 that viruses were separated from non-viruses and defined as infectious particles containing only one type of nucleic acid, devoid of metabolism, unable to grow and to divide and reproduced from their genetic material only.

Within a few years, the main problems posed by oncogenic viruses, if not solved, were correctly posed. Among them was the problem of repression and derepression of viral functions in transformed cells.

Repression and derepression of viral functions

Ahlström and Andrewes [16] had discovered, in 1938, that Shope's rabbit fibroma, a benign local infection, can be made active and generalized by tar or carcinogenic hydrocarbons. "Time and experiences will show — wrote Andrewes in August 1950 [17] — whether this finding has any bearing on the power of chemical carcinogens to evoke cancer, whether in fact they can perchance be acting by upsetting an equilibrium between a tumor virus and its host cell." A few months earlier, in April 1950, Duran-Reynals [1] had written: "All in all, it seems extremely probable that viruses are the proximal cause of the tumors resulting after injection of chemicals." A most brilliant intuition!

In fact, in that very year 1950, it was shown that UV light induces the "unmasking" of the prophage, that is induces the vegetative phase which culminates in the production of virions. And the hypothesis was proposed in 1953 (A. Lwoff [18]) that the neoplastic potentiality of a cell was perpetuated in the form of the genetic material of a virus and that carcinogenic agents act by inducing the expression of the potentialities of the viral genetic material, expression which would culminate in the formation of new viral particles.

A meeting on Oncogenic Viruses was held in Rye in 1960. The discussion led to the following statements: "We are obviously dealing here with repression and "derepression" of viral functions, and we have to conclude that, from a practical point of view, a virogeny-like situation does exist."

"From a theoretical point of view, virogeny, the situation homologous to lysogeny, would imply a complete repression and also the attachment of the genetic material of the tumor virus to a specific receptor of the cell, whether chromosomal or not" (Lwoff [19]).

It is known that in numerous virus transformed or malignant cells, a number of viral functions are not expressed. For example, viral proteins are not synthesized in the germinative layer of the papillomatous skin nor in the SV40 transformed cells. The non-expressed viral functions are induced by a variety of factors: differentiation in the case of the skin cells; fusion with the permissive cells in the case of SV40 transformed cells.

In order to account for data concerning the mammary tumor viruses, Bentvelzen [20] has been led to postulate the existence of a repressor and also of mutations of regulator and operator genes.

Cassingena and Tournier [21] have shown that the extract of SV40 transformed cells contains something which acts as a repressor. It decreases the plaque count, decreases the fraction of infected permissive cell synthesizing viral proteins, and decreases the infectivity of viral DNA. The infectivity is restored with trypsin. The activity of the extract of transformed cells is suppressed by trypsin. Moreover, the extract of *permissive* cells neutralizes the effect of the extract of *transformed* cells. *The extract of permissive cells also induces the vegetative phase of the virus in SV40 transformed cells.* The extract of non-permissive cells is devoid of inducing activity. Finally, the extract of SV40 transformed cells acts only on SV40 and not on polyoma or other viruses. The extract of polyoma transformed cells acts only on polyoma virus. Things happen as if the extract of a *virus transformed cell* would contain something which inhibits some viral functions, this inhibition being specific. Things happen also as if the extract of permissive cells would contain something which inactivates the factor responsible for inhibition. The simplest hypothesis is that the substance which inhibits viral functions is a repressor.

Whatever the case might be, inhibition and induction of viral functions is one of the key problems facing viral oncologists. Physical and chemical carcinogens induce the vegetative development of the bacteriophage in lysogenic bacteria. X-rays induce the formation of the virions of the leukemia and of the mammary carcinoma viruses.

On March 31, 1971, an anonymous correspondent of *Nature* [22] suggested that there is no counterpart to an immunity factor — that is to a repressor — in transformed cells. It is true that the existence of a repressor in transformed cells had not been demonstrated. Yet, one should not ignore that viral functions can be specifically inhibited and induced.

Is the oncogenic power of an oncogenic virus a property of the virus?

Another question concerning oncogenic viruses is still posed nowadays: is the oncogenic power of an oncogenic virus a property of the virus? This question might seem strange, for the fact that a virus is able to induce a cancer is today out of the question. So, what to do when one dislikes oncogenic viruses? Simply to decide that the viral genes are not responsible for malignant transformation. The virus is oncogenic because it transduces cellular genes. This hypothesis was discussed by Hieger [23] in 1961 and was proposed again by an anonymous correspondent of *Nature* [24], who, on March the 17th, 1971, writes the following: "A devil's advocate might these days well argue that spontaneous cancer has nothing to do with viruses and even in animals is not a virus disease. It is possible, for example, to put together a not entirely implausible case that those animal tumor viruses, which now provide a livelihood to so many people, are the creation of unnatural rather than natural selection. ... Is it unreasonable to suggest that the initial transformation to malignancy has nothing at all to do with virus infection? All the subsequent manipulations of the tumor cells may result in the selection of a virus which is tumorigenic because it has picked up from the tumor cells in which it multiplied the cellular genes capable of causing transformation."

The difficulty is that many oncogenic viruses are not oncogenic to their natural host. So, it would be necessary to admit that before they can transform the cell they infect, their genome has to be reinforced by some cellular genes capable of causing transformation. Are these genes coming from the normal cells of the natural host, or from the normal cells which are going to be transformed? Of course, the viral genes responsible for transformation have to come from somewhere but this does not mean that the transduction hypothesis is acceptable.

The development of our knowledge concerning mammary cancer

In view of the fact that we are celebrating for Professor Otto Mühlbock, an historical survey of the development of mouse mammary carcinoma is not out of place.

In 1936, Bittner [25] recognized that a milk adjuvant was instrumental in the development of cancer. The adjuvant was later on called milk influence, milk factor, milk agent. In 1944, Bittner considered that the influence is probably a colloid of high molecular weight. That very same year, Andervont and Bryan [25] showed that the agent elicits the production of antibodies, a characteristic of known tumor viruses. And in 1952, Andervont [27] concludes firmly that the milk influence is a virus, and added: "Such a virus fulfills the requirements for the virus theory of cancer to a considerable extent, insofar as this type of tumor in this species is concerned." But, in 1957, Bittner [28], fully aware of the virus-like characteristics of the milk factor, still calls it "influence".

"For the development of mammary carcinoma in virgin and breeding females three agents usually must be present and active," claims Bittner:

"(a) an active mammary tumor milk influence which is generally transferred by nursing,

(b) hormonal stimulation of the mammary tissue resulting in growth suitable for the cancerous change,

(c) an inherited susceptibility to the development of spontaneous mammary tumors which may be transmitted by males and females of the susceptible stock."

What is the relation of these three factors? In 1939, Lacassagne [29], who had shown that estrogens can induce mammary cancer in the male mouse, writes an extensive paper on the relationships of hormone and mammary cancer. Although Lacassagne quotes Bittner's papers, no reference is made to the milk factor. Bittner [30] considers in 1942 the three influences: milk inciter, genetic inciter and estrogen inciter as complementary factors. Duran-Reynals [1] expressed a slightly different opinion in 1950: "The hormone just prepares the ground for a virus present in the milk and other body fluids or tissues in the proper genetic background." Thus, Bittner proposes a balanced concept according to which the genetic, the hormonal and the viral factors, play an equal role. Lacassagne ignored the virus and made the hormone responsible for the mammary cancer. Duran-Reynals took the emphasis off the hormone.

Yet, it was discovered by Otto Mühlbock [31], in 1956, that hundred per cent of supposedly virus free mice develop mammary cancer after implantation of the hypophysis. The obvious conclusion was that the hormonal factor is a primary one in the development of mammary cancer and that therefore, in mice carrying the virus, the virus is only an accelerator or an intensifier. At the 1957 meeting of the New Academy of Sciences, Andervont [7] also accepts the existence of mouse strains devoid of the mammary tumor virus and writes: ". . . The fact remains that the presence of the virus is not essential for the production of breast cancer. Chemical carcinogens are also able to induce these tumors in strains of mice that, under normal conditions, develop few breast tumors and do not harbor the virus."

The real question now is the very existence of virus-free mice. If they do

exist, can a cancer develop as a result of the action of estrogens or of carcinogens? I confess that I have been unable to form an opinion.

Let us nevertheless consider the problem of the relative roles of the hormone
and of the virus in transformation. The experiments of Rhim and co-workers
[32], although they deal with carcinogens, are worth reporting. Rat embryonic
cells are not transformed either by dimenthylbenzanthracene nor by the
Rauscher virus alone. Yet, if both factors are allowed to act simultaneously, the
cells are transformed. Here, like in the mouse mammary tumor, both agents
seem to be complementary. Now, the carcinogen alone and the virus alone can
transform mouse cells. Why embryonic rat cells do require both agents is not
clear. Anyhow, in that particular case, the carcinogen and the virus are both
essential and complementary.

If mammary cancer can develop in a virus free mouse, then the virus would
not be necessary. But when the virus is present it seems to play an important
role. Is is now clear that hormones which control the development and
differentiation of the mammary gland also controls the development of the
virus. The action on the virus could of course be indirect, that is mediated by
the cell. Whatever the case might be, the development of our knowledge
concerning the mammary tumor virus shows that the value of an opinion does
not lie so much in its correctness as in its power to act as a catalyst for
experimental work. Even if the hypothesis is wrong, good experiments
necessarily lead to the right conclusions. Moreover, anyone can have the right
idea whereas only few are able to perform good experiments. This is especially
true in the field of mammary carcinoma.

Finally, I may add a few words on the interaction between host and viral
genomes.

Everybody knows that a proviral phase probably exists for some DNA
oncogenic viruses, especially the Simian Virus 40. So far as RNA oncogenic
viruses are concerned, the history begins in 1962 with Temin [33], who proposed
the hypothesis that oncogenic RNA viruses are reproduced in the form of a
provirus, that is of DNA integrated with a cellular chromosome. A few years
later, in 1968, Bentvelzen [20] studies the transmission of the nodule inducing
virus and of the Mühlbock virus and concludes that the two viruses, in their
strain of origin, are replicated and transmitted as a provirus. Finally, in 1970,
Hanafusa and Myamoto [34] show that the factor Chf could be the genome of
an avian leukosis virus integrated within a cellular chromosome.

Thus, it appears probable that within a few years the existence of a provirus
of DNA and of RNA oncogenic viruses will be demonstrated. The problem of
the inhibition and induction of viral functions of course remains. This is to my
mind one of the key problems of cancer research.

References

[1] F. Duran-Reynals, Am. J. Med. 8 (1950) 490.
[2] A. Borrel, Bull. Inst. Pasteur 5 (1907) 593, 641.
[3] Viruses and cancer, In: Virus Diseases, Cornell Univ. Press, 1943, p.147.
[4] C.P. Rhoads, Ann. N.Y. Acad. Sci. 54 (1952) 872.
[5] L. Gross, Ann. N.Y. Acad. Sci. 54 (1952) 1184.
[6] L.W. Law, Ann. N.Y. Acad. Sci. 68 (1957) 616.
[7] H.B. Andervont, Ann. N.Y. Acad. Sci. 68 (1957) 649.
[8] J.B.S. Haldane, Nature 182 (1933) 265.
[9] A. Haddow, Nature 154 (1944) 194.
[10] F.M. Burnet, Principles of animal virology, Academic Press, N.Y., 1955.
[11] R.N. Salaman, The potato's influence in shaping society, 1952.
[12] J.J. Bittner, Cancer Res. 2 (1942) 710.
[13] F.M. Burnet and M. McKie, Australian J. Exptl. Biol. Med. Sci. 6 (1929) 277.
[14] E. Wollman and E. Wollman, Compt. Rend. Soc. Biol. 124 (1937) 931.
[15] F. Duran-Reynals, Virus-induced tumors and the virus theory of cancer, In: The physiology of cancer, F. Hamburger and W.H. Fishman (eds.), Hoeber-Harper, N.Y., 1953, p. 298.
[16] C.G. Ahlstrom and C.H. Andrewes, J. Pathol. Bacteriol. 47 (1938) 65.
[17] C.H. Andrewes, Brit. Med. J. 14 (1950) 81.
[18] A. Lwoff, Bacteriol. Rev. 17 (1953) 271.
[19] A. Lwoff, Cancer Res. 20 (1960) 820.
[20] P. Bentvelzen, Genetical control of the vertical transmission of the Mühlbock mammary tumor virus in the GR mouse strain, Hollandia, Amsterdam, 1968.
[21] H.G. Suarez, G.E. Sonensheim, R. Cassingena and P. Tournier, In: The biology of oncogenic viruses, L.G. Silvestri (ed.), North-Holland Publishing Company, Amsterdam, 1971, p.1; and personal communication.
[22] Anonymous, Nature New Biology 230 (1971) 129.
[23] I. Hieger, Carcinogenesis, Academic Press, N.Y., 1961.
[24] Anonymous, Nature New Biology 230 (1971) 65.
[25] J.J. Bittner, Ann. N.Y. Acad. Sci. 68 (1957) 636.
[26] H.B. Andervont and W.R. Bryan, J. Natl. Cancer Inst., 5 (1944) 143.
[27] H.B. Andervont, Ann. N.Y. Acad. Sci. 54 (1952) 1004.
[28] J.J. Bittner, Ann. N.Y. Acad. 68 (1957) 636.
[29] A. Lacassagne, Am. J. Cancer 37 (1939) 414.
[30] J.J. Bittner, Cancer Res. 2 (1942) 710.
[31] O. Mühlbock, Adv. Cancer Res. 4 (1956) 371.
[32] J.S. Rhim, M. Vass and H.Y. Cho, Int. J. Cancer 7 (1971) 65.
[33] H.M. Temin, Cold Spring Harbor Symp. Quant. Biol. 27 (1962) 407.
[34] H. Hanafusa, T. Hanafusa and T. Miyamoto, In: The biology of oncogenic viruses, L.G. Silvestri (ed.), North-Holland Publishing Company, Amsterdam, 1971, p. 170.

Part 2

GENERAL ASPECTS

GENETIC FACTORS IN TUMORIGENESIS

W.E. HESTON
Laboratory of Biology, National Cancer Institute
Bethesda, Md., U.S.A.

Because of the warm friendship I have enjoyed with Professor Otto Mühlbock over these many years and the excellent working relationship between the Netherlands Cancer Institute and both the Jackson Laboratory where I started in cancer research and the National Cancer Institute where I have been these many years, I was very pleased to accept the invitation to take part in this conference.

I have been asked to help build a foundation for this meeting by reviewing some of the studies of the past that have directed the thinking and progress of research leading up to the present conference.

Medical research progresses in waves, and today viruses are riding the crest of the wave of cancer research. Three to four decades ago the genetics of the host was on the crest of the wave and virus was a forbidden word in cancer research. In our institute Dr. Ray Bryan was permitted to work on the Rous sarcoma virus only if he called it chicken tumor agent I. The present conference is going to make it clear that the greater advances in cancer research in the future are going to be made at the union of the host genome and the virus.

This conference has been in the process of development for over 60 years. Bashford [1,2] and Murray [3] published in the Proceedings of the Royal Society of London in 1909 and 1911 results from their breeding experiments which revealed that female mice in whose ancestry cancer of the mammary glands occurred not farther back than grandmothers were more liable to develop mammary cancer than were those in whose ancestry cancer was more remote. In 1924 Lynch [4] published the results from her crosses between females of a high mammary cancer strain with males from a low mammary cancer strain. She observed a higher incidence in females from the backcross of the F_1 to the high tumor strain than in those of the F_2 generation, indicating the effect of genetic factors.

During this interim there had been the running debate between Slye [5]

13

arguing that cancer as a single disease was inherited as a simple recessive trait, and Little [6] who recognized much greater complexity. Slye was at a disadvantage because she did not inbreed her strains of mice and she lost the debate, whereas Little had foreseen that in order to analyze any trait as complex as cancer one would have to have controlled genetic material. He had started inbreeding his strains and with them he was able to substantiate his claims. It was the development of these inbred strains of mice by Little, Strong, and others that gave the impetus for the surge in research on the genetics of cancer in the decades to follow.

Lung tumors

The best tumor for classical genetic analysis has been the lung tumor of the mouse. The genetic influences are evident and the picture is not complicated by hormonal factors. If there is a virus involved in lung tumors it must be so intimately associated with the genome that thus far we have not been able to identify it. Furthermore, lung tumors can be induced by a host of chemical carcinogens and this does not alter the genetic picture. These induced tumors appear as discrete nodules that can be counted accurately giving a quantitative measure of response so advantageous in genetic analyses.

Bittner [7] observed that his strain A mice that had been inbred by Strong had a high incidence of lung tumors. He crossed his high lung tumor strain A with the low lung tumor strain C57BL and obtained results that suggested single dominant factor inheritance. The incidence of lung tumors in the F_1 was approximately that in strain A and the incidence in the F_2 was approximately ¾ of that in strain A. This work was done carefully, the numbers were large and the average ages at which the animals were autopsied were recorded.

Andervont [8] obtained results for chemically induced lung tumors which would seem to substantiate Bittner's conclusions but he recognized that there was variation in latent period and great variation among the inbred strains in response to the carcinogen indicating more complex inheritance. Lynch [9] observed that the number of induced tumors occurring in each animal was also influenced by genetic factors.

A rather extensive analysis of the inheritance of both spontaneous and dibenzanthracene-induced lung tumors was carried out in my own laboratory (Heston [10, 11]) with crosses between susceptible strain A and the resistant strain C57L. When response was measured in terms of the number of induced tumor nodules in the lung the results were typical of quantitative inheritance involving multiple genes. The mean response of the F_1 mice was intermediate between that of the parent strains; the mean response of the F_2 was likewise intermediate but with greater variation than that of the F_1's; the mean of the mice resulting from backcrossing the F_1 to strain A was intermediate between that of the F_1 and of A; and the mean of the backcross of the F_1 to strain C57L was intermediate between the F_1 and C57L. When response was measured in terms of latent period similar results were obtained. From the excess of variation in the F_2 over that in the F_1 it was estimated that at least 4 pairs of genes must be involved.

When age was controlled the results for spontaneous pulmonary tumors were similar to those for the induced tumors. At a given age the incidence of lung tumors in the F_1 was intermediate to that of strain A and of strain C57L and the incidence in the C57L backcross was intermediate between that of the F_1 and the C57L. This indicated that more than one pair of genes were involved also in the development of spontaneous lung tumors, which gave an explanation of why there could be strains of mice with intermediate incidences of lung tumors as well as those with high and low incidences.

Thus far, there have not been conclusive data for the identification and location of a specific gene for lung tumors. Tatchell [12] believed she had evidence for such a gene in linkage group VII and she designated the gene as *tu*, but her conclusion was based on coupling data and was never confirmed by repulsion data. Bloom and Falconer [13] postulated a lung tumor resistant gene *ptr* by which A and C57BL differed but this has never been located in a linkage group.

Effects of specific known genes

Many known genes have been shown to either increase or decrease the occurrence of lung tumors [14]. Hairless in linkage group III has been associated with a decrease in lung tumors. Lethal yellow and viable yellow, alleles in group V, increase lung tumors. Vestigial tail, shaker-2 and waved-2 in group VII have been associated with a decrease in lung tumors. Fused in group IX, obese in group XI, and flexed-tail in group XIV have been associated with a decrease in lung tumors. The gene for dwarf inhibits lung tumors. It appears that these results represent the effect of the genes tested rather than linkage with a tumor gene, and that this effect is in some way related to the effect of the gene tested on normal growth, for these genes tend to effect normal growth in the same direction that they effect susceptibility to lung tumors [15].

Similar linkages have been observed by a number of other investigators between these and other genes and other kinds of tumors. MacDowell *et al.*

[16] showed that dilution in linkage group II was associated with leukemia, and Law [17] showed that flexed-tail was likewise associated with leukemia. The latter undoubtedly was a pleiotropic effect since flexed-tail is known to have an influence on the hemopoietic system. Murphy [18] reported linkage between the steel locus and leukemia, and Meier et al. [19] have shown that hairless is associated with susceptibility to leukemia. Recently Deringer [20] has reported that lethal yellow increased susceptibility to reticular neoplasms. Bittner [21] linked brown with mammary tumors and we [22] found that obese reduced mammary tumors probably through its effect upon endocrine secretion. Brown [23] also has been linked with gastric tumors. Steel has been used by Stevens [24] to increase the testicular teratomas that occur in his strain 129 mice. Both lethal yellow and viable yellow increase the occurrence of hepatomas [25] but they also increase liver size [26]. Obese [22] also increases hepatomas. Lethal yellow [27] increases induced skin tumors.

One of the most remarkable effects of a specific gene is that of viable dominant spotting on ovarian tumors [28]. The introduction of this gene can increase the incidence of ovarian tumors from 0 to 100%, the sequence of changes in the ovary being similar to those following irradiation. The dwarf gene that stops normal growth at about 8 to 11 days causes a drastic inhibition of tumors [29]. The only tumors I have ever known to occur in a dwarf mouse were a few chemically induced lung tumors and they did not grow beyond barely visible size.

Reports later at this conference undoubtedly will be concerned with linkage between some of these genes or others and specific oncogenic viruses. I am sure that Meier and his coworkers think the association with the hairless gene is between this gene and the leukemia virus. Later in this conference others will discuss the relationship between histocompatibility genes of the mouse and the leukemogenic viruses.

Induced subcutaneous tumors

In early studies of subcutaneous tumors induced with dibenzanthracene, Andervont [30] mated the highly susceptible strain C3H to the more resistant strains Y and I and observed that in each case the susceptibility of the F_1 was intermediate to the two parent strains. He concluded that if susceptibility to the carcinogen has a genetic basis it is probably due to the influence of multiple factors. Burdette [31] measured the susceptibility of strains C3H and JK, and their F_1 hybrids to the induction of subcutaneous tumors with methylcholanthrene. He observed that C3H was more susceptible than JK and that the F_1

was intermediate, as Andervont had found. He concluded that the results were compatible with the existence of more than one gene for susceptibility to induced tumors, at least one of which is dominant and at least one of which is recessive. An alternative postulate from these data could have been a single pair of genes with incomplete dominance had it not been for the wide variation in a number of inbred strains tested.

Leukemia

Early studies on the genetics of leukemia in mice were carried out particularly by MacDowell and coworkers, and by Cole and Furth. From hybridization studies between their high-leukemia strain AKR and their low-leukemia strain Rf, Cole and Furth [32] concluded that leukemia was inherited probably as a multiple factor character. In the various crosses the common logarithm of the percent leukemia was a simple function of the percent heredity from the AKR strain.

The experiment of MacDowell and coworkers [33] designed to show with progeny tests whether there was a clear cut segregation of genes for leukemia in the backcross generation stands as a classic genetic study of cancer. The experiment was started by mating a single male of the high-leukemia strain C58 to 3 females of the low-leukemia strain StoLi. Seven of their F_1 sons were backcrossed to 18 StoLi females. Fifty males from this backcross born between June 30, 1937 and July 13, 1937 were the subjects of this study. The reassortment of genes in these 50 males was indicated by the segregation of the 3 pairs of coat color genes by which the parent strains differed. The question was whether by breeding tests, i.e., by incidence of leukemia in their progeny, these males would be shown to be intrinsically uniform or diverse in regard to the tendency to leukemia. On September 21, 1937 each of the 50 males was mated to 10 StoLi females in the second backcross. I clearly recall hearing on a visit with MacDowell his recounting how these 500 StoLi females that were from inbred generations 41 to 43 and had been born between April 12 and July 21, 1937, were mated with the males in such a way as to distribute equally among the males any possible differences in the females. Females were placed with males only when in estrus, an extra box being maintained for those not in estrus, and the females were isolated when vaginal plugs were found. Four hundred Bagg Albino foster nurses were standing by to nurse second backcross litters so their mothers could be remated on the day of parturition. MacDowell practically lived in the animal room, as only he would have done, to see that the experiment would be carried out controlled in the most minute detail.

The 50 second backcross families from these 50 males varied in number from 49 to 56, totalling 2,677 animals on which diagnoses were made and the incidence of leukemia in each family determined. The results indicated that the problem was more complex than had been anticipated. The incidence of leukemia in the 50 families ranged from 0 to 42.8 %, and instead of the families grouping as would be expected from segregation of a single pair or a few pairs of genes, there was a fairly symmetrical frequency distribution with the modal class at 17 to 20%. Detailed analyses of the data revealed certain extrinsic influences despite the great care with which the experiment was conducted, but since the variation between families transcended the variation caused by these influences it could be concluded that the 50 backcross fathers were genetically diverse as the result of the segregation of genes influencing the incidence of leukemia.

Gross' observation in 1951 [34] of the transmission of mouse leukemia by cell-free extracts inoculated into newborn mice followed by the discovery of the Moloney virus and other leukemogenic viruses shifted the emphasis from the genotype of the host to the virus. Law and Moloney [35, 36] noted in reciprocal hybridization studies that the Moloney virus was transmitted principally through the maternal line, if indeed at all through the male and in foster-nursing studies it was shown to be transmitted readily by the milk. This was in sharp contrast with the leukemias of the high-leukemia strains such as C58 and AKR which had always been seen to pass as readily through the male as through the female. This suggested that any leukemogenic virus in these high-leukemia strains must be very closely associated with the host genome. Thus, we have the link connecting the early work of Cole and Furth, and of MacDowell and coworkers with the present conference.

Mammary tumors

Soon after the Jackson Laboratory had become established in its new location at Bar Harbor, Maine, in 1929, the staff set up crosses between high- and low-mammary tumor strains that they had developed by that time. The high-tumor strain DBA was crossed with the low-tumor strain C57BL and also with a line of *Mus bactrianus*. High-tumor strain A was crossed with low-tumor strain CBA(X) and high-tumor strain C3H(Z) was crossed with low-tumor strain I. As was the usual practice in any genetic experiment at that time, reciprocal crosses were made. The significant outcome of these crosses, the results of which could be tabulated some 3 years later, was the difference between the reciprocal hybrids. The mammary tumor incidence of the F_1 coincided with that of the maternal strain [39].

At the same time Korteweg [38] who was then director of the Netherlands Cancer Institute and who had obtained breeding stock of Little's strains DBA and C57BL, was also making crosses between these high- and low-tumor strains and was also including the reciprocal cross. His data, like the Jackson Laboratory data, showed a difference between the reciprocal F_1 females, the incidence of mammary tumors in the F_1 being like that of the maternal strain.

Since the chromosomes of the reciprocal females were identical (although the reciprocal males would have differed in their sex chromosomes) the influence passed from the mother causing the daughter to develop mammary cancer, had to be extrachromosomal. Thus, in these two laboratories on opposite sides of the Atlantic, an extrachromosomal factor in mammary tumors of the mouse had been discovered. This was a very significant event in the chain of events leading to the conference we are holding today. The first virus to be universally accepted as a tumor virus was discovered by geneticists using genetic techniques.

Through his foster-nursing studies, Bittner [39] was able to show that the extrachromosomal factor causing mammary tumors in mice was an agent transmitted through the milk and he promptly named it the milk factor or milk agent. But throughout his scientific career Bittner never lost sight of the genetics of the host. In all of his papers he emphasized the importance of the three factors, the genetic constitution of the host, the hormonal influence, and the milk agent.

In 1942 Bittner [40] published incidences of mammary tumors in the high-tumor strain A, in the low-tumor strain C57BL, and in their F_1 and F_2 generations that suggested dominant single gene inheritance. The incidence in the females of the F_1 generation that received the milk agent approached 100% being comparable with the incidence in the high-tumor strain A, and that in the F_2 females with the agent was approximately 75%. The incidence in the backcross to the resistant parent strain was approximately 50%. The average age at which the tumors appeared in both the F_1 and F_2 females was greater than that in strain A which is important since, as he also showed, mice which developed tumors at an early age had progeny with a higher incidence of mammary tumors than mice born to mothers that developed their tumors at a later age.

In 1945 we [41] published the results of a study designed to ascertain whether or not there was gene control over the mammary tumor virus. High-tumor strain C3H females were outcrossed to low-tumor strain C57BL males and the resulting F_1 females were backcrossed to males of each parent strain. This resulted in two groups of backcross females that should have received the virus in equal amounts and should have been equal in respect to any other maternal influences since both groups had F_1 mothers. They differed in that the group with C3H fathers would be expected to have on the average 75% susceptible strain chromatin, whereas the group with the C57BL fathers would have an average of 25 % susceptible strain chromatin. Both groups were then tested with foster-nursed uniform (B x C3H)F_1 females to see if this difference in genotype would result in a difference in quantity or quality of virus as detected in the mammary tumor incidences of the two groups of test females. The results indicated that there was genetic control over the propagation and transmission of the virus, for the difference between the test groups was statistically significant. Thus, we had reached another step in the development of the subject of our present conference.

These results, published in 1945, stimulated considerable thought regarding the intimate relationship of this agent or virus to the host cell. The virus was viewed more as an integral part of the cell. It was looked upon somewhat as a plasmagene of Darlington, the Kappa factor of Sonneborn, or the transmissible mutagen of Murphy. Questions were raised as to whether it could arise by mutation of some part of the cell, as to how many genes were involved in controlling it, and as to whether the virus could be eliminated solely by altering the genotype of the host and if so, would it be brought back? A very extensive study involving several series of backcrosses was then undertaken to attempt to answer these questions [42].

In one series in which susceptible strain C3H females were outcrossed to resistant strain C57BL males and this was followed by a series of backcrosses to the resistant strain males, we observed that by building up a background of C57BL genotype the virus was eliminated and this was accomplished by the third backcross generation. The fact that this was done so quickly indicated that there were relatively few genes controlling the virus and suggested that there might be only one. By the time this information was obtained the series had reached the seventh backcross generation.

We then started backcrossing to susceptible strain C3HfB males to see if by reconstituting susceptible strain C3H genotype the virus would appear again. Some mammary tumors did appear in the females of this series but it was obvious that they were not due to the usual mammary tumor virus and were then considered to be the result of the susceptible genotype alone, a conclusion we were later to modify.

For a second series we started by outcrossing C57BL females to C3HfB males and backcrossing to C3HfB males to see if the virus would arise in the presence of the susceptible strain C3H genotype. Again a few tumors arose, but there was no evidence of the usual mammary tumor virus and we again interpreted their cause as simply the susceptible strain genotype.

For a third series we started with C57BL females and outcrossed to C3H males and this was followed by a series of backcrosses to C3H males. Here we obtained evidence that the usual mammary tumor virus was occasionally transmitted by the male, as has been reported elsewhere, and as a result of such an infection a high-mammary tumor line would arise.

We [43] then obtained further evidence on the number of genes involved in the control of the virus by producing 76 first backcross females [(C3HB x B)BC] that were not only tested for their ability to transmit the virus but were also bred to produce a second backcross generation, the females of which were in turn tested with foster-nursed test females. The results failed to show single gene segregation. Instead, the data suggested that the MTV can be propagated in the presence of one or more of several genes. There was also evidence that females able to transmit the virus vary in quantity or quality of virus produced, presumably due to the numbers of genes they had favoring the propagation of the virus.

In the early work with the mammary tumor virus it was generally assumed that by removing the virus through foster-nursing on a resistant strain the mammary tumors would be practically eliminated. We were, therefore, rather surprised when our C3HfB line derived in 1945 by foster-nursing a cesarean born litter of C3H on a strain C57BL female had an incidence of mammary tumors approaching 40% in breeding females, although the tumors came up at an advanced age [44]. We interpreted these tumors as resulting from the high genetic susceptibility of strain C3H together with the hormonal stimulation resulting from having litters and not the result of the virus. This interpretation was supported by reciprocal crosses between the C3HfB line and strain C57BL that showed that whatever was causing the tumors was transmitted as readily by the male as by the female parent [45]. The incidences of mammary tumors in the reciprocal F_1 females were practically identical although the incidence for each group was somewhat less than that in the C3HfB females.

Such an interpretation had to be modified when we sent our C3HfB line to the laboratory in Berkeley and the staff there found type B particles in the mammary tumors that arose in the line [46]. While these looked like the usual MTV particle the virus was different in that it was transmitted more as genes are transmitted, i.e., by the male as readily as by the female. Thus, the concept of the NIV was born. This was another prominent stepping stone in the development of the present conference. A mammary tumor virus that was transmitted more as a genetic factor had been discovered.

More recently Vlahakis and I [47] have developed the strain C3H-A^{vy}fB which is like C3HfB except that it has the A^{vy} gene that is known to increase the occurrence of mammary tumors. Females of this C3H-A^{vy}fB strain have the surprisingly high incidence of mammary tumors of 90% at an average age of 15 months and the factor causing this high incidence is transmitted by either parent. Both reciprocal F_1 hybrids between C3H-A^{vy}fB and BALB/c have incidences of mammary tumors in the vicinity of 90 % with that of those with BALB/c mothers being even slightly higher than that of those with C3H-A^{vy}fB mothers. B particles that are surely NIV have been seen in the tumors. BALB/c females that were fostered in C3H-A^{vy}fB had a low incidence of mammary tumors, no higher than would be expected in BALB/c females, thus failing to give evidence that the NIV was being transmitted through the milk. In addition, immunologic tests for the virus in C3H-A^{vy}fB milk samples have for the most part been negative. Thus, we have a line with a very high incidence of mammary tumors due to a virus that is transmitted more as a genetic factor.

This, then, brings us to the heart of the present symposium. The genetics of experimental tumors has progressed into the area of viruses only to come back to a union of the virus and the host genome. The situation in strain C3H-A^{vy}fB is in many respects like that in Mühlbock's strain GR [48] on which so much exciting work has been done in his laboratory. I am sure this work will be described in detail by others in this symposium. Results with GR and other strains have stimulated Bentvelzen in developing his concept of genetical transmission of the GR mammary tumor virus incorporated in the genome of the host as a provirus [49]. Now similar concepts are held by others in regard to other oncogenic viruses. We look forward to a thorough discussion of these and related exciting areas of research in the subsequent sessions of this conference.

Summary

Genetic factors in tumorigenesis have been studied since the turn of the century but the development of the inbred strains of mice by Little, Strong, and others initiated a surge of investigation in this area. Initial segregation ratios suggested simple dominant inheritance for lung tumors and mammary tumors. Subsequent work, however, has indicated more complex multiple-factor inheritance for not only lung and mammary tumors but also for induced subcutaneous sarcomas and leukemia. Many known genes have been associated with the occurrence of a number of kinds of neoplasms, but in many of these cases the relationship appears to be the effect of the specific gene rather than true linkage. During the last two decades genetic control of the oncogenic viruses, the subject of the present conference, has been the most interesting and probably most fruitful segment of the investigation of the genetics of cancer.

References

[1] E.F. Bashford, Proc. Roy. Soc. Med. 2 (1909) 72.
[2] E.F. Bashford, Proc. Roy. Soc. London 81 (1909) 310.
[3] J.A. Murray, Proc. Roy. Soc. London 84 (1911) 42.
[4] C.J. Lynch, J. Exp. Med. 39 (1924) 481.
[5] M. Slye, J. Cancer Res. 10 (1926) 15.
[6] C.C. Little, J. Cancer Res. 12 (1928) 30.
[7] J.J. Bittner, Public Health Rept. U.S. 53 (1938) 2197.
[8] H.B. Andervont, Public Health Rept. 53 (1938) 232.
[9] C.J. Lynch, Proc. Soc. Exp. Biol. Med. 43 (1940) 186.
[10] W.E. Heston, J. Natl. Cancer Inst. 3 (1942) 69.
[11] W.E. Heston, J. Natl. Cancer Inst. 3 (1942) 79.
[12] J.A.H. Tatchell, Nature 190 (1961) 837.
[13] J.L. Bloom and D.S. Falconer, J. Natl. Cancer Inst. 33 (1964) 607.
[14] W.E. Heston, Proc. Intern. Genet. Symp., Tokyo, Kyoto, 1956. Cytologia (1957) 219.
[15] W.E. Heston, M.K. Deringer, I.R. Hughes and J. Cornfield, J. Natl. Cancer Inst. 12 (1952) 1141.
[16] E.C. MacDowell, J.S. Potter and M.J. Taylor, Cancer Res. 5 (1945) 65.
[17] L.W. Law, J. Natl. Cancer Inst. 12 (1952) 1119.
[18] E.D. Murphy, In: The Jackson Laboratory, 40th Annual Report, Bar Harbor, Maine (1968-1969) pp. 29.
[19] H. Meier, D.D. Meyers and R.J. Huebner, Proc. Natl. Acad. Sci. USA 63 (1969) 759.
[20] M.K. Deringer, J. Natl. Cancer Inst. 45 (1970) 1205.
[21] J.J. Bittner, Research Conf. on Cancer (1944) Washington, D.C., A.A.A.S. (1945) 63.
[22] W.E. Heston and G. Vlahakis, J. Natl. Cancer Inst. 29 (1926) 197.
[23] L.C. Strong, J. Natl. Cancer Inst. 5 (1945) 339.
[24] L.C. Stevens and J.A. Mackensen, J. Natl. Cancer Inst. 27 (1961) 443.
[25] W.E. Heston and G. Vlahakis, J. Natl. Cancer Inst. 40 (1968) 1161.
[26] G.L. Wolff, Cancer Res. 30 (1970) 1722.
[27] G. Vlahakis and W.E. Heston, J. Natl. Cancer Inst. 31 (1963) 189.
[28] E.S. Russell and E. Fekete, J. Natl. Cancer Inst. 21 (1958) 365.
[29] F. Bielschowsky and M. Bielschowsky, Brit. J. Cancer 14 (1960) 195.
[30] H.B. Andervont, Public Health Rept. 53 (1938) 1665.
[31] W.J. Burdette, Cancer Res. 3 (1943) 318.
[32] R.K. Cole and J. Furth, Cancer Res. 1 (1941) 957.
[33] E.C. MacDowell, J.S. Potter and M.J. Taylor, Cancer Res. 5 (1945) 65.
[34] L. Gross, Proc. Soc. Exp. Biol. Med. 78 (1951) 342.
[35] L.W. Law, Proc. Soc. Exp. Biol. Med. 111 (1962) 615.
[36] L.W. Law and J.B. Moloney, Proc. Soc. Exp. Biol. Med. 108 (1961) 715.
[37] Jackson Laboratory Staff, Science 78 (1933) 465.
[38] R. Korteweg, Nederlandsch Tijdschrift voor Geneeskunde 78 (1934) 240.
[39] J.J. Bittner, Am. J. Cancer 97 (1939) 90.
[40] J.J. Bittner, Cancer Res. 2 (1942) 540.
[41] W.E. Heston, M.K. Deringer and H.B. Andervont, J. Natl. Cancer Inst. 5 (1945) 289.
[42] W.E. Heston, M.K. Deringer and T.B. Dunn, J. Natl. Cancer Inst. 16 (1956) 1309.
[43] W.E. Heston, G. Vlahakis and M.K. Deringer, J. Natl. Cancer Inst. 24 (1960) 721.

[44] W.E. Heston, M.K. Deringer, T.B. Dunn and W.D. Levillain, J. Natl. Cancer Inst. 10 (1950) 1139.

[45] W.E. Heston and M.K. Deringer, J. Natl. Cancer Inst. 13 (1952) 167.

[46] D.R. Pitelka, H.A. Bern, S. Nandi and K.B. deOme, J. Natl. Cancer Inst. 33 (1964) 867.

[47] G. Vlahakis, W.E. Heston and G.H. Smith, Science 170 (1970) 185.

[48] O. Mühlbock, Europ. J. Cancer 1 (1965) 123.

[49] P.A.J. Bentvelzen, Genetical control of the vertical transmission of the Mühlbock mammary tumor virus in the GR mouse strain. Hollandia, Amsterdam, 1968.

SOME CHARACTERISTICS OF TUMOR ANTIGENS OF VIRUS-INDUCED NEOPLASTIC CELLS AND THEIR ROLES IN ONCOGENESIS

Lloyd W. LAW

Laboratory of Cell Biology, National Cancer Institute, Bethesda, Md., U.S.A.

Introduction

Tumor antigens (TA) of diverse types have now been described in many populations of neoplastic cells. These TA are identified by immunologic reactions of diverse types. One class of antigen referred to as tumor-specific transplantation antigen (TSTA) occurs on the cell membrane and is detected by classical transplantation rejection procedure in syngeneic hosts. These were first detected in carcinogenic hydrocarbon-induced anaplastic sarcomas of inbred strains of mice [1] but are now known to be present on neoplastic cells of many species and to be induced by several different chemical carcinogens [2, 3]. In contrast to the TSTA of neoplasms induced by the DNA- and RNA-oncogenic viruses, each carcinogen-induced neoplasm appears to have individually distinct antigens whereas the TSTA of virus-induced neoplasms cross-react within each group.

It should be recognized that it is most difficult to distinguish between the acquisition of new (qualitative) antigens, TSTA on the cell surface or the development of these as a result of a change in the profile of already existing histocompatibility isoantigens. Thus, long-transplanted carcinogen-induced neoplasms used principally in detecting antigenic changes present an enigma. At least in viral-induced neoplasms the TSTA at any time can be shown to retain their virus-specific nature and this is probably a distinctive character suggesting that these are not isoantigens.

This discussion will describe some tumor antigens of virus-induced neoplasms studied in our laboratory, and attempt to assess their interrelations and their biologic roles, particularly of the TSTA, in the induction and repression of neoplasms.

25

Antigens of oncogenic DNA and RNA viruses

The oncogenic virus systems best studied fall into separate patterns relative to the nature of the tumor antigens detected and the techniques used for their study. The DNA viruses such as polyoma, SV40 and the adenoviruses, usually induce neoplasms *in vivo* and *in vitro* that do not produce infectious virus. The antigens of these neoplasms that are therefore not antigens of the mature virion but nevertheless are most likely specified by viral genetic material perpetuated in the neoplastic cells, fall into two classes: those detected by classical serologic methods and called T- or neo-antigens and confined to the nucleus, principally, and those detected by transplantation-rejection procedures in syngeneic hosts and termed tumor specific transplantation antigens (TSTA). These two methods appear to be detecting different classes of antigen and no close biologic relationships exist between the two. The T- or neo-antigens detected by complement fixation (CF), immunofluorescence (IF) or immunodiffusion techniques show no intrinsic relationship to tumors or oncogenesis. These latter antigens are detectable in *in vivo* infections where tumors do not develop and in early *in vitro* lytic infections with these DNA viruses. In contrast, as will be discussed later, TSTA is a major determinant in the induction or repression of DNA virus-induced neoplasms [4].

The structure of oncogenic RNA viruses and their manner of replication differ strikingly from the DNA viruses. Since there is usually continued production of infectious virus in neoplastic cells induced by these viruses, it has been extremely difficult to distinguish the various antigens so far detected from viral antigens.

The best studied tumor antigens are those found in the leukemias of rodents produced by several leukemogenic viruses. A number of antigenic systems, principally those expressed on the cell surface, have been defined. Some of these antigens now appear to be distinct from virion antigens and may be considered as TSTA as will be discussed later. The continued production of infectious virus by neoplastic cells induced by the oncogenic RNA viruses leads to viral antigen incorporation into the membrane. Thus, a study of cell surface determinants on leukemic cells, and probably on other neoplastic cells induced by RNA viruses, may indeed be in some experimental situations a study of viral-surface antigens. This possibility is reinforced by recent reports of "artificial heterogenization" or antigenic conversion of some transplantable tumors [5, 6].

Specific surface antigens found on leukemic cells induced by the murine leukemogenic viruses (MuLV) fall into several distinct systems [7]: The G-antigen found in Passage A (Gross) virus induced and many spontaneous leukemias and also in normal tissues of high-leukemic strains, the FMR-antigen found on leukemic tissues induced by Friend, Moloney and Rauscher viruses and E found in certain C57BL leukemic cells. The relationship of these antigens detected by means of cytotoxic and immunofluorescence tests on living cells to the infectious virus is not clear. They may indeed represent virion antigens except in the case of the type specific, soluble G-antigen. The relationship of virus-specific cell surface antigens demonstrable by tumor rejection to the above-defined antigens and to virion antigens is not known. It is assumed by some investigators that the antigens detected by cytotoxicity assays represent virus-specific transplantation antigens (TSTA). However, it may be pointed out that in the well-defined H-2 system of the mouse it is not known whether the antigen specificities detected by cytotoxicity assays always represent transplantation rejection (histocompatibility) specificities.

Group-specific and type-specific soluble antigens of murine leukemogenic viruses have been detected through the use of several serologic techniques [8]. These antigens represent virion antigens or structural viral antigens. The development of these techniques has provided important information relating to viral leukemogenesis and may be extended to tumors induced by other oncogenic viruses.

The murine leukemogenic-sarcomogenic virus complex may provide a model to distinguish the various classes of RNA virus-specific antigens. Some neoplasms produced in heterologous hosts, the rat and hamster, as well as in the homologous host, the mouse, by MSV do not produce infectious virus but do contain defective virus, free of envelope antigens. Three such neoplasms also give evidence for the existence of TSTA, thus allowing distinction of virion from nonvirion antigens. These will be considered in some detail later.

TSTA detected in certain breast adenocarcinomas induced by MTV in inbred mice have been described through the use of classical transplantation-resistance tests. As in the case of leukemias and other solid tumors induced by MuLV and by MSV, these transplantable adenocarcinomas continue to produce infectious virus and distinction between the effects of virion antigen and of new surface antigens of the TSTA type, specified by MTV, is difficult to make. Nevertheless, several recent reports suggest the existence of common antigens among a group of transplanted adenocarcinomas (probably representing MTV) and in addition antigens specific for the neoplasms [9,10]. Table 1 lists some common antigens of different types detected in neoplastic cells induced by the several oncogenic viruses.

Table 1
Occurrence in several systems of virus-specific tumor and cellular antigens.

Virus	Classes of antigens		
	TSTA	Other antigens	Virion antigens
(DNA)			
Polyoma virus	+		–
SV40 virus	+	T-antigens	–
Adeno (12, 18, etc.) virus	+		–
Shope papilloma virus	+ (?)		?
(RNA)			
Leukemogenic viruses (MuLV)	+ (?)	Detected by cytotoxicity assay, immunofluorescence; type and group specific internal antigens	+
Murine sarcoma virus (MSV)	+ (?) and +	Internal cytoplasmic	+ and –
Mammary tumor virus (MTV)	+ (?)	Detected by immunodiffusion and immunoprecipitation	+
Rous virus (SR)	+	–	–

There is some evidence to indicate, using tumors of the hamster induced by different "strains" of polyoma virus, that there is not always a common antigenicity of TSTAs. The polyoma viruses of different origins were shown to induce TSTAs with differing antigenicities [11].

TSTAs designated in the tables as + (?) represent systems in which infectious virus continues to be released from the tumors employed and may not, therefore, represent new cell-surface antigens. In the case of the Shope papilloma-carcinoma system, in which an increased regression rate of primary virus-induced papillomas occurs, infectious DNA can nevertheless be isolated from the benign and neoplastic lesions.

Cross reactions among the leukemogenic viruses (MuLV) have been studied using soluble antigens or transplantation rejection procedures. Type A (Gross) appears antigenically distinct from the Friend–Moloney–Rauscher (FMR) group and the Graffi and Rich viruses appear as distinct antigenic classes. Friend and Rauscher viruses differ from the other MuLV in that they induce erythroblastosis in mice.

Membrane antigens in addition to TSTAs have been described in tumor cells induced by SV40 and by polyoma viruses and termed S antigens. These have been detected by the indirect membrane fluorescent technique. One of these, the (SV40 induced) S antigen, does not appear to be TSTA [12].

Biological significance of tumor antigens

The precise roles that the above-described antigens play in the actual process of viral oncogenesis has not been determined. Though TSTA are detected using transplantable tumors there is now direct evidence that the immune reactivity of the host towards TSTA determines the probability of the development of primary tumors. This will be discussed using the polyoma virus-mouse system. However, the role of T-antigens detected by serologic means (CF, IF) in cells infected with the DNA viruses is not so clear. It does appear that these antigens, as well as the TSTA, are coded by the viral genome or a portion of it. Particularly the serologically detectable antigens therefore become extremely important diagnostic tools in searching, for example, for viruses in human neoplasms, although such searches to date have not yielded significant information [13]. This is possible because the different antigens of virus-induced tumors by any single virus are identical or closely related serologically, as far as is known. The intracellular localization of the neo-antigens suggests that they have little immunologic significance as far as defense mechanisms of the host are concerned.

The neo- or T-antigens may also be considered as disturbing mitotic regulation by facilitating DNA synthesis since they are actually induced early in the acute infectious cycle, although T-antigen is not known to be identical with any of the enzymes involved in DNA syntheses. The possibility that T-antigens interfere with normal regulatory cell processes seems likely.

It is possible that the antigens detected in neoplasms induced by the leukemogenic viruses, by MTV, and by MSV (murine sarcoma virus) represent viral structural antigens. The significance of these in oncogenesis is not known, but their localization at the cell surface makes them potentially significant in relation to contact inhibition, cell division, and immunologic reactions.

Determination of the mechanisms responsible for the induction of the several types of tumor antigens, including TSTA, must await the development of knowledge of the chemical nature of these antigens. It seems reasonable to assume at least in some instances that viral genetic material maintained in the neoplastic cell is responsible for TSTA and its specificity. This evidence will be discussed in the SV40 virus experimental system. In considering mechanisms of induction of tumor antigens, the characteristics of TL-antigens as found in some leukemias are of interest [14]. This most probably reflects "gene activation" which is invariable in some types of leukemogenesis. Although there is a connection between "activation" of TL-genes and leukemogenesis, the TL-antigens on the cell surface (detected by cytotoxicity assay) is not the character responsible for the malignant behavior of these leukemic cells, nor do TL-antigens act as TSTA.

Experimental models in the study of tumor antigens. Polyoma virus-induced neoplasia and TSTA

There is good evidence obtained from model systems to suggest strongly that immunologic surveillance is operating to delay and prevent tumor induction, that this surveillance is mediated principally by cellular immune mechanisms and that the immune system may be augmented or interfered with to influence the tumor surveillance efficacy. Polyoma virus-induced tumor cells, free of intact virus, are antigenic [15]. They contain a virus-specific "new" cellular TSTA antigen that is stable and heritable and which is found to be effective in "sensitizing" immunologically competent mice to reject transplants of polyoma tumors. It was of interest therefore to attempt to utilize this antigenic difference between tumor and normal host cells, as a means of controlling the development of virus-induced neoplasms *in the autochthonous host*. The results which follow show that this can be done in a syngeneic system, in a very effective manner.

Upon inoculation into newborn mice of certain strains, polyoma virus multiplies to high titer in many organs, produces an antiviral antibody response, and, after a fairly short latent period, induces neoplastic growths principally in the salivary glands but in other tissues as well. Most neoplasms that arise are epithelial in origin. C57BL, strain A and C3H/Lw mice, however, are strikingly resistant to the oncogenic effects of the virus introduced during the neonatal period and behave as adult animals of susceptible strains despite the fact that polyoma virus again multiplies to high titer and antiviral antibodies are produced. That resistance to polyoma viral oncogenesis is related to defense mechanisms operating at the level of the intact organism is shown by the ability of virus to transform organ explants of both resistant strain C57BL and A salivary tissues to neoplastic growths [16].

The animal with a deficient immune mechanism is useful for studies of host resistance to spontaneous and experimentally induced neoplasms. Surgical removal of the thymus in the neonatal period or use of immunosuppressant antilymphocyte serum, ALS, completely eliminates the capacity of immunized C57BL mice to reject syngeneic polyoma tumors [17].

Table 2 shows the results of tumor induction by polyoma virus in C57BL mice normally resistant to the oncogenic effects of polyoma virus.

The effectiveness of sensitized lymphoid cells administered to the animal after viral infection in preventing the origin of frank neoplasms adds further weight to the significance of TSTA and the immunologic status of the host in the control of neoplastic growths. Resistance to the induction of polyoma tumors can be transferred in the same way as homograft immunity, by the

Table 2
Polyoma-induced neoplasms in normally resistant C57BL mice following thymectomy.

Strain	Group	Age at virus infection (days)	Tumor incidence*	Latent period (months) Mean	Range
C57BL	Thymectomized (3 days)	4−7	18/26 (73%)	2.5	2−4.5
	Thymectomized (3 days)	14−18	21/42 (50%)	3	2.5−4
	Controls	4−18	0/54		
	Controls	4−7	0/37		

*Number of mice with tumors/number injected with virus.
LID_1 polyoma virus, 2×10^6 plaque-forming units used for infection.

Table 3
Prevention of polyoma virus-induced neoplasms in thymectomized C57BL strain mice.

Group	Treatment*	Number mice tumorous/ number mice
Thymectomized	None	61/80 (77%)
	Sensitized syngeneic cells $(1−2 \times 10^6/g)$	0/39
	Sensitized syngeneic cells $(1−2 \times 10^3/g)$	7/24
	Thoracic duct cells (sensitized syngeneic)	0/8
	Non-sensitized syngeneic cells	14/28
	X-rayed syngeneic cells	9/11
	Sensitized allogeneic cells (C3H)	8/10
	Serum from hyperimmunized mice	17/23
Intact	None	0/67 (0%)

*Mice thymectomized at 3 days of age. Polyoma virus inoculated at 7 days of age at a concentration of 2×10^6 pfu. Thoracic duct cells inoculated at the reduced concentration of 4×10^4 cells/g body weight of recipient. Intravenous inoculations of all cells done in 0.2

injection of cells from lymphoid organs. The results recorded in table 3 are in accord with the thesis that immunity is of the homograft rejection type and is transferrable by sensitized lymphoid cells that seed out, become established and function in the recipient. In summarizing the results it is clear that certain stringent criteria must be met in adoptive immunity:[1]

(1) Nonsensitized lymphoid cells were not effective in preventing tumor induction when transferred at 30 days after virus infection.

(2) "Sensitization" of lymphoid cells was achieved either by homologous virus or by the use of allogeneic (C3H) polyoma tumor cells (free of infectious virus) but containing TSTA.

(3) The effective cell is probably the long-lived, small circulating lymphocyte since thoracic duct (TD) cells obtained within the first 24 hours of drainage were effective whereas TD cells from thymectomized mice did not prevent tumor induction.

(4) Sensitized allogeneic cells were ineffective. It is therefore surprising to note the effectivenenss of sensitized allogeneic and even of xenogeneic lymphoid cells in inhibiting the growth of primary sarcomas in the rat [18].

(5) Serum obtained from those mice providing effective sensitized lymphoid cells did not reduce the incidence of neoplasms.

(6) Irreversible damage from 5000 r X-irradiation to sensitized lymphoid cells prevented the transfer of immunity.

(7) The repression of polyoma virus-induced neoplasms was long lasting. Only two of 57 C57BL mice observed throughout life developed neoplasms [19].

These results suggest the existence of a very strict limitation on attempts to control neoplastic growths in the primary host since genetic differences between recipient and donor would preclude effective adoptive immunity. It has been shown, however, that if histocompatibility differences are weak, transfer of sensitized lymphoid cells between inbred strains, e.g., between C3H/Bi and C3H/Lw, was effective in preventing polyoma virus-induced neoplasms, provided that the susceptible strain (C3H/Bi) was first made

---

[1] Many previous studies refer to the effectiveness of passive transfer of immunity by lymphoid cells. These experiments, which entail mixing of neoplastic target cells and lymphoid cells prior to transfer to a syngeneic host, are misleading in that they may in fact represent "neutralization." They fail to satisfy the criteria for adoptive immunity.

---

ml volume at 30 days post-virus infection. Neoplasms were principally of the salivary glands and the latent period ranged from 2 to 6 months. Lymphoid cells were ordinarily obtained from the spleen and the concentration of cells was $1\text{-}2 \times 10^6/g$ body weight unless otherwise stated. Lymph node cells were equally effective. Assuming that 70 percent of splenic cells are lymphoid in origin and that 10 percent are sensitized, repression of neoplasms to a considerable degree was therefore achieved with as few as 2000 cells.

tolerant to the histocompatibility antigens of the resistant strain (C3H/Lw) [20].

The TSTAs described for other DNA virus-induced neoplasms, e.g., those induced by SV40 and the adenoviruses, are in all likelihood functionally similar to those found in polyoma virus-induced neoplasms and repression of neoplasms in the autochthonous host may indeed be achieved in a similar manner as suggested by published reports [21,22].

SV40 virus-induced neoplasms and tumor antigens

Our continuing efforts to study well-defined TSTA is in the direction of solubilizing and purifying these. This depends upon the development of a reliable *in vitro* method for detecting TSTA and for continuous monitoring of the steps during purification procedures. Polyoma virus-induced neoplastic cells of several lines have not been effective "target cells" for example in *in vitro* cytotoxic assays. We have, therefore, used SV40 virus-transformed cell lines, adapted to tissue culture, that are lysed by humoral antibodies specific for SV40 virus and for the SV40 TSTA [23]. SV40 tumor specific transplantation antigens, TSTA, were initially demonstrated by resistance to SV40 tumor transplants in adult hamsters immunized with SV40 virus or with SV40 transformed cells. Several features of the SV40 TSTA are known: (1) it is specific; human, hamster and mouse neoplastic cells share TSTA capable of stimulating transplantation resistance to SV40 induced tumors, (2) TSTA is distinct from T and S antigens, (3) TSTA is associated with cell membranes as will be shown later, and (4) it is probably coded for by the viral genome as suggested by data presented later.

Two cell lines, SV.AL/N of A strain origin and mKSA (Tu5) of BALB/c strain origin have been shown by appropriate tests to express their respective TSTA and T antigens. These ^{51}Cr-labeled target cells are selectively killed in the presence of specific antibody and complement. Inhibition of cytotoxicity can, therefore, be used to measure in a precise manner the antigen concentration and specific activity of the different SV40 transformed cell lines.

The cytotoxic effects of sera obtained from AL/N mice immunized with SV40 transformed neoplastic cells (SV.AL/N cells), from non-immunized syngeneic controls and from hyperimmune allogeneic donors $(C^3)^2$ are shown in fig. 1. Direct serum titration was against SV.AL/N target cells. This assay

[2] This antiserum is directed against the H-2 alloantigenic specificities 1 and 3 and detects specific histocompatibility antigens expressed on AL/N and BALB/c target cells.

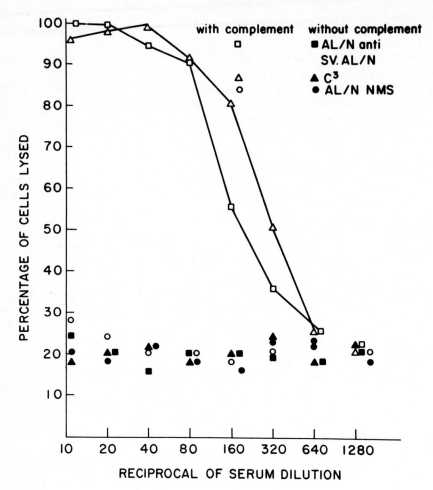

Fig. 1. Titration of sera against ^{51}Cr-labeled SV.AL/N target cells containing TSTA. 25 μl volumes of sera and 0.05 ml target cells (5×10^4) were added to each tube and incubated for 45 min at 37° C. 0.05 ml fresh-frozen rabbit serum (1/4) was added where indicated and incubation continued for 90 min at room temperature.

allows simultaneous identification of cellular histocompatibility (H) antigens and TSTA.

The specificity of the cytotoxic reaction as being directed against SV40-induced neoplastic cells is shown in fig. 2. Both SV.AL/N and mKSA ^{51}Cr-labeled cells were lysed whereas normal syngeneic lymph node cells (AL/N) and a polyoma virus transformed AL/N line (Py.AL/N) were not. On

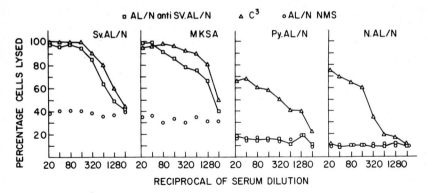

Fig. 2. Titration of sera with labeled SV40 transformed cells: SV.AL/N and mKSA and with normal syngeneic lymph node cells, N.AL/N and polyoma virus-transformed cells, Py.AL/N. Sera of 3 types: □ - □ from hyperimmunized syngeneic AL/N mice given SV.AL/N cells, ○ - ○ from non-immunized AL/N mice and △ - △ alloimmune serum (H-2.1 and H-2.3 specificities).

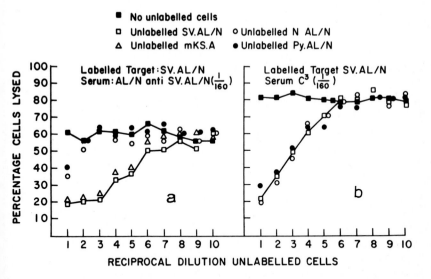

Fig. 3. (a) Inhibition of cytotoxicity using unlabeled cells. Labeled SV.AL/N target cells incubated with a fixed aliquot of AL/N anti-SV.AL/N serum (diluted 1/160) and varying numbers of unlabeled SV.AL/N cells = □ - □, Py.AL/N cells = ● - ●, normal AL/N cells = ○ - ○ or no cells = ■ - ■ (b). As in 3a except alloantiserum (H-2.1 and H-2.3) diluted 1/60 used. Background lysis was 20% in both A and B.

the other hand an alloantiserum against H-2 specificities was cytotoxic for each of the four targets used.

The results of inhibition by antigens of cytotoxicity using SV40 transformed target cells are shown in fig. 3a. Suitably diluted unlabeled cells of the four types: SV.AL/N, mKSA, Py.AL/N and normal AL/N lymph node cells were incubated with anti-SV.AL/N serum diluted 1/160. Following addition of standard amounts of labeled SV.AL/N cells (SV40 transformed) and rabbit complement, the assay for cytotoxicity was completed. Both SV40 transformed lines (containing SV40 specific TSTA) inhibited cytotoxicity with a far greater efficiency than either of the control cell lines. Fig. 3b shows the results using a built-in positive control for this system. Alloantiserum was used diluted 1/160 rather than the hyperimmune SV.AL/N antiserum. In this case all of the cell lines inhibited cytotoxicity with equal efficiency.

We have recently observed that crude membrane preparations and crude soluble extracts (after papain digestion) of SV.AL/N cells are capable of inhibiting the specific cytotoxic effects directed by SV40 specific humoral antibody against SV40 transformed target cells [24]. These results as well as our previous observations showing that H-2 specificities are separable from non-H-2 specificities by G-150 Sephadex fractionation of soluble antigenic preparations [25] indicate in a positive manner the likelihood of further purification of TSTA.

It is obvious that the cytotoxic inhibition assay allows precise quantitation of surface antigen concentration on intact cells or on various subcellular fractions. A major problem encountered, however, is selection and adaptation of neoplastic cells, fibroblastic in nature, to be used as effective target cells.

Interrelationships of SV40 tumor-specific surface (TSS) antigen, T-antigen, tumor-specific transplantation antigen (TSTA) and surface (S) antigen

Wright [26] in this laboratory has studied the relationships of the several antigens detected on/in SV40-induced neoplastic cells. Hamster embryonic cell lines developed by Diamondopoulos et al. [27] were used. The four cell lines shown in table 4 originated from the same pool of hamster embryonic tissues. Each line is tumorigenic and had been tested in vivo for the presence of SV40-specific TSTA. Two of these lines (1808 and a cloned derivative 2952) contain both T and S antigens. A third line, 1807, contains only the S antigen. The fourth line, 1809, obtained from cells never exposed to SV40 virus, transformed spontaneously, and lacks both T and S antigens. Only the T+S+ lines (2952 and 1808) contain viral-specific nucleic acids and also express SV40 specific TSTA.

Table 4

Interrelations of tumor antigens of hamster embryonic cell lines.

Cell line	Description	SV40 antigens			Contains SV40 specific	
		T	S	TSTA	RNA	DNA
1808	Embryonic hamster, transformed after exposure to SV40 virus (non-virus releaser)	+	+	+	+	+
2952	Clone established from 1808 at 43rd passage level	+	+	+	+	+
1807	Embryonic hamster, transformed after exposure to SV40 virus (non-virus releaser)	−	+	−	−	−
1809	Embryonic hamster, spontaneously transformed	−	−	−	−	−

(Data of P.W. Wright.)

Using the cytotoxic assay of ^{51}Cr-labeled hamster target cells described above and a hyperimmune antiserum, anti-SV.AL/N from mice, it was shown that the two cell lines, 2952 and 1808, were sensitive to the serum. These two lines contain the T, S and TSTA antigens (see table 4). These observations were supported by quantitative absorption experiments, that is, only the T+, S+ lines, 2952 and 1808, could efficiently reduce the activity of the anti-SV.AL/N serum. This set of experiments shows that: (1) The surface antigens detected by cytotoxicity probably are identical with TSTA, (2) virus genetic material must be present in transformed cells for the expression of TSTA and T antigens, (3) surface antigen appears unrelated to either TSTA or T antigen and is not dependent upon SV40 genetic material for expression. The relationship of viral genetic material to TSTA has not been determined.

Though viral genetic material present in the neoplastic cell is necessary for expression of TSTA, it is not known whether this codes for a new protein present on the cell membrane or whether it changes the profile of existing histocompatibility antigens. An answer to this question, however, may be possible using the cytotoxicity inhibition system described above with inbred mouse strains where distinctions are likely possible between new surface antigens and histocompatibility isoantigens.

Tumor antigens and immune responses in neoplasms induced by RNA oncogenic viruses

Neoplasms induced by RNA viruses of the avian and murine leukemia-sarcoma complexes and by the murine mammary tumor virus (MTV) have yielded extensive information of various tumor antigens principally because they lend themselves to serologic analysis. Several types of antigens have been described for the leukemias using *in vitro* and serologic techniques [8]: (1) cell-surface antigen (detected by cytotoxic assays), (2) type-specific soluble antigen (detected by immunofluorescence), (3) viral antigen (detected by neutralization of infectivity) and (4) group-specific (gs) soluble antigen (detected by complement fixation). TSTAs have also been demonstrated using tests of resistance to transplanted leukemias in virus-immunized recipients. G-antigens found in Gross virus-induced neoplasms are distinct from those found in the FMR group (Friend, Moloney, Rauscher leukemogenic viruses). In view of the failure of any single laboratory to employ a broad spectrum of immunologic procedures to assay antisera and viral and tumor antigens, the interrelationships of these various antigens have not been established.

A most obvious source of tumor antigens of the several types in RNA tumors is infectious virus or a structural part of the virus since productive nonlytic infection of the tumor cells continues indefinitely in contrast to DNA oncogenic viruses. Thus, expression of TSTA (homologous transplantation antigens) could be an expression of replicating, intact, infective virus incorporated in the cell membrane. The following results show, however, that TSTAs of some RNA virus-induced tumors are of nonvirion origin, but are nevertheless specified by the virus inducing the neoplasm.

MSV-induced tumors and their antigens

Neoplasm XM-1 is a transplantable hemangiosarcoma induced in a $(BC3H)F_1$ mouse by the murine sarcoma virus, MSV, an MLV pseudotype of the Moloney isolate. Originally this tumor was an "atypical granuloma" the typical tumorous growth induced by MSV in mice that released infectious MSV and was transplantable only to thymectomized or to X-irradiated syngeneic recipients. From the fifth transplant generation, however, it assumed the behavior of a true neoplasm and was transplantable to and grew progressively in immunologically competent syngeneic mice. Numerous critical assays from this time through the fortieth transfer generation have failed to reveal the presence of infectious MSV or of MLV and assays were negative for group-specific antigen

Table 5

Results of syngeneic transplantation of neoplasm XM-1 (hemangiosarcoma) into recipients immunized with MSV-pseudotype viruses and with MLV and RLV.

Group	Number mice	Number with progressively growing tumors	Mean age at death in days and range
Immunized with			
(1) MSV(MLV)*	50	8 (19.4%)	73 (37–120)
MLV	17	5	43 (30–70)
(2) MSV(RLV)	28	19 (74.4%)	40 (20–50)
RLV	11	10	51 (28–87)
No immunization			
(3) (Litter mates)	85	66 (77.6%)	33 (17–48)

*Three weekly immunizations with tumor challenge two weeks later were more effective than one immunization: only 1/29 resulted in progressive growth with three immunizations whereas 7/21 progressive growths were obtained following a single immunization with 0.5×10^4 FFU of MSV(MLV). Immunizations with MLV, MSV(RLV) and with RLV were done once a week for three weeks with challenge of XM-1 cells done subcutaneously two weeks after the last immunization. Mice immunized as in (1) above did not resist a polyoma virus-induced tumor.

Table 6

Characteristics of neoplasm XM-1 and of several *in vitro* derived clones.

	Cells neoplastic	MSV[1]	Presence of: Defective MSV	MLV[2]	TSTA[3]
XM–1	+	–	+	–	+
Clone { H–1	+	–	–	–	+
H–14	+	–	–	–	+
H–11	–	–	–	+	+
#60	+	–	–	+	–

[1] Presence of MSV detected by focus formation on mouse embryo cells. Also negative following density gradient banding by H^3-uridine labeling.
[2] Detected by syncitial cell formation with XC cells and mouse embryo cells.
[3] Detected by both immunosensitivity and immunogenicity assays except clone H-11.
(Data of S.S. Chang and L.W. Law.)

(gs). Nevertheless, XM-1 does contain "defective" MSV genome as revealèd by rescue experiments and contains type C particles [28].

The immunosensitivity of XM-1 is shown in table 5. The pseudotype virus MSV (MLV), or MLV alone, adequately immunized adult $(BC3H)F_1$ mice to grafts of 1-5 x 10^6 neoplastic cells. Surprisingly, the pseudotype virus MSV(RLV) of similar concentration and RLV alone provided little, if any, immunity to XM-1. The immunizing capacity of MSV(MLV) and of MLV in contrast to a minimal or no immunizing effect of MSV(RLV) was somewhat unexpected. Excellent cross reactivity between MLV and RLV in virus neutralization and transplantation studies, using leukemic cells, have been recorded and they have been considered to belong to the same serotype. Nevertheless, since the XM-1 neoplasm was originally induced by the MSV(MLV) pseudotype virus, it must be considered that the TSTA on XM-1 cells may indeed be MSV(MLV) specific.

XM-1 tumor cells are immunogenic. Surgical removal of progressively growing tumors initially inoculated into foot pads produced a state of immunity to subsequent challenge. If grafting of XM-1 was delayed to 3 weeks or longer after surgical removal, a striking enhancement of tumor growth occurred. It has not been determined as yet if this represents a specific and immunologic phenomenon.

Through adaption of XM-1 to tissue culture, it was possible to obtain individual clones. The characteristics of these in the various assays, in comparison with the parental *in vivo* passaged XM-1, are shown in table 6. Tumor #60 represents clone H-14 following 6 consecutive passages *in vivo* in $(BC3H)F_1$ recipients.

Although XM-1, the parental line, contained "defective" MSV none of the clones yielded rescued virus using highly concentrated RLV. Tumor #60, though derived from an MLV-free clone (H-14), nevertheless acquired MLV in *in vivo* passage, but appears to have lost its TSTA. Some preliminary conclusions can be drawn from these data:

(1) The presence of a "defective" MSV genome apparently is not necessary for the expression of TSTA (nor is the presence of infective MSV or MLV necessary).

(2) Since TSTAs are virus specific, RNA viral material must exist in some form in the neoplastic cells.

(3) The neoplastic state (see clones H-1 and H-14) may be maintained without detectable MSV, MLV or "defective" MSV.

Two other "non-releaser" neoplasms show properties similar to XM-1: MSB-1 of epithelial cell origin induced by MSV(MLV) in a BN strain rat (29) and PD_4-T_1 induced *in vitro* by infecting PD_4 strain hamster embryo cells with

Table 7

Induction of resistance to transplantation of PD_4-T_1 tumor cells in syngeneic hamsters pretreated with X-irradiated PD_4-T_1 cells.

Challenge levels	Normal controls	Immunization[1] with PD_4-T_1
4×10^3	5/5 (8)[2]	0/3 (−)
4×10^2	5/5 (11)	0/4 (−)
4×10	3/5 (14)	0/4 (−)
Total	13/15	0/11

[1] Hamsters received three inoculations of 2-14 x 10^6 irradiated (15,000 r) PD_4-T_1 cells, s.c., 2 weeks apart, and were challenged with viable cells 1 month later.
[2] Progressively growing tumors/total inoculated (mean latency period to tumor detection in days).

Table 8

Characteristics and properties of PD_4-MSV(H) and PD_4-T_1 hamster tumor cells.

Assay	Results	
	PD_4-MSV(H)	PD_4-T_1
TD 50 in syngeneic PD_4 hamsters	1 to 4×10^4 cells	2 to 4×10^2 cells
Electron microscopy	Positive for type C virus particles	Negative for type C virus particles
Complement fixation with anti-MSV sera	Positive	Negative
Infectivity of tissue culture and freeze-thaw supernatant of cells	Foci	No foci
Oncogenicity of lethally X-irradiated (15,000 r) cells in newborn BALB/c mice	Tumors (MSV +)	No tumors
Density gradient banding by ^{3}H-uridine labeling	Peak at 1.17	No peak
Recovery of leukemia virus by MSV genome rescue	Positive	Negative
Genome rescue	Not tested	Positive with RLV
Immunofluorescene	Positive	Negative

(Data of J. McCoy, R.C. Ting, D.L. Morton and L.W. Law.)

the Harvey isolate of MSV, H-MSV [30]. Both of these neoplasms are virus-free as detected by all available critical assays, yet both contain defective MSV rescuable by leukemogenic helper viruses.

Neoplasm PD_4-T_1, a fibrosarcoma, was derived from passage *in vivo* in PD_4 strain hamsters and is a variant of the parental PD_4-MSV(H) tissue-culture grown line. PD_4-T_1 has a tumor associated transplant antigen (TSTA) as revealed in table 7, and shows cross-reactivity with a transplant antigen of the parental line. The parental line in contrast to the variant subline releases infective MSV and MLV and also shows the presence of antigens detected by immunofluorescence and complement fixation and induces high levels of neutralizing antibodies; thus it would appear that these assays are detecting virion antigens that in all probability are unrelated to the TSTA. A comparison of some of the characteristics of the non-releaser variant, PD_4-T_1, and of the parental line, PD_4-MSV(H), is shown in table 8.

The results obtained to date, therefore, with these three RNA virus-induced but "non-releaser" neoplasms show that where TSTAs are detectable these virus-specific antigens are distinct from viral antigens and are analogous to the transplantation antigens specified by DNA oncogenic viruses.

Probable influence of tumor antigens on the induction and repression of lymphocytic neoplasms

The suppression of immune reactions has helped to analyze their role in the induction and control of neoplastic growths. The frequency of those neoplasms which contain virus-specific or tumor-specific transplantation antigens (TSTA) usually is increased strikingly in animals rendered immunologically defective by neonatal thymectomy, treatment with ALS and in some instances by X-irradiation [19]. On the other hand, immune deficiencies do not always influence the frequency or latent period of neoplasms known to contain tumor-specific TA; for example, chemically-induced primary fibrosarcomas and mammary tumor virus-induced tumors of the mouse appear not to be susceptible to ALS or to neonatal thymectomy [19].

Heterologous antilymphoid sera have been shown to be effective suppressants of cell-mediated immune responses such as skin graft or tumor rejection and of delayed hypersensitivity reactions. Processes that lead to humoral antibody production are also sensitive to ALS but may have unusual time-dependent relationships to antigen administration. ALS has been reported to increase the frequency and shorten the latent period of neoplasms induced by polyoma, adeno-12 and murine sarcoma (MSV) viruses [31]; one regimen of treatment with ALS produced localized reticulum cell sarcomas following infection with a leukemogenic virus (MLV) [32]. This neoplasm has been observed with high frequency in man bearing kidney transplant and given immunosuppressants, including ALS [33].

In many of the tumor systems, referred to above, cell-mediated immune response elicited by tumor specific transplantation antigens (TSTA) appear to be involved; however, preliminary evidence suggests a role of humoral antibodies in susceptibility and resistance of neoplasms induced by the RNA leukemogenic-sarcomagenic viruses.

The relationship was explored between immunologic reactivity, using ALS as an immune suppressant, and the induction and repression of lymphocytic neoplasms in adult BALB/c mice infected with the murine leukemogenic virus,

Table 9

Influence of different regimens of ALS-treatment on MLV-induced lymphocytic neoplasms in 12 week BALB/c mice.

Group	No. exps.	Treatment with ALS at days:	Total ALS	No. leukemia No. mice		Latent period (months)
(a)	6	−7, +7	0.2 ml	28/41 (70%)		3.2 (2.2−4.0)
(b)	1	−7, +4	0.2 ml	7/8		3.0 (2.8−3.3)
(c)	1	−3, −1	0.2 ml	4/6		4.0 (3.5−4.5)
(d)	2	−7, +7, +9, +11, +13, +15	0.6 ml	8/8	(87%)	2.8 (1.5−3.8)
I (e)	2	−7, −4, −2	0.3 ml	15/16		3.5 (3.0−5.0)
(f)	1	−7, −4, 1, 0	0.4 ml	5/8		2.5 (2.0−3.5)
(g)	1	−11, −9, −7	0.3 ml	8/8		2.7 (2.0−3.5)
(h)	1	+7, +10, +13	0.3 ml	1/8	(19%)	4.0
(i)	1	+14, +17, +20	0.3 ml	2/8		5.0, 7.0
II	8	MLV only	−	2/73 (2.7%)		4.0, 5.0
III	5	ALS only	0.2 to 0.6 ml	1/48 (2%)		3.0

MLV inoculated intraperitoneally on day 0; infectivity titer of standardized preparation as determined by syncytial cell formation with XC and mouse embryo cells was $1 \times 10^{4.5}$/ml.

MLV. The induction of lymphocytic neoplasms in the mouse is a thymus-dependent mechanism and removal of the thymus inhibits leukemogenesis simply by removal of the non-lymphoid elements that provide for the conversion from a normal to a leukemic cell. Thus, the role of immune suppression here could not be studied by surgical thymectomy.

Different regimens of treatment with ALS were employed and attempts to reverse the effects of ALS were made using adoptively transferred syngeneic sensitized and non-sensitized lymphoid cells at different concentrations and timing.

By reference to table 9 it may be seen that 12-week-old pathogen-free BALB/c strain mice resist the leukemogenic effects of intraperitoneally injected MLV, group II. The different schedules of subcutaneously injected ALS provided a striking sensitivity to the leukemogenic virus, provided at least one treatment of ALS was administered prior to virus. The reduced effect of ALS administered beginning 7 days after virus infection (group I, h and i) has been observed also in this laboratory using MSV(MLV) in the induction of solid tumors in BALB/c mice. Generalized lymphocytic leukemia was detected as early as 1½ months after MLV infection in these adult mice and death followed

Table 10

Adoptive immunity to MLV-induced leukemia in ALS-treated BALB/c mice (ALS given on days -7, -4, -1 and MLV on day 0).

Group	A		B	
	No. leuk. Total no.	(latent period)	No. leuk. Total no.	(latent period)
Non-sensitized lymphoid cells	8/40	(4.1 months)	23/28	(3.5 months)
Sensitized lymphoid cells	20/21	(1.8 months)	–	
None	23/32	(2.8 months)	19/21	(2.5 months)

Intravenous inoculations of 25-60 x 10^6 lymphoid cells of splenic origin were made in the period from 3 to 10 days after the last ALS treatment in group A, whereas inoculations were given in group B at less than 3 days or at 14 days after ALS. Totals of 5 separate experiments. Sera from those donors providing normal lymphoid cells that reversed sensitivity to virus did not influence reactivity nor did sera from hyperimmunized BALB/c donors; these latter sera had high levels of anti-MSV neutralizing antibodies.

usually in 2 weeks. ALS alone (group III) was ineffective; previously normal rabbit serum (NRS) was observed not to influence MLV induction of lymphocytic leukemia. All six ALS preparations used in this study were found to be immunosuppressive.

If ALS is inactivating or removing those lymphoid cells concerned with the establishment of immune competence, it should be possible to replace those components removed by ALS and thus restore the immune response and as a consequence, prevent leukemogenesis. This has been accomplished successfully in restoring the capacity to reject allogeneic skin grafts and in restoring the response to sheep erythrocytes [34,35]. By reference to table 10 it may be seen that intravenously inoculated lymphoid cells of splenic origin from 12-20 week old syngeneic BALB/c donors were capable of restoring the capacity to resist the oncogenic effects of MLV provided adoptive transfer was done in the period from 3 days to 10 days after the last ALS treatment. Presumably, lymphoid cells inoculated at 2 days or earlier were inactivated by residual ALS while it was too late for those immunocompetent cells administered beyond 10 days to prevent emergence of transformed cells. Dosage of lymphoid cells as well as time was a critical factor in succesful adoptive transfer; not shown in table 10 is the lack of restorative capacity of 10×10^6 lymphoid cells transferred during the sensitive period 3 to 10 days after the last ALS injection.

These results, reestablishing resistance to the leukemogenic effects of virus by adoptive immunity, support the concept that the immunosuppressive effect of ALS is directly responsible for the observed increased susceptibility.

It was expected that lymphoid cells from "immunized" syngeneic donors would be more effective than lymphoid cells from non-immunized donors in reestablishing resistance to MLV leukemogenesis. This indeed has been the experience in adoptive transfer experiments in mice bearing neoplasms with polyoma-specific tumor antigens as previously discussed and with carcinogen-induced neoplasms. On the contrary, putatively sensitized lymphoid cells from BALB/c donors may have enhanced leukemogenesis.

The virus used for immunization, MSV(MLV), is known to provide adequate immunity against the transplantation of an MLV-induced transplantable leukemia containing TSTA and against a transplantable MSV(MLV)-induced hemangiosarcoma [28]. Previous work has also shown that MSV and MLV share common antigens. Sensitized lymphoid cells used in this study were always obtained from hyperimmunized syngeneic donors from 2 weeks to 4 months after the last immunization. We have no good explanation for the reduced capacity of these lymphoid cells of splenic or lymph node origin to reverse susceptibility to MLV. These cells retain their capacity to initiate *in vitro* cytotoxic reactions and to provide strong graft versus host reactions.

The immunosuppressive effect of ALS as shown in these studies in all probability allows cells converted to neoplasia by virus to survive; these cells are so highly antigenic that they would be eliminated in the normal animal. MLV is known to induce resistance against the transplantation of lymphoma cells carrying the corresponding antigen in BALB/c mice. Thus, as with DNA virus-induced neoplasms, immune suppression and tumor antigens of the transplantation type (TSTA) appear to be major determinants in tumor induction with an RNA virus, MLV. That this is so is seen in the lack of increased susceptibility in those animals rendered tolerant at birth to virus or to new virus-specified cellular antigens [36]. In this situation immunosuppression would be expected to have a negligible influence.

The reversal of susceptibility in ALS-treated BALB/c mice by adoptive transfer of syngeneic adult normal lymphoid cells probably represents replacement of those immune elements removed by ALS. Critical factors in the reversal were both timing and concentration of the adoptive transfer cells.

ALS appears to remove selectively or inactivate those cells concerned with the establishment and maintenance of immunocompetence but to be relatively ineffective against cells of lymphoid origin susceptible to transformation by MLV from the normal to the neoplastic state.

The model system described here lends itself to studies of the mechanisms concerned with susceptibility and resistance to lymphoid neoplasms induced in the primary host.

Discussion and summary

Knowledge now becoming available concerning the diverse new antigens of neoplastic cells induced by DNA and RNA oncogenic viruses will hopefully lead to answering questions as to their origin and biologic significance.

Many cell surface antigens have been identified. Those (TSTA) detected by transplantation rejection and specified by DNA oncogenic viruses are most likely major factors in the *in vivo* behavior of neoplastic cells *in the primary host* and are capable of evoking immune response of the homograft type that hold in check or eliminate foci of neoplastic cells. The effective immune reaction is cellular in nature and directly related to lymphoid cells.

The TSTAs specified by RNA oncogenic viruses appear to be analogous to the DNA virus-specified antigens in those instances discussed here, principally using "non-releaser" MSV-induced neoplasms, where distinctions could be made between TSTA and virion antigens. This does not rule out the likelihood that viral surface antigens, of virus-induced leukemic cells for example, also function as TSTA.

Effective surveillance mechanisms are suggested as being operative in primary hosts in the elimination of newly arisen neoplastic cells containing new cell-surface antigens (TSTA) in the polyoma virus- and MLV-(leukemia) model systems. In both systems surveillance is mediated principally by cellular immune mechanisms amenable to interference by immunosuppressive procedures.

Where neoplastic cells (apart from those of lymphoid origin) containing strong virus-specific TSTA are adaptable to *in vitro* assays, as for example in simple, rapid, quantitative cytotoxicity-inhibition assays, TSTA may be measured directly as in the SV40 virus-induced neoplasms described. This reliable *in vitro* method thus allows for further progress in the analysis and characterization of TSTA and for attempts at solubilization and chemical purification.

References

[1] R.T. Prehn, Fed. Proc. 24 (1965) 1018.
[2] R.W. Baldwin and C.R. Barker, Int. J. Cancer 2 (1967) 355.
[3] H.J. Rapp, W.H. Churchill, B.S. Kronman, R.T. Pulley, W.J. Hammond and T. Borsos, J. Natl. Cancer Inst. 41 (1968) 1.
[4] L.W. Law, R.C. Ting and E. Leckband, Proc. Natl. Acad. Sci. U.S. 57 (1967) 1068.
, [5] V.P. Hamburg and G.J. Svet-Moldowsky, Nature 203 (1964) 773.
[6] B. Stück, L.J. Old and E.A. Boyse, Nature 202 (1964) 1016.
[7] L.J. Old and E.A. Boyse, Fed. Proc. 24 (1965) 1009.
[8] L.J. Old, E.A. Boyse, G. Geering and H.F. Oettgen, Cancer Res. 26 (1968) 1288.
[9] D.C. Morton, G.F. Miller and D.A. Wood, J. Natl. Cancer Inst. 42 (1969) 289.
[10] J. Vaage, Nature 218 (1969) 102.
[11] J.D. Hare, J. Virol. 1 (1967) 905.
[12] S.S. Tevethia, M. Katz and F. Rapp, Proc. Soc. Exp. Biol. Med. 119 (1965) 896.
[13] W.P. Rowe and A.M. Lewis, Jr., Cancer Res. 28 (1968) 1319.
[14] E.A. Boyse, L.J. Old and E. Stockert, *In:* P. Grabar and P.A. Miescher, Immunopathology 4th International Symp. (Basel: Schwabe and Co., 1965) p. 23.
[15] K. Habel, Cancer Res. 28 (1968) 1825.
[16] C.J. Dawe, L.W. Law and W.P. Rowe, Pathol. Biol. 9 (1961) 711.
[17] L.W. Law, Trans. Proc. 2 (1970) 117.
[18] P. Alexander, E.J. Delorme and J.G. Hall, Lancet 1 (1966) 1186.
[19] L.W. Law, Cancer Res. 29 (1969) 1.
[20] L.W. Law, Life Sci. 8 (1969) 1079.
[21] B.E. Eddy, G.E. Grubbs and R.D. Young, Proc. Soc. Exp. Biol. Med. 117 (1964) 575.
[22] H. Goldner, A.J. Girardi, V.M. Larson and M.R. Hilleman, Proc. Soc. Exp. Biol. Med. 117 (1964) 851.
[23] P.W. Wright and L.W. Law, Proc. Natl. Acad. Sci. U.S. 68 (1971) 973.
[24] E. Appella, P.W. Wright and L.W. Law, unpublished data.
[25] S. Strober, E. Appella and L.W. Law, Proc. Natl. Acad. Sci. U.S. 67 (1970) 765.
[26] P.W. Wright, Nature 233 (1971) 18.
[27] G.Th. Diamandopoulos, S.S. Tevethia, F. Rapp and J.F. Enders, Virology 34 (1968) 331.
[28] L.W. Law and R.C. Ting, J. Natl. Cancer Inst. 44 (1970) 615.
[29] R.C. Ting, Proc. Soc. Exp. Biol. Med. 126 (1967) 778.
[30] J. McCoy, R.C. Ting, D.L. Morton and L.W. Law, (1972) in press.
[31] L.W. Law, R.C. Ting and A.C. Allison, Nature 220 (1968) 611.
[32] A.C. Allison and L.W. Law, Proc. Soc. Exp. Biol. Med. 127 (1968) 207.
[33] C.F. McKhann, Transplantation 8 (1969) 209.
[34] R.H. Levey and P.B. Medawar, Proc. Natl. Acad. Sci. U.S. 58 (1967) 470.
[35] W.S. Martin and J.F. Miller, J. Exp. Med. 128 (1968) 855.
[36] L.W. Law, Fed. Proc. 29 (1970) 171.

REPLICATION OF ONCORNAVIRUSES

L. MONTAGNIER[1]
Fondation Curie, Institut du Radium, 91-Orsay, France

As the subject has been extensively reviewed in past years (see for instance ref. [1]), this paper will be restricted to the most recent molecular aspects of the replication of oncogenic RNA viruses (oncornaviruses) [2].

In 1969, at the 4th Symposium on Comparative Leukemia Research, I discussed three possible mechanisms for the perpetuation of the genome of oncornaviruses [3].

(1) The RNA–DNA–RNA hypothesis, first proposed by Temin [4];

(2) The orthodox model: like the RNA of non-oncogenic viruses, the viral RNA is replicated by specific RNA replicases through complementary copies;

(3) The built-in theory; a portion (or the totality) of the viral genes is already present in the cellular genome, and viral infection derepresses them by a mechanism of gene amplification. This theory could be viewed as an extrapolation of the oncogene theory of Huebner and Torado [5].

None of these models was experimentally established at that time, but some predictions could be made, which have been recently confirmed. In particular, the finding of enzymes associated with virions of non-oncogenic viruses and the lack of effect of some inhibitors of protein synthesis at the first step of infection, led to the prediction that if hypothesis 1 was right, a polymerase capable of synthesizing DNA on RNA templates, might be present in the virions.

Moreover, the isolation of thermosensitive mutants has ruled out the variant of hypothesis 3, which assumed that the totality of viral genome would have been present in cells before infection.

As I hope to show, there may be some truth in each of these three models. Actually, a combination of the three mechanisms seems to give a good account

[1] The author wishes to thank Drs. Baluda, Beaudreau, Biswal, Cavallieri, Duesberg, Gallo, Hanafusa, Riman, Temin, Todaro, Vigier and Vogt for letting him know in advance their unpublished work, and Miss P. Allin for many helpful suggestions.

49

of the extreme complexity and variety of the facts known about these viruses. This complex scheme may be in turn only a simplified reflection of the control mechanisms normally operating in eukaryotic cells for the expression and transfer of genetic information.

Before going into speculations, let us recall briefly the facts which have to be taken into account anyway, and their possible interpretations. Only positive results will be examined.

1. Components associated with, or present in the virions

1.1. Envelope components
Because of their size, their complex structure, their way of formation by budding of the plasma membrane, it is not surprising that many components,

Table 1
Components of oncornavirions.

	Location	Origin
ATPase [6] Ribonuclease [7] DNA endonuclease [8]	Adsorbed on the surface of virions	Cellular
Part of cell coat [9] Part of plasma membrane Virus-specific glycoproteins (viral type specific antigen) [10, 11]	Components of the outer envelope	Cellular and viral
Transfer RNA [12, 13] Ribosomal RNA [13, 14] 7S RNA [15] DNA [16, 17]	Found inside the virions	Cellular
RNA dependent DNA-polymerase [18-20] DNA replicase [17, 21, 22] DNA endonuclease [22] DNA exonuclease [8] DNA ligase [8]	Associated with nucleo-capsid	Mainly viral with cell participation?
RNA (10^7 to $1,2.10^7$) [23] Core proteins (including group specific antigen) [11, 23-26]	Components of the nucleocapsid	

including cell components, have been found in purified preparations of virions (table 1). The difficulty lies in separating those which are outside the membrane envelope from those which are inside, and in the latter, those which are accidentally incorporated from those which play a role in viral replication. Treatment of virions with low doses of pronase seems to free the virions from external nucleases [8,27]. A moderate treatment with non-ionic detergents disrupts the outer envelope and releases the nucleocapsid [28].

Although no cell surface antigen has been found associated with virions, there is little doubt that the virion envelope contains some components of the cell plasma membrane and is surrounded with a mucopolysaccharide layer similar or identical to the cell coat: the viral surface adsorbs the dye ruthenium red to the same extent as the cell coat [9].

Analysis of the proteins of purified RSV virions has also revealed the existence of at least two viral glycoproteins, which could be identified as the type-specific viral antigen. Since this antigen reacts with the neutralizing antibodies, they are probably located at the surface. This antigen varies with the virus strain and is therefore virus-coded [10,11].

1.2. Nucleic acids present in the virions

The only nucleic acid large enough to encode the viral genetic information is the large RNA component, whose molecular weight is in the order of 10^7 daltons. However, several other nucleic acid molecules have been repetitively found associated with virions, and they seem to be inside rather than outside the viral envelope [13]. They are:

Transfer RNA molecules; methylation and labeling experiments have shown that these molecules are of cellular origin. Interestingly, the proportion of individual species differs from that of the bulk of transfer RNAs contained in the cell [12, 13].

Another fraction of small RNA arises probably from the breakdown of the large RNA components [29]. However, a 7S RNA, G-C rich, has also been found in RSV virions [15]. It seems to differ from similar species existing in uninfected cells.

The 28S and 16S species of ribosomal RNAs have also been found [14] in variable quantities; this is not surprising, since ribosomes have been found associated with the plasma membrane [30].

Finally, labeling with [^{3}H-methyl] thymidine has allowed the detection of small amounts of DNA [16,17]. The size of this DNA is small (4-7S); at least one fraction is G-C rich. No association of this DNA with the large RNA component could be found. The origin and function of this DNA is not known. It cannot be excluded that it might serve as a primer for the DNA polymerase present in virions, at least in the *in vitro* reaction.

Framingham State College
Framingham, Massachusetts

Structure of the large RNA component.   Treatment by heat or by agents disrupting hydrogen bonds irreversibly dissociates the viral RNA into several pieces of similar size, suggesting that they were not covalently bound before extraction [31,32]. According to another interpretation [33], these changes may reflect the loss of a peculiar secondary structure which maintains a very compact configuration of the native RNA in intact virions. This possibility is remote, since electron microscopy of the extracted RNA has shown some RNA molecules with a length corresponding to a molecular weight of 10^7 [34,35], together with shorter fragments arising from ribonuclease-induced breaks or from dissociation into subunits. Assuming the extracted RNA to consist of several pieces, it remains to be proven that they exist as such in intact virions, since breaks in definite regions of viral RNA could result from the action of the ribonuclease present inside the virion (fig. 1).

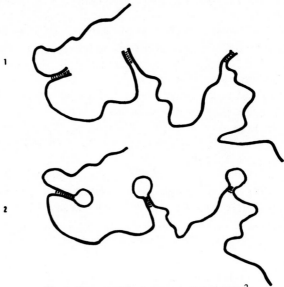

Fig. 1. Two possible structures of viral RNA.[2]

A subunit structure would have some important consequences for the replication and the genetics of oncornaviruses. As we have previously suggested [32], each unit may be replicated and translated independently, as is the case

[2] Note added in proof: Since heat dissociation of the 65 S RNA releases also transfer-like RNA molecules (E. Erikson and R.L. Erikson, J. of Virology 8 (1971) 254), a third structure is possible, in which the RNA subunits are held together by such small RNA molecules.

for myxovirus and reovirus RNA subunits. The formation of recombinants by exchange of subunits is predicted by this model, and this is compatible with recent work on mutants [36,37]. Along the same line, an interesting finding has been made recently by Duesberg and Vogt [38]. In the avian virus group, the RNA of transforming (sarcomagenic) viruses is slightly larger than that of leukosis viruses, as evidenced by differences in electrophoretic mobilities. The origin of this difference lies in the size of the subunits upon dissociation by heat; two classes of subunits were found in transforming viruses, while leukemia viruses lacked the larger component. Some of the non-transforming mutants of SR-RSV, induced by hydroxylamine treatment of the virions, also have an RNA smaller than the untreated virus [39].

If these results would apply to other groups of oncornaviruses, particularly the murine leukemia sarcoma complex, they could strongly suggest that the transforming ability of sarcoma viruses is encoded in a piece of RNA which is lacking in leukemia viruses. As we have previously suggested on the basis of radiobiological data [32], this piece of RNA, as well as the information for viral production, may belong to distinct subunits, replicating independently. As a corollary of this assumption, a mechanism must exist to ensure normally a correct assembly of the units into the nucleocapsid, and eventually replace a lacking subunit by one of the other type. As suggested by Pons [40] for the subunits of influenza RNA, the proteins of the core could serve as a backbone for this assembly.

1.3. Internal proteins of the virions
In recent studies of the proteins of RSV, several proteins of the nucleocapsid have been separated, two being tentativily identified as the group-specific antigens [23]. The polymerase activity was found to be distinct from these proteins, and to be, from the view point of quantity, a minor component of the virion [41].

2. DNA is involved

Historically, studies with actinomycin D and DNA synthesis inhibitors gave the first indication that DNA synthesis and DNA transcription were involved in the initial events of viral RNA replication (see for review [1,42,43]).

2.1. Effects of actinomycin D
   Low doses of actinomycin D (and low doses of UV light) irreversibly inhibit virus replication during the early phase sensitive to DNA inhibitors, and

reversibly once the infection is established. This was interpreted as meaning that cellular DNA transcription or perhaps that of a proviral DNA was required. Yet, some other interpretations cannot be ruled out. First, the early action of the inhibitor can be explained by its effect on cell division, which is required for the establishment of infection. Secondly, the continuous inhibitory effect of actinomycin D could be due to its known action on the synthesis of ribosomal RNA precursors in the nucleolus; it should be pointed out that synthesis of myxovirus RNAs which is known to proceed without a DNA intermediate is also inhibited by the drug at the beginning of infection [43,44].

The sensitivity of viral RNA synthesis to actinomycin D may simply reflect its intranuclear location; there is evidence suggesting that the passage from nucleus to cytoplasm and the translation of some new nuclear messenger RNAs need the concomitant synthesis of ribosomal precursors in the nucleolus [45]. If replication of viral RNA in the nucleus is mediated by a shortlived replicase, the synthesis of which (in the cytoplasm) depends on the translation of a nuclear m-RNA (cellular or viral) and therefore is controlled by nucleolar activity, the replication of viral RNA itself will be controlled by this activity. Thus, in agreement with this hypothesis, replication of picornavirus, which is purely cytoplasmic, is generally insensitive to actinomycin D. That of myxoviruses, which may take place in either the nucleus or the cytoplasm (there is a nuclear replicase activity as well as a microsomal-bound activity [46]), will be more or less sensitive to the drug, depending on the prominence of one location over the other. Replication of oncornaviruses is perhaps exclusively intranuclear.

2.2. Requirement for DNA synthesis

The use of various inhibitors of DNA synthesis have shown that cell DNA synthesis (S phase) [42] and also mitosis [47, 48] were required for the establishment of infection. More recent experiments with inhibited cells (blocked in G1) have suggested that a specific DNA synthesis was also required, independently of that required for the entry of the cell into the S phase. If such cells are infected in the presence of the thymidine analog, 5-BUdR, and then exposed to visible light in order to induce breaks in the DNA which has incorporated the analog, virus production is inhibited, although the subsequent entry of cells into the S phase is not impaired [49,50]. These results could be interpreted in three ways:

(1) A proviral DNA is made soon after infection, and its further integration in the cell genome would require the entry into S phase [47]. However, the requirement for cell mitosis is not explained.

(2) There is a requirement for a function appearing in a cellular organelle (mitochondria?) only when its DNA is replicating. Synthesis of mitochondrial

DNA is in some cases not synchronized with that of nuclear DNA [51], and therefore may occur in the G1 phase.

(3) The infecting virions are able to trigger a limited duplication (amplification) of a specific region of the cell genome coding for a nuclear membrane site (even though the bulk of the cell genome is not replicated) although optimum conditions for this amplification may occur during the S phase. The expression of these genes subsequent to their amplification will take place only after cell division, at the time of reconstruction of the nuclear membrane.

It has recently been found that in cells where the replication of a given oncornavirus has already been established, infection by another strain of virus (of a different subgroup in order to avoid early interference) still requires a specific DNA synthesis [52,53]. According to the third interpretation, this would suggest that the number of nuclear sites for RNA replication is a limiting factor, and that synthesis of new sites for the second virus requires further gene amplification.

3. Effects of inhibitors of protein synthesis

The initial phase of infection (that sensitive to DNA inhibitors) is not sensitive to antibiotics which interfere with the translation of RNA on ribosomes (puromycin, cycloheximide) [42,54]. This result led to the suggestion that a pre-existing cellular enzyme or a virion enzyme would carry out the initial step of replication [3,4,55].

It should be noted, however, that (a) mitochondrial protein synthesis is not inhibited by cycloheximide [56], and (b) two recent reports [57,58] which await confirmation, indicate that chloramphenicol, a specific inhibitor of protein synthesis in prokaryotes and mitochondria, also inhibits RSV replication.

4. DNA polymerase activity associated with virions

The initial work of Temin and Mizutani [18] and of Baltimore [19] on virus RNA-instructed DNA polymerase has been followed by an impressive burst of research extending their findings, but showing also that the significance of the enzyme for viral replication was not as clear as it was believed initially, *viz.* that of a virus-specific "reverse transcriptase".

It is probably too early to draw any conclusion regarding the actual function of this enzyme in viral replication; however, the following features of this enzyme can be considered as established.

4.1. Occurrence of the enzyme

The enzyme has been found in all the oncornaviruses where it has been looked for: avian sarcoma and leukosis viruses (the presence of the enzyme in the naturally occurring leukosis virus (RIF) has not been reported),murine leukemia and sarcoma viruses, murine and rat mammary tumor viruses, hamster, cat leukemia and sarcoma viruses, and a viper C-type virus [59,60].

The non-oncogenic RNA viruses (nothing is known about DNA viruses) lack the enzyme, with three, perhaps four exceptions. These are the two "slow viruses", Visna virus [60-62] and the slow pneumonia forming virus [63]; the group of "foamy virus" widely spread in mammals (simian, feline, bovine and hamster) which causes formation of syncytia in cultured cells [64]. None of these viruses is known to be oncogenic.[3] However, Visna virus seems to be related to the oncornaviruses by the structure of its virion and the size of its RNA [62].

The association of the enzyme with oncornaviruses has prompted several groups to search for a similar activity in cells in which similar viruses may exist in a cryptic form, leukemic cells for instance. Similar polymerase activities were found in white blood cells from leukemic patients [66-68], but later improved technique allowed its detection in established lines derived from embryonic tissues, including normal human diploid lines [69]. The lower activity initially found in normal cells could be due to technical reasons, since recently Penner and coworkers [70] have found an equally high activity in normal lymphocytes stimulated by phytohemagglutinin. The enzyme has not been reported in differentiated tissue of adult organisms.

At the present time, it is not clear whether or not the enzyme found in leukemic cells is the same and has the same template requirements as that found in oncornaviruses, and whether or not that of normal cells is identical to that found in tumor cells.

4.2. Template requirements

It is established that the enzyme contained in oncornaviruses can use some sequences of the large viral RNA of the nucleocapsid as template, since soon after the beginning of the reaction a DNA copy is found associated with the viral RNA [71]. Upon denaturation, this DNA can be rehybridized with the viral RNA. After longer incubation, the DNA product is always small (4-7S) so that the question is raised whether this is due to a natural property of the enzyme, or is caused by the breakdown of the template RNA to small pieces by ribonuclease, so that only the piece having the proper recognition site will be

---

[3] Note added in proof: Recently, Takemoto and Stones [65] have shown that Visna and slow pneumonia forming viruses could induce morphological transformation of murine cells.

copied. However, a very long incubation time (19 hr) allowed Duesberg and Canaani [72] to obtain a DNA product, which made the viral RNA 75% RNase resistant under hybridization conditions, thereby showing complementarity with a major part of the sequences of this RNA.

It was recently found by Duesberg *et al.* [41] that RSV-RNA is a good template for the solubilized enzyme (freed from its endogenous template), but only in the native state; previous heating of the RNA, which may destroy either the subunit association or a peculiar secondary structure, resulted in the loss of template activity. This would suggest that the enzyme can recognize only specific helical regions of viral RNA. Indeed, work with synthetic polymers has shown that single-stranded ribopolynucleotides were poor templates for the polymerase preparations, with the exception of poly rC. In contrast, several double-helical copolymers, such as dC:rG and rA:rU or dA:rU, dT:rA are much better primers than RNA [73]. Ribosomal RNA and transfer RNA are used by the polymerase contained in extracts of leukemic cells [66], but this exception confirms the rule, since precisely these RNAs have a high degree of secondary structure.

It should be emphasized, that a polymerase preparation from *E.coli*, presumably the Kornberg enzyme, can also use double-helical copolymers and ribosomal RNA as templates [74-77]. Moreover, traces of added DNA stimulate the template activity of RNA [76]. Therefore, these *in vitro* studies shed no light on the actual template for these enzymes *in vivo*[4].

4.3. One or two enzymes?

In addition to the formation of DNA—RNA hybrid, the endogenous polymerase of oncornavirions subsequently makes double-stranded DNA, probably from the DNA strand which has been displaced from the hybrids [78] or from the hybrid itself [79]. While added viral RNA has no stimulatory effect on preparations not freed from the endogenous viral RNA [80], addition of DNAs from exogenous sources, particularly G-C rich DNAs, stimulates the synthesis of DNA by the enzyme preparation [17,21,22].

Moreover, by using specific inhibitors, it was possible to delineate the two reactions. Derivatives of rifampycin (particularly dimethyl-N-rifampycin) inhibit selectively the RNA-stimulated reaction [81], while actinomycin D (at high doses) inhibits the DNA-stimulated reaction [82].

---

[4] Note added in proof: It has been recently shown that the virion enzyme requires a primer (an oligodeoxyribonucleotide) in order to transcribe single-stranded ribopolynucleotides [120]. In the endogenous reaction (inside virions), the natural primer seems to be a small piece of RNA, covalently linked to the DNA product and hydrogen-bonded to the large viral RNA component [121]. The template activity of heat-denatured viral RNA can be restored by adding an oligodeoxyribonucleotide as primer [122].

These results suggest either that two distinct enzymes are present in the virions, or that a single enzyme has two distinct binding sites, one for ribonucleotide templates, and another for DNA remplates. Favoring a single enzyme with two sites is the finding [41] that the DNA-stimulated activity could not be separated from the activity stimulated by viral RNA, using the solubilized RSV enzyme.

4.4. Location of the enzyme inside the virions

In nearly all instances the enzyme activity did not appear unless the intact virions were treated with non-ionic detergents. Since this treatment disrupts the outer envelope and releases the nucleocapsid this suggests that the enzyme(s) was associated with the latter component. This was confirmed by equilibrium density analysis, which showed that most of the enzymatic activity accompanied the nucleocapsid component [28, 83].

However, the enzyme is distinct from the major proteins of the nucleocapsid, including the group-specific antigen, since (a) antibodies against purified gs antigen did not inhibit the enzyme activity [84], (b) a defective RSV mutant lacking the polymerase still induced the gs antigen [36] and (c) the enzyme activity could not be identified with any of the RSV capsid proteins [41].

4.5. Origin and possible role of the virion enzyme in viral RNA replication

Three possibilities have to be considered.

(a) The enzyme is of cellular origin and has no key role in viral replication.

(b) The enzyme acts as a reverse transcriptase, making a whole DNA copy of the large viral RNA.

(c) The enzyme is essential for the initiation of viral replication and acts as an agent for amplification of certain cellular genes.

The constant association of the enzyme with infective virions and its absence in a non-infectious mutant of RSV [36] seems to eliminate the first hypothesis. However, this hypothesis should not be completely excluded, since several reports [58,85] have suggested a possible association of viral nucleocapsid and virions of RSV with mitochondria. Since an action of viral genes on the cell membrane is likely, this action could also alter the mitochondrial membranes [86], and consequently some mitochondrial proteins, including a DNA polymerase, could be released and subsequently be absorbed to the viral nucleocapsid. It would be interesting therefore to compare the template requirements of the mitochondrial DNA polymerase of infected cells with the polymerase of oncornavirions.

Since alterations of mitochondria are a feature common to many tumors, the mitochondrial origin of the enzyme would also explain its appearance or its higher activity in leukemic cells.

The aforementioned RSV mutant may lack the polymerase activity because of its inability to undergo, an early interaction with mitochondria or to alter cellular membranes, including mitochondrial membranes.

A critical evidence for hypothesis 2 would be the isolation from infected cells of DNA–RNA intermediates, or virus-specific DNA of the size of the viral RNA, or of its subunits. Thus far, the search for such intermediates, which is technically difficult, has been unsuccessful. Data suggesting a mechanism of gene amplification for the maintenance of transformed characters will be discussed elsewhere [87].

5. Homology of viral RNA sequences with cellular DNA

The search for a homology between viral RNA and DNA of virus-transformed cells was originally undertaken to seek a confirmation of the provirus hypothesis. If the proviral DNA is integrated into cellular DNA, it should be detectable by specific hybridization with the viral RNA. Such homology was readily obtained, but was also found in uninfected cells of the same species [88,89], and in cells from other species of vertebrates [89].

The homologous region has a peculiar base composition, which does not reflect the base composition of viral RNA. It seems likely, as pointed out by Harel [90], that the viral RNA possesses one or several relatively short sequences, homologous to repetitive sequences of the cellular DNA. However, these results do not exclude a more specific homology due to the presence of a whole viral provirus. Indeed, Baluda and associates [91] have shown that AMV- or RSV-infected cells do contain more homologous sequences to AMV-RNA than do uninfected cells, by using hybridization techniques which seem to overcome difficulties arising from unspecific hybridization.[5] Although the base composition of the hybridized sequences was close to that of whole viral RNA [92], it is not yet possible to decide whether this increased homology means that all viral sequences are present in the cellular DNA, or, alternatively, arise from the duplication of cellular genes bearing a sequence homologous to a portion of viral RNA.

6. Genetic analysis of viral functions; isolation of viral mutants

6.1. Naturally defective mutants
It was known for several years that avian leukosis viruses could serve as helper

[5] Note added in proof: Similar results have been obtained by Rosenthal *et al.* [123].

for the Bryan strain of Rous sarcoma virus, by wrapping the nucleocapsid of this virus in their own envelope (phenotypic mixing). The question as to whether or not the sarcoma virus was completely defective for the synthesis of its envelope components has been clarified by several recent studies [93-96], which have also led to the discovery of an endogeneous defective helper virus. Results can be summarized as follows. The Bryan strain of Rous sarcoma virus RSV(O) lacks the information for some envelope components. However, if it is grown in chick embryo cells of the C/O genotype, complete virus is produced. Two virus types could be distinguished: RSVβ(O) which is infectious, and RSVα(O) which is not infectious for any known type of avian cells unless it is associated with a helper leukosis virus. If the same experiment is done with cells of the C/O' genotype, even the RSVβ(O) virions are not infectious for any known type of avian cell. Presumably, non-infective virions lack some envelope component(s) essential for their penetration into the cells. The RSVβ(O) virus produced under these conditions can still infect and transform chicken cells, if it is incorporated artificially into these cells in presence of inactivated Sendai virus. However, RSVα(O) is neither infectious nor transforming under the same conditions. C/O cells have the gs antigen before infection, while C/O' have not and the factor which allows C/O cells to produce infectious RSVβ(O) can be transfered and propagated in C/O' cells by means of a leukosis virus. Therefore, this factor, called chf [94] (chick cell-associated helper factor) behaves as an endogeneous defective leukosis virus. Its defectiveness seems to lie in the assembly of complete virions from nucleocapsid and envelope precursors, since in the presence of a non-defective leukosis virus, whole virions (RAV60) are produced [96].

A similar defective helper virus has been found by Vogt and Friis [95] in C/A chick cells, which also contain the gs antigen. The factor is transmissible to similar cells which normally lack the gs antigen. Another defect is probably common to the endogenous chf and RSVα(O), since no infectious virus was formed when these two agents were both present in the same cell. This defect may be related to the absence of a functional DNA-polymerase in the virions of RSVα(O), no such activity having been found in RSVα(O) virions [36].

These studies have shown that, first, defective RSV can be rescued by non-defective viruses, not only at the stage of virion morphogenesis (phenotypic mixing), but also at the level of earlier functions by complementation. Secondly, since RSVα(O), once incorporated into a permissive cell, is transforming, the gene inducing the polymerase activity is not necessary for the maintenance of transformation.

6.2. Radiation-induced defective mutants

Defective mutants of the Schmidt-Ruppin strain of RSV have been obtained artificially by means of γ-irradiation [97], UV light [98] and hydroxylamine [99]. Two classes of mutants can be distinguished. (i) Mutants able morphologically to convert chick cells, but which are not able to reproduce [97,98]. The transformation state induced by some of these mutants seems to be unstable [98]. (ii) Mutants able to reproduce, but having lost their transforming activity [97-99] (NT(γ), table 2).

Table 2
Characteristics of some mutants of RSV.

Virus strain	Poly-merase	GS antigen	Viral envelope proteins	Assembly of virion compo-nents	Transformation Morphology	Growth in agar	Ref.
RSV-SR	+	+	+	+	+	+	
RAV	+	+	+	+	−	−	
RSVβ(O)	+	+	−	+	+	+	[36, 94]
RSVα(O)	−	+	−	+	+	+	[36, 94]
Chf	−?	+	+	−	−	−	[36, 94]
NT (γ)	+	+	+	+	−	−?	[97]
TS75	−?	−?	+	+	+	+	[103]
TS149	+	+	−	−?	−	+	[103]
T1	+	+	+	+	−	−	[100]
FU 19	+	+	+	+	−	?	[102]

This dissociation of the two functions, transformation and virus reproduction, led to the suggestion that they were coded by independent fractions of the viral genome [32,97].

6.3. Conditional mutants

Recently several thermosensitive mutants of RSV have been obtained by means of mutagenic agents [100-102]. Some of them (T1, FU 19) are unable to transform the infected cells at the nonpermissive temperature, though they can replicate normally (table 2). In cells transformed at the permissive temperature, some of the transformation characters are under the permanent control of the thermosensitive viral function, since a shift to the non-permissive temperature allows the cell to recover normal growth properties, and a shift from non-permissive to permissive temperature can "retransform" them; both processes occur in a few hours after the shift, do not require cell division and are insensitive to actinomycin D. The process of "detransformation" is also insensitive to inhibitors of protein synthesis, while the second process is sensitive (Vigier and Biquard, personal communication). An important conclusion from these studies is that some of the transformation characters (which also condition tumorigenicity) are dependent on the continuous action of virus-coded protein(s). Another mutant isolated by Vogt and coworkers [103] (TS149) is unable to produce complete virions and to transform, while the production of gs antigen and of viral RNA seems to be normal.

At the present time, only one mutant defective for an early function of replication has been isolated (TS75) [103]. It is clear that the isolation of such mutants may play a decisive part in investigations of the process of viral replication, particularly in elucidating the role of the DNA polymerase.

Table 2 summarizes the characteristics of some of the RSV mutants we have just discussed.

7. Findings supporting an RNA–RNA replication

To establish this mechanism, which is used by non-oncogenic RNA viruses, at least two kinds of evidence have to be brought forward.

(a) Isolation of intermediate forms of replicating RNAs: double-stranded replicative form, replicative intermediate, and (or) complementary single-stranded RNA.

(b) Isolation of a virus-specific RNA–RNA replicase. A non-mendelian transmission of genetic viral information will also support this mode of replication.

The first type of investigations has been complicated by the finding of small amounts of double-stranded RNA of high molecular weight in uninfected cells [104]. This RNA does not increase significantly upon infection of chick cells by RSV, and in another system, rat liver, we have shown that at least one part hybridizes to repetitive sequences of cell DNA, and therefore has a cellular origin [105]. This does not exclude the possibility that a minor fraction of this RNA is virus specific. Indeed, complementary sequences of MSV-RNA have been found in nuclei of a rat cell line transformed by MSV and continuously producing virus [106]. The size of this RNA is that of a subunit of viral RNA and duplexes formed with viral RNA have the expected size for a replicative form of one subunit.

The existence of complementary sequences is not sufficient *per se* to prove a self-replication of RNA. An alternative hypothesis is that they arise from symmetric transcription of both strands of cell DNA, as we have suggested for rat liver double-stranded RNA [105].

7.1. RNA replicases

A replicase activity stimulated by addition of RNA has been found in myeloblasts transformed by AMV [107], but the product was not well characterized. Similar replicase activity may exist also in uninfected cells as suggested by several recent reports of RNA-dependent polymerase activities in leukemic cells [108], macrophages [109], plants [110] and bacteria [111].

A self-replication mechanism of a viral RNA would not exclude a RNA–DNA–RNA mechanism. It is conceivable that once the proviral DNA is transcribed into viral RNA, this RNA is replicated by a cellular replicase. Such a mechanism may be a normal process in uninfected cells for the duplication of certain species of messenger RNAs; for instance, when a rapid production of a given protein in large amounts is required (immunoglobulin, excretory proteins, etc.).

8. Vertical transmission

Vertical transmission from one generation of animals to another is a major feature of oncornaviruses. Since the subject will be extensively discussed in this Symposium, I shall comment only on the possible molecular mechanisms of this transmission.

Since C-type particles have been found in reptiles and higher vertebrates (see for review [112]), a strictly vertical transmission would imply a very accurate mechanism for maintenance of viral replication through the evolutionary emergence of higher vertebrates. Obviously, the best mechanism to match this requirement, especially for a silent (not expressed) transmission such as that postulated by Huebner and associates [112], is the integration of a proviral DNA in the cellular genome.

A prediction of this model is that the viral information will be transmitted as a mendelian factor. The finding that the transmission of gs antigen in chickens follows the mendelian pattern [113], together with the finding that it is associated with the presence of an endogenous defective ALV [95,96], and also studies of the vertical transmission of the GR strain of MTV [114], seem to confirm this prediction.

However, there is an alternative interpretation compatible with an RNA-RNA replication. The replication rate of a selfreplicating viral RNA in the cell nucleus may be controlled by one or several cellular genes (see *infra*). If the replication rate is low, but sufficient to insure that every cell will receive at least one template, the viral genome would be transmitted without sign of expression (no gs antigen). At higher rates, the number of viral copies would be

64   L. Montagnier

sufficient to go through the nuclear membrane and be expressed in the
cytoplasm.

A variant of this hypothesis is that a second set of cellular genes controls the
translation of viral RNA. In either case, transmission of the gs will be
apparently mendelian. A similar gene control may also exist for the production
of complete virions at the level of production or assembly of the viral envelope
components. Since the cellular control is quantitative, a prediction of this
model is that there may be various intermediate cases of cells with low levels of
viral expression and cells with high levels, depending on the number of RNA
templates. Supporting experimental evidence is yielded by *in vitro* studies of
hamster cells transformed by the SR-strain of RSV. A clone of transformed
cells' was passaged many times and subsequently subcloned. Some subclones
were found to be rich in gs antigen while the RSV genome could be rescued by
co-cultivation with chicken cells. Some other clones were poor in gs; the virus
was difficult to rescue in such cells, even under optimum conditions for
heterokaryon formation. Still other clones were gs⁻ and the virus could not be
rescued [115]. The reversion observed by MacPherson in hamster cells
transformed by another stock of SR-RSV can be explained in the same way
[116].

In contrast, there are cases of oncornavirus-transformed cells in which the viral
genome has never been lost, even upon repeated cloning [49,117]. They may
correspond to a higher rate of replication of viral RNA.

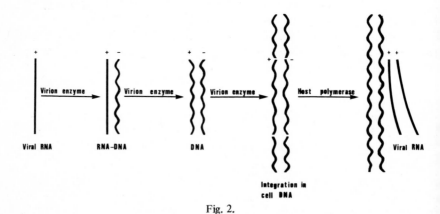

Fig. 2.

Figs. 2, 3 and 4. Two possible schemes of viral RNA replication. (2) The RNA-DNA-RNA
mechanism, with integration into cellular DNA. (3 and 4) The RNA-RNA mechanism, with
cellular DNA amplification.

9. Synthesis

Most, if not all the results that we have examined are compatible with the provirus hypothesis of Temin. The main point of this theory is based on the reverse transcription of the RNA viral genome into DNA, which could later on be integrated in the cell (fig. 2). The isolation from oncornaviruses of a DNA polymerase which could, *in vitro*, use viral RNA as template, strongly supports this point, but at the present time there is no unequivocal evidence that the enzyme acts as a reverse transcriptase in infected cells. That the polymerase is

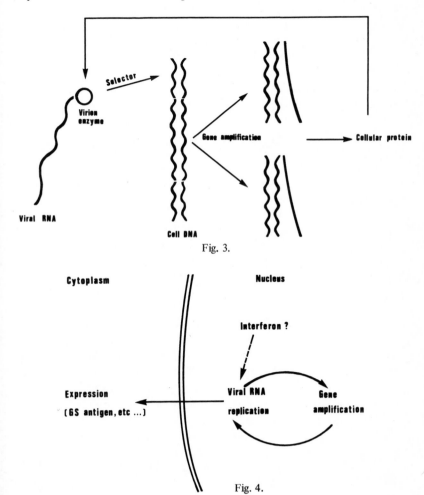

Fig. 3.

Fig. 4.

used *in vivo* is suggested, but not completely established, by the absence of infectivity in a virus mutant with no detectable polymerase activity.

The only evidence for the integration of a proviral DNA lies in the hybridization experiments of Baluda and coworkers, although they do not say whether all viral sequences are present or not.

As we have pointed out, a self replication mechanism of viral RNA may follow the integration of viral DNA, and its transcription into RNA. An objection to this model has been raised by Rubin [118]. If integration is an obligatory step for virus replication and transmission its vertical transmission should always follow the mendelian pattern. This is not so, since the transmission of RSV in chickens is maternal, and never occurs in the male. It could be argued, however, that for unknown reasons, viral genes are repressed in the male germ line, and cannot subsequently be derepressed in the embryo.

Although next months' new discoveries may make the attempt obsolete, I would like to challenge this theory by another one, which also seems to accommodate the facts presently known.

9.1. An alternative hypothesis

It is based on one of the possible mechanisms of cell differentiation, *i.e.* gene amplification. The quantitative control of gene expression — transcription and translation — would depend primarily on the selective duplication of gene sequences in the DNA, perhaps according to the mechanism suggested by Callan [119]. I postulate that the initiation of viral RNA replication depends on a cell function which is normally not expressed, and that expression requires gene amplification. Selection of the region to be expressed will require specific recognition of a replicator site in the DNA by small molecules acting as "selector". Small DNA or RNA molecules are likely candidates for this function. Association of the selector with a DNA replicator region will allow formation of a complex with a site on the nuclear membrane. According to the replication theory, this will trigger the duplication of the DNA sequences under the control of the replicator, by a specific polymerase. A loop of DNA containing the duplicated "slave" copies will result, and this loop will be transcribed by the cellular transcriptase (fig. 3). Such duplications will normally take place in G_1 or at the beginning of the S phase, and slave copies will be destroyed at the next mitosis, because the compact structure of the coiled chromosome cannot accommodate the loops.

I also postulate that some sequences of viral RNA (those which are homologous with repetitive sequences of DNA) can act as selector, and that the viral polymerase will act for the specific duplication of the DNA region(s) recognized by the selector.

Expression of the amplified genes will give information required for the initiation of viral replication. This cellular information is unlikely to be the RNA replicase itself. If this were the case, it would be difficult to explain why infection by a second virus requires a new cycle of gene amplification, since the enzyme would already be present. More likely, it may be a specific site required for the attachment of the replicating complex of viral RNA.

It can be seen that when the replication is already established, the viral replicative complex and the cell amplification system, together form a positive feed-back system, which can be perpetuated indefinitely (fig. 4). Similar circuits may be established for the maintenance of differentiation characters.

A regulation of such systems is obviously needed; endogenous interferon may have the function of controlling the replication rate of viral RNA.

The present hypothesis does not exclude the possibility that reverse transcription of a whole viral genome could occasionally occur and lead to integration of the proviral DNA. But this mechanism would not regularly be required for the initiation of viral replication.

I have already mentioned the possibility that mitochondria may be involved in the replication of oncornaviruses. A functional role for mitochondria in viral replication will of course deeply modify the concepts elaborated in the two preceding theories. Undoubtedly, further work will throw light on this intriguing question.

References

[1] P. Vigier, *In:* J.L. Melnick, Progress in medical virology, vol. 12, (Karger, Basel 1970) 240.
[2] R.C. Nowinski, L.J. Old, N.H. Sarkar and D.H. Moore, Virology 52 (1970) 1152.
[3] L. Montagnier, *In:* R.M. Dutcher, Comparative Leukemia Research 1969, Bibl. Haemat. 36 (Karger, Basel, 1970) 45.
[4] H.M. Temin, Natl. Cancer Inst. Monograph 17 (1964) 557.
[5] R.J. Huebner and G.J. Todaro, Proc. Natl. Acad. Sci. U.S. 64 (1969) 1087.
[6] G. De-The, J. Natl. Cancer Inst. Monograph 17 (1964) 651.
[7] M. Rosenbergova, F. Lacour and J. Huppert, Compt. Rend. Acad. Sci., Paris 260 (1965) 5145.
[8] S. Mizutani, H.M. Temin, M. Kodama and R.T. Wells, Nature New Biology 230 (1971) 232.
[9] H.R. Morgan, J. Virol. 2 (1968) 1133.
[10] P.H. Duesberg, G.S. Martin and P.K. Vogt, Virology 41 (1970) 631.
[11] P.P. Hung, H.L. Robinson and W.S. Robinson, Virology 43 (1971) 251.
[12] J.W. Carnegie, A.O.'C Deeny, K.C. Olson and G.S. Beaudreau, Biochim. Biophys. Acta 190 (1969) 274.
[13] J.M. Bishop, W.E. Levinson, N. Quintrell, D. Sullivan, L. Fanshier and J. Jackson, Virology 42 (1970) 182.

[14] T. Obara, D.P. Bolognesi and H. Bauer, Int. J. Cancer 7 (1971) 535.

[15] J.M. Bishop, W.E. Levinson, D. Sullivan, L. Fanshier, N. Quintrell and J. Jackson, Virology 42 (1970) 927.

[16] W.E. Levinson, J.M. Bishop, N. Quintrell and J. Jackson, Nature 227 (1970) 1023.

[17] J. Riman and G.S. Beaudreau, Nature 228 (1970) 427.

[18] H.M. Temin and S. Mizutani, Nature 226 (1970) 1211.

[19] D. Baltimore, Nature 226 (1970) 1209.

[20] S. Spiegelman, A. Burny, M.R. Das, J. Keydar, J. Schlom, M. Travnicek and K. Watson, Nature 227 (1970) 563.

[21] S. Spiegelman, A. Burny, M.R. Das, J. Keydar, J. Schlom, M. Travnicek and K. Watson, Nature 227 (1970) 1029.

[22] S. Mizutani, D. Boettiger and H.M. Temin, Nature 228 (1970) 424.

[23] P.H. Duesberg, H.L. Robinson, W.S. Robinson, R.J. Huebner and H.C. Turner, Virology 36 (1968) 73.

[24] A. Gregoriades and L.J. Old, Virology 37 (1969) 189.

[25] W. Schäfer, F.A. Anderer, H. Bauer and L. Pister, Virology 38 (1969) 387.

[26] S. Oroszlan, C.L. Fisher, T.B. Stanley and R.V. Gilden, J. Gen. Virol. 8 (1970) 1.

[27] J. Huppert, F. Lacour, J. Harel and L. Harel, Cancer Research 26 (1966) 1561.

[28] B.I. Gerwin, G.J. Todaro, V. Zeve, E.M. Scolnick and S.A. Aaronson, Nature 228 (1970) 435.

[29] W.S. Robinson and P.H. Duesberg, *In:* Y. Ito, Subviral carcinogenesis, (Aichi Cancer Center, Nagoya 1966) p.3.

[30] M.C. Glick and L. Warren, Proc. Natl. Acad. Sci. U.S. 63 (1969) 563.

[31] P.H. Duesberg, Proc. Natl. Acad. Sci. U.S. 60 (1968) 1511.

[32] L. Montagnier, A. Golde and P. Vigier, J. Gen. Virol. 4 (1969) 449.

[33] J.P. Bader and T.L. Steck, J. Virol. 4 (1969) 454.

[34] N. Granboulan, J. Huppert and F. Lacour, J. Mol. Biol. 16 (1966) 571.

[35] T. Kakefuda and J.P. Bader, J. Virol. 4 (1969) 460.

[36] H. Hanafusa and T. Hanafusa, Virology 43 (1971) 313.

[37] T. Graf, 6th Meeting of the European Tumor Virus Group, Bad Wimpfen, 1971.

[38] P.H. Duesberg and P.K. Vogt, Proc. Natl. Acad. Sci. U.S. 67 (1970) 1673.

[39] D.P. Bolognesi and T. Graf, Virology 43 (1971) 214.

[40] M.W. Pons, Current Topics Microbiol. 52 (1970) in press.

[41] P.H. Duesberg, K.V.D. Helm and E. Canaani, Proc. Natl. Acad. Sci. U.S. 68 (1971) 747.

[42] J.P. Bader, *In:* J.S. Colter and W. Paranchych, The molecular biology of viruses (Academic Press, New York–London, 1967), p.697.

[43] L. Montagnier, *In:* L.V. Crawford and M.G.P. Stoker, The molecular biology of viruses (Cambridge University Press, 1968) p. 125.

[44] D.P. Nayak, *In:* R.D. Barry and B.W.J. Mahy, The biology of large RNA viruses (Academic Press, London–New York, 1970) p.371.

[45] H. Harris, E. Sidebottom, D.M. Grace and M.E. Bramwell, J. Cell Sci. 4 (1969) 499.

[46] B.W.J. Mahy, *In:* R.D. Barry and B.W.J. Mahy, The biology of large RNA viruses (Academic Press, London–New York, 1970) p.392.

[47] H.M. Temin, J. Cell, Physiol. 69 (1967) 53.

[48] H. Yoshikura, J. Gen.Virol. 8 (1970) 113.

[49] H.M. Temin, *In:* R.D. Barry and B.W.J. Mahy, The biology of large RNA viruses (Academic Press, London–New York, 1970) p.233.

[50] P. Balduzzi and H.R. Morgan, J. Virol. 5 (1970) 470.

[51] M.M.K. Nass, Science 165 (1969) 32.

Replication of oncornaviruses 69

[52] P.H. Duesberg and P.K. Vogt, Proc. Natl. Acad. Sci. U.S. 64 (1969) 939.
[53] P. Vigier, Compt. Rend. Acad. Sci., Paris 270 (1970) 1192.
[54] H.M. Temin, *In:* L.G. Silvestri, The biology of Oncogenic Viruses, (North-Holland, Amsterdam, 1971) p. 176.
[55] M. Green, Ann. Rev. Biochem. 39 (1970) 702.
[56] J. Loeb and B. Hubby, Biochim. Biophys. Acta 166 (1967) 745.
[57] N.J. Richert, J.D. Hare and P.C. Balduzzi, Proc. Bacteriol. (1971) 222.
[58] O. Mach and J. Kara, Folia Biol. 17 (1971) 65.
[59] M. Hatanaka, R.J. Huebner and R.V. Gilden, Proc. Natl. Acad. Sci. U.S. 67 (1970) 143.
[60] J. Schlom, D.H. Harter, A. Burny and S. Spiegelman, Proc. Natl. Acad. Sci, U.S. 68 (1971) 182.
[61] L.B. Stone, E. Scolnick, K.K. Takemoto and A.A. Aaronson, Nature 229 (1971) 257.
[62] F.H. Lin and H. Thormar, J. Virol. 6 (1970) 702.
[63] K.K. Takemoto, C.F.T. Mattern, L.B. Stone, J.E. Coe and G. Lavelle, J. Virol. 7 (1971) 301.
[64] W.P. Parks, G.J. Todaro, E. Scolnick and S.A. Aaronson, Nature 229 (1971) 258.
[65] K.K. Takemoto and L.B. Stones, J. Virol. (1971) 770.
[66] R.C. Gallo, S.S. Yang and R.C. Ting, Nature 228 (1970) 927.
[67] A.A. Kiessling, G.H. Weber, A.O. Deeny, E.A. Possehl and G.S. Beaudreau, J. Virol. 7 (1971) 221.
[68] W.W. Ackermann, W.H. Murphy, B.A. Miller, H. Kurtz and S.T. Barker, Biochem. Biophys. Res. Commun. 42 (1971) 723.
[69] E.M. Scolnick, S.A. Aaronson, G.J. and W.P. Parks, Nature 229 (1971) 218.
[70] P.E. Penner, L.H. Cohen and L.A. Loeb, Biochem. Biophys. Res. Commun. 42 (1971) 1228.
[71] M. Rokutanda, H. Rokutanda, M. Green, K. Fujinaga, R.K. Ray and C. Gurgo, Nature 227 (1970) 1026.
[72] P.H. Duesberg and E. Canaani, Virology 42 (1970) 783.
[73] S. Spiegelman, A. Burny, M.R. Das, J. Keydar, J. Schlom, M. Travnicek and K. Watson, Nature 228 (1970) 430.
[74] S. Lee-Huang and L.F. Cavalieri, Proc. Natl., Acad. Sci. U.S. 50 (1963) 1116.
[75] L.F. Cavalieri and E. Carroll, in press.
[76] L.F. Cavalieri and E. Carroll, Biochem. Biophys. Res. Commun. 41 (1970) 1055.
[77] P.J. Cassidy, J. Biol. Chem. 241 (1966) 2173.
[78] K.F. Manly, D.F. Smoler, E. Bromfeld and D. Baltimore, J. Virol. 7 (1971) 106.
[79] L. Fanshier, A.X. Garapin, J. McDonnell, A. Faras, W. Levinson and J.M. Bishop, J. Virol. 7 (1971) 77.
[80] G.S. Beaudreau and J. Riman, Compt. Rend. Acad. Sci., Paris 271 (1970) 1728.
[81] M. Green, M. Rokutanda, K. Fujinaga, H. Rokutanda, C. Gurgo, R.K. Ray and J.T. Parson, *In:* L.G. Silvestri, The biology of oncogenic viruses (North-Holland, Amsterdam, 1971) p.193.
[82] J.P. McDonnell, A.C. Garapin, W.E. Levinson, N. Quintrell, L. Fanshier and J.M. Bishop, Nature 228 (1970) 433.
[83] J.M. Coffin and H.M. Temin, J. Virol. (1971) in press.
[84] S.A. Aaronson, W.P. Parks, E.M. Scolnick and G.J. Todaro, Proc. Natl. Acad. Sci. U.S. 68 (1971) 920.
[85] L. Gazzolo, G. De-The, P. Vigier and P.S. Sarma, Compt. Rend. Sci., Paris 268 (1969) 1668.

[86] A.S. Levine, R. Petraitis and J. Green, Nature 192 (1961) 1271.

[87] L. Montagnier, H. Collandre, J. Gruest and G. Torpier, In: Proceedings of the First International Conference on Cell Differentiation (Munksgaard, Copenhagen, 1972), in press.

[88] L. Harel, J. Harel, F. Lacour and J. Huppert, Compt. Rend. Acad. Sci., Paris 263 (1966) 616.

[89] M. Yoshikawa-Fukada and J.D. Ebert, Proc. Natl. Acad. Sci. U.S. 68 (1971) 743.

[90] J. Harel, L. Harel, F. Lacour and G. Frezouls, In: Défectivité, démasquage et stimulation des virus oncogènes (Ed. CNRS 1969) p. 103.

[91] M.A. Baluda, In: Replication and persistence of the RNA oncogenic viruses (Proc. Tenth Intern. Cancer Congress, Houston, in press).

[92] M.A. Baluda and P.D. Markham, Nature New Biology 321 (1971) 90.

[93] R.A. Weiss, J. Gen. Virol. 5 (1969) 511.

[94] H. Hanafusa, T. Miyamoto and T. Hanafusa, Proc. Natl. Acad. Sci. U.S. 66 (1970) 314.

[95] P.K. Vogt and R.R. Friis, Virology 43 (1971) 223.

[96] T. Hanafusa, H. Hanafusa and T. Miyamoto, Proc. Natl. Acad. Sci. U.S. 67 (1970) 1997.

[97] A. Golde, Virology 40 (1970) 1022.

[98] K. Toyoshima, R.R. Friis and P.K. Vogt, Virology 42 (1970) 163.

[99] T. Graf, H. Bauer, H. Gelderblom and D.P. Bolognesi, Virology 43 (1971) 427.

[100] G.S. Martin, Nature 227 (1970) 1021.

[101] K. Toyoshima and P.K. Vogt, Virology 39 (1969b) 930.

[102] J.M. Biquard and P. Vigier, Compt. Rend. Acad. Sci. Paris 271 (1970) 2430.

[103] R.R. Friis, K. Toyoshima and P.K. Vogt, Virology 43 (1971) 375.

[104] L. Montagnier, Compt. Rend. Acad. Sci. Paris 267 (1968) 1417.

[105] L. Harel and L. Montagnier, Nature New Biology 229 (1971) 106.

[106] N. Biswal and M. Benyesh-Melnick, Proc. Natl. Acad. Sci. U.S. 64 (1969) 1372.

[107] K.F. Watson and G.S. Beaudreau, Biochem. Biophys. Res. Commun. 17 (1969) 925.

[108] I. Watanabe and I. Haruna, Acta Heamatol. Japonica 12 (1969) 99.

[109] V. Neuhoff, W.B. Schill and D. Jacherts, Hoppe-Seyler's Z. Physiol Chem. 351 (1970) 157.

[110] S. Astier-Manifacier and P. Cornuet, Biochim. Biophys. Acta 232 (1971) 484.

[111] B.G. Louis and P.S. Fitt, Biochem. J. 121 (1971) 629.

[112] R.J. Huebner, G.J. Todaro, P.S. Sarma, J.W. Hartley, A.E. Freeman, R.L. Peters, C.E. Whitmore, H. Meier and R.V. Gilden, In: Défectivité, démasquage et stimulation des virus oncogènes (Ed. CNRS, 1969) p. 33.

[113] F.E. Payne and R.C. Chubb, J. Gen. Virol. 3 (1968) 379.

[114] P. Bentvelzen and J.H. Daams, J. Natl. Cancer Inst. 43 (1969) 1025.

[115] P. Vigier and G. Bataillon, Virology (1971) in press.

[116] I. MacPherson, Science 148 (1965) 173.

[117] D. Simkovic, J. Svoboda and N. Valentova, Folia Biol. 9 (1963) 82.

[118] H. Rubin, In: Replication and persistence of the RNA oncogenic viruses (Proc. Tenth Intern. Cancer Congr., Houston, in press).

[119] H.G. Callan, J. Cell. Sci. 2 (1967) 1.

[120] D. Baltimore and D. Smoler, Proc. Natl. Acad. Sci. U.S. 68 (1971) 1507.

[121] I.M. Verma, N.L. Meuth, E. Bromfeld, K.F. Manly and D. Baltimore, Nature New Biology 233 (1971) 131.

[122] P. Duesberg, K.V.D. Helm and E. Canaani, Proc. Natl. Acad. Sci. U.S. 68 (1971) 2505.

SYMMETRY OF THE NUCLEOCAPSID OF
THE ONCORNAVIRUSES*

Nurul H. SARKAR, Dan H. MOORE and Robert C. NOWINSKI

Institute for Medical Research, Copewood Street, Camden, N.J. 08103

and the

McArdle Laboratory for Cancer Research, Madison, Wis. 53706, U.S.A.

1. Introduction

Viruses have been classified on the basis of their genetic constituents as RNA and DNA viruses. The next division is based on the symmetry of the viral architecture, particularly the symmetry of the nucleocapsid structure. Nucleocapsids are described as having either cubic or helical symmetry. Most virions are found in one or the other of these groups, with some exceptions. However, the symmetry of the oncornaviruses has been described as uncertain by Wilner [1], or complex by Fenner [2]. In the past there have been some suggestions as to the possible helical nature of the nucleocapsid structure of the leukemia viruses by Vogt [3], and De Thé and O'Connor [4] but nothing definitive has been stated. More recently, Sarkar and Moore [5] formally proposed that the nucleocapsid of the mouse mammary tumor virus was helical. Subsequently this idea was supported by Thomas *et al.* [6] and Nowinski *et al.* [7].

In this communication we review the various structures that have been found by others and by us in oncornaviruses of the chicken, mouse, and cat and attempt to interpret these findings in terms of the possible structure of the nucleocapsid of this virus group.

2. Methods and materials

The following viruses were purified by density-gradient centrifugation in sucrose: AvLV, from the plasma of chicks infected with avian myeloblastosis virus; MuLV, from the plasma of mice infected with Rauscher leukemia virus,

*This study was supported by USPH Grants CA-08740 and CA-0874A from National Institutes of Health and Grant-in-Aid Contract M-43 from the State of New Jersey.

and also from a tissue culture line of the murine L1210 ascites leukemia; MuMTV, from the milk of RIII mice; and FeLV, from a tissue culture line of feline fibroblasts infected with this virus. The viral band (density 1.15-1.16 g/ml^3) was separated, diluted with phosphate buffered saline (PBS) pH 7.4, and pelleted by ultracentrifugation. The pellet was resuspended in a small volume of PBS. Purified virions were also treated with Tween 80-ether and the nucleoids were isolated. Untreated virions, as well as nucleoids, were examined in the electron microscope after being negatively stained with phosphotungstic acid (PTA) at pH 7.0.

3. Results and discussion

The majority of virions that are penetrated by PTA show spherical nucleoids with no apparent symmetry (fig. 1). In a small percentage of virions and isolated nucleoids obtained after detergent treatment of the virus two distinctive structures are found: (a) single strands, 30-50 Å in diameter (fig. 5); and (b) paired strands, 70-90 Å in diameter (figs. 3, 4 and 6). In some cases the paired strands are seen connected by periodic bridges, 63 Å apart (fig. 4), or the two strands are twisted around each other to make a double helical structure with a pitch of 126 Å (fig. 2). The strands contain subunit structures. It should

---

Figs. 1-6. Nucleocapsid structure of the oncornaviruses. The virions were negatively stained with sodium phosphotungstate, pH 7.0.

Figs. 1 and 2. Mouse mammary tumor viruses. Both the particles show the characteristic surface projections and spherical nucleocapsid. The details of the internal structure of the nucleocapsid cannot be discerned in fig. 1, except for its thread-like appearance. A short segment of double helical structure (80 Å in diameter) can be seen in fig. 2. (arrow). (Fig. 1, x 300,000; fig. 2, x 360,000.)

Figs. 3 and 4. Rauscher leukemia virus. Paired strands with subunit structures are clearly seen on the perimeter of the nucleoids. These paired strands have been considered as helical structures. The periodic crossings of the helix are particularly clear in fig. 4 (arrows). (Fig. 3, x 420,000; fig. 4, x 450,000.)

Fig. 5. Feline leukemia virus. The nucleocapsid of a feline leukemia virus shows a single strand 30 Å in diameter (follow the arrows). (x 300,000.)

Fig. 6. L1210 ascites tumor cells. Paired strands are well resolved around the periphery of the nucleoid of a virus isolated from L1210 ascites tumor cells. Note the similarity of the paired strands with those in figs. 3 and 4. (x 360,000.)

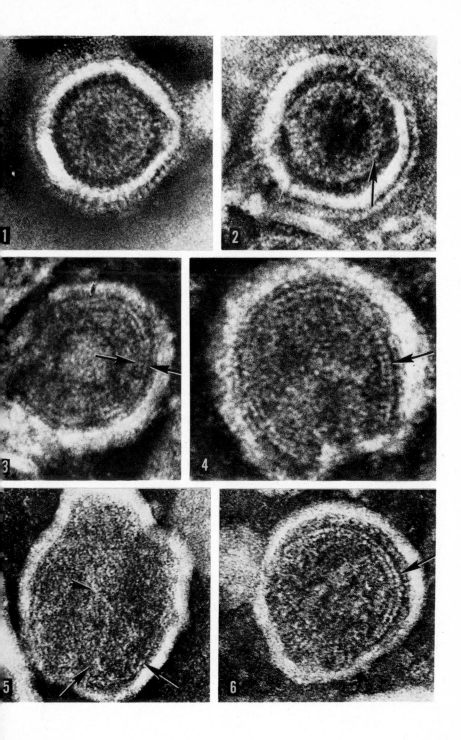

be emphasized that in most cases the paired strands are always found at the periphery of the nucleoid.

Besides the results reported here, previously published micrographs show both single strands (see fig. 13 of ref. 8; fig. 6 of ref. 5; fig. 5 of ref. 9; figs. 5-8 of ref. 7); double strands in the paired form (see figs. 22 and 24 of ref. 4; fig. 6a of ref. 10; figs. 8 and 9 of ref. 11; fig. 2D of ref. 12); and double helical configurations (see fig. 26 of ref. 4; figs. 4a,b,c,e and 5 of ref. 5; and fig. 9 of ref. 7).

On the basis of these observations there are three alternatives for the nucleocapsid symmetry: (a) the large concentric two-ring structure could be assembled from stacked small rings of diameter 70-90 Å; (b) the annular ladder-like structure could be a single helix that is held in an unusual configuration that suggests cross-striations between two strands; or (c) the annular ladder-like structure could be a double helix compressed along its length which in two dimensional view appears as two strands connected by periodic bridges (fig. 4). The stacked ring arrangement of the nucleocapsid structure would be expected to yield small rings (70-90 Å in diameter) upon disruption. However, the findings of 30-50 Å strands excludes this interpretation. The possibility for a single helix held in an unusual configuration also does not appear likely. It is difficult to imagine the conformation of a single helix that would give the appearance of ladder-like structures or the appearance of two strands twisted around each other (rope-like arrangement of strands). Thus, the only alternative left is to assume that the basic structure of the nucleocapsid is a double helix. Compression along the length of the helix would give the ladder-like appearance, whereas separation of the strands would yield single helices and/or single strands. From these considerations we favor the hypothesis that the nucleocapsid is a double helix of nucleoprotein; however, the possibility of a single helix cannot be definitively ruled out at this time.

The hollow spherical structure of the nucleoid of budding virions observed in thin sections and the finding of helical segments only at the periphery of the nucleoid suggest that the nucleocapsid helix is supercoiled as a hollow sphere in the immature virion.

3.1. A model of the nucleocapsid

According to our measurements, the mean diameter of the single strands is 30 Å and that of the double helix is 80 Å. Repeated crossings of the helix are at 63 Å intervals; thus, if the helix were single-stranded the pitch would be 63 Å, whereas if the helix were double-stranded the pitch would be 126 Å. Based on these measurements we have constructed three-dimensional scale models of the nucleocapsid of the oncornaviruses, containing either a single or a double helix. The double-stranded helix with a pitch of 126 Å contains the same length of

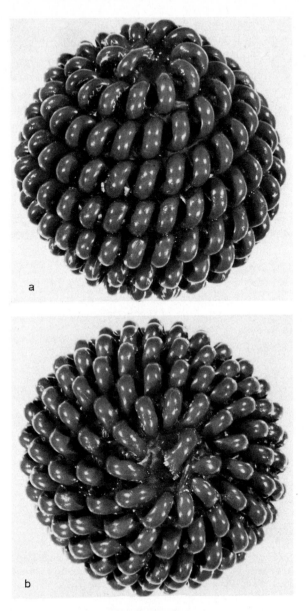

Fig. 7. Photograph of a scale model of the nucleocapsid of the oncornaviruses. A nucleo-protein strand (3 mm in diameter) is coiled with a pitch of 6.3 mm in a single helical structure of diameter 8 mm. The 8 mm helix is supercoiled about a spherical structure 47 mm in diameter; the resultant diameter (measured from two opposite midpoints of the coiled structure) of the nucleocapsid is therefore 55 mm. (a) Horizontal view, (b) Polar view. This model accommodates a strand 3.7 meters in length.

nucleoprotein as does the single helix with a pitch of 63 Å. A photograph of a single-stranded helical model is presented in fig. 7. The scale of the model was 1 mm = 10 Å, or a final magnification of 1×10^6. The model contains 9 coils of a single-stranded nucleocapsid helix, and if reduced to scale would accommodate a nucleoprotein strand 3.7μ length. Thus the viral RNA would have an estimated molecular weight of 3.7×10^6 daltons, corresponding to a 36S RNA strand. This estimated molecular weight of the oncornavirus RNA agrees with the values calculated by Sarkar and Moore [13] from the measurements of the lengths (by electron microscopy) of the RNA molecules, and by Lyons and Moore [10] from chemical determinations. It should be mentioned, however, that the estimated size of the RNA is based solely on model building. Certainly, latitude must be considered for errors inherent in such an analysis. Nevertheless, in our attempts at model building, we have not been able to assemble a 60-70S RNA molecule into a nucleocapsid of the described symmetry.

3.2. Morphogenesis of the oncornaviruses

The proposed model explains the morphogenesis of the oncornaviruses, particularly the development of the crescent in the leukemia-sarcoma particles and the morphological transition of the freshly-budded virion into B or C type particles (fig. 8).

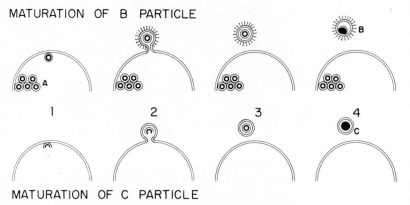

Fig. 8. Schematic representation of the morphological development of the type B and C particles. A type A particle (top fig.) inside the cytoplasm is shown at the periphery of the cell. As it starts budding, it acquires spikes from the cell membrane. Stage 3 shows a freshly budded immature B particle. At stage 4 the mature particle exhibits a condensed, eccentric nucleoid. Type C particles also bud from the cell. The nucleocapsid starts forming a double shelled structure immediately below the site of viral budding (stage 1). Thin-section electron microscopy shows this as a crescent-like structure. As the budding of the membrane continues, the crescent enlarges (stage 2) until it forms a hollow sphere (stage 3). In the extracellular particle the hollow spherical nucleoid undergoes a rapid structural transition to yield a condensed nucleoid (stage 4).

In the case of C particles, if we assume that the supercoiling of the nucleocapsid is initiated near the cell membrane and proceeds perpendicular to the cell surface, then in thin-section electron microscopy a crescentlike structure would be observed (stage 1, fig. 8). The inner ring of the crescent corresponds to the nucleocapsid, while the outer ring corresponds to the nucleoid capsule, which is assembled co-ordinately with the nucleocapsid. Ultimately a complete nucleoid is formed as a hollow sphere inside which may be trapped cellular material. At this stage the morphology of the nucleoid of the C particle is similar to that of the nucleoid of the B particle (cytoplasmic A particle). Thus, the structure of the nucleoid of immature MuMTV and of type C particles (stage 3, fig. 8) is consistent with what one could expect to find assuming the proposed model.

In budding virions the structural integrity of the supercoiled nucleocapsid is maintained by interactions between the protein subunits of the neighboring strands, which in turn are under the influence of the microenvironment of the virion. As soon as the virus is budded into the extra-cellular space the microenvironment is changed; as a result, the interaction between the protein subunits is altered and the hollow-spherical nucleocapsid collapses. This is a random process, since in thin-sections of both type B and C particles the nucleoids do not necessarily show a circular profile. Furthermore, the intensity of the staining of the nucleoid by uranyl acetate and lead citrate is not uniform and varies from particle to particle; this suggests different degrees of condensation and orientation of the structural elements of the nucleocapsid.

3.3. Difficulties in finding helical structures

As has been discussed above, the mature oncornavirus is a degenerate form in respect to symmetry of the nucleocapsid (i.e. the nucleocapsid is disrupted into randomly oriented nucleoprotein strands and only rare helical segments remain). According to our model, only that turn of the nucleocapsid coil which is in the equatorial plane of the nucleoid (fig. 7a) would be observed. Upon drying on the grid the most equatorial coil of the nucleocapsid would correspond to its periphery. Thus, the nucleocapsid must be oriented on the grid in such a way that the equatorial coil is parallel to the plane of the grid for the helical nature of the nucleocapsid to be observed. Coils away from the equatorial plane would not be resolved due to superimposition of coils above and below it. The probability of such preferred orientation of the nucleocapsid on the grid must be small.

Our model predicts that the helical symmetry would be best seen in only the most peripheral positions of the nucleoid and this is indeed what is actually observed.

3.4. Considerations of the models of the nucleocapsids proposed by others

Kakefuda and Bader [14] have proposed a model for the nucleocapsid of murine leukemia virus in which they considered RNA as the only constituent of the nucleocapsid. In their model naked RNA is coiled into a primary helix of diameter 160 Å, which in turn is supercoiled into a hollow spherical structure that is retained by an intermediate membrane. Several pertinent questions can be raised about this model. (a) How would the RNA by itself maintain such a large helical structure? Furthermore, what interactions are there in naked RNA that could account for the extensive supercoiling? (b) It has been established by many authors [15-18] that the group-specific antigen in the oncornaviruses is a component of the viral nucleocapsid. If so, this model fails to explain the presence of the group-specific antigens. (c) The dimensions of the nucleocapsid helix (160 Å in diameter) is not compatible with a supercoiled spherical structure, as only 3-4 turns could be envisaged. (d) Finally, the explanation for the collapse of the hollow sphere by temperature-dependent scissions is not in agreement with the extraction of 60-70S RNA from purified mature virions (both type B and C particles). Although the basic symmetry of their model in terms of a hollow coiled sphere is similar to our model, the dimensions and chemical constitution of the nucleocapsid helix differ.

Another model for the structure of the nucleocapsid of oncornaviruses has been proposed by De Thé and O'Connor [4]. They conceived their model on the basis of the findings of two-ring structures that surround a central mass in the nucleocapsid of murine leukemia virus. They proposed that the morphological transition of these viruses occurs when the rings collapse and fuse with the inner mass. Reappraisal of these micrographs (see fig. 24, for example), however, shows that the two rings are actually a single helical structure which is usually observed at the periphery of the nucleoid. In general, our morphological data agree with that of De Thé and O'Connor [4], but our proposed model differs from their model due to different interpretations of the electron microscopic findings.

5. Summary

Negative staining of the oncornaviruses and isolated nucleoids reveals two essential structures in the nucleocapsid: a) *single strands* (30-50 Å in diameter) that were presumed to be nucleoprotein; and b) closely associated *double strands* (70-90 Å in diameter) coiled in a helical nucleocapsid. The helical nucleocapsid segments are generally observed at the periphery of the nucleoid. This finding, as well as hollow-spherical symmetry of the nucleoid observed in thin-section of budding virions, suggests that the nucleocapsid of a freshly budded oncornavirus is supercoiled as a hollow sphere. This symmetry is considered *transient,* as the nucleocapsid of an extracellular virus undergoes a conformational rearrangement (uncoiling and condensation) and only rare helical segments remain. Thus we propose that the nucleocapsid of the oncornaviruses is helical and that these viruses should be classified as "helical viruses" with regard to the symmetry.

References

[1] B. Wilner, A classification of the major groups of human and other animal viruses. (Burgess Pub. Co., 1969) p. 150.
[2] F. Fenner, The biology of animal viruses. (Academic Press, New York 1968) p. 73.
[3] P.K. Vogt, *In:* Advances in virus research. (Academic Press, New York 1965) II. p. 294.
[4] G. de Thé and T.E. O'Connor, Virology 28 (1966) 713.
[5] N.H. Sarkar and D.H. Moore, J. Microscopie 7 (1968) 539.
[6] J.A. Thomas, E. Hollande, M. Henry and M. Ducros, Compt. Rend. Acad. Sci., Paris 269 (1969) 2471.
[7] R.C. Nowinski, L.J. Old, N.H. Sarkar and D.H. Moore, J. Virol. 42 (1970) 1152.
[8] R.F. Zeigel and F.J. Rauscher, J. Natl. Cancer Inst. 32 (1964) 1277.
[9] J. Calafat and P. Hageman, Virology 38 (1969) 364.
[10] M.J. Lyons and D.H. Moore, J. Natl. Cancer Inst. 35 (1965) 549.
[11] J.D. Almeida, A.P. Waterson and J.A. Drewe, J. Hygiene 65 (1967) 467.
[12] B.I. Gerwin, G.J. Todaro, V. Zeve, E.M. Scolnick and S.A. Aaronson, Nature 228 (1970) 435.
[13] N.H. Sarkar and D.H. Moore, J. Virol. 5 (1970) 230.
[14] T. Kakefuda and J.P. Bader, J. Virol. 4 (1969) 460.
[15] A. Gregoriades and L.J. Old, Virology 37 (1969) 189.
[16] W. Schäfer, F.A. Anderer, H. Bauer and L. Pister, Virology 38 (1969) 387.
[17] M.A. Fink, L.R. Sibal, N.A. Wivel, C.A. Cowles and T.E. O'Connor, Virology 37 (1969) 605.
[18] R.C. Nowinski, N.H. Sarkar, L.J. Old, D.H. Moore, D.I. Scheer and J. Hilgers, Virology 46 (1971) 1.

Part 3

GENETIC FACTORS IN ONCOGENESIS BY AVIAN TUMOR VIRUSES

THE BIOLOGY OF AVIAN TUMOR VIRUSES AND THE ROLE OF HOST CELL IN THE MODIFICATION OF AVIAN TUMOR VIRUS EXPRESSION*

J. SVOBODA

Institute of Experimental Biology and Genetics
Czechoslovak Academy of Sciences
Prague 6, Flemingovo 2, Czechoslovakia

Avian oncogenic viruses, containing high-molecular weight RNA [1,2] and, according to recent findings, also a specific DNA [3,4], represent one of the best known families of oncogenic viruses. They have been collectively called the avian leukosis complex and individual members of this complex are the etiological agents of individual forms of leukemias and sarcomas.

These viruses have identical structures. They consist of a lipoprotein envelope and nucleoid, containing the virus genome. Between the envelope and the nucleoid an inner membrane is detectable [5,6]. The internal part of the virion also contains the group-specific antigen (gs antigen) [7-9], which is common to all viruses of the avian leukosis complex. The typical property of these viruses is that they mature by budding on the cell membrane and are usually present in clusters here.

Of all these viruses, chicken sarcoma viruses, particularly Rous sarcoma virus (RSV), have been studied in greatest detail. Extensive information on RSV has been obtained thanks to a quantitative tissue culture test developed by Temin and Rubin [10]. This test makes it possible to titrate RSV *in vitro* on the basis of its ability to change morphologically (or to transform) chicken fibroblasts and to stimulate the proliferation of such transformed cells. By isolating the virus from individual groups of transformed cells called "foci" it was possible to isolate the progeny of one infectious virus particle and in this way to obtain clones of the virus.

In experiments with the cloned viruses it was shown that one type of the virus is sufficient to transform chicken fibroblasts with sarcoma virus. Temin [11] isolated mutants of RSV which produce a specific type of morphological transformation, i.e. formation of round or fusiform transformed cells.

*This investigation was aided by a grant from the Jane Coffin Childs Memorial Fund for Medical Research (U.S.A.)

Classification of the avian tumor viruses

Generally the avian leukosis complex represents a group of closely related viruses. Nevertheless, there are distinct differences between these viruses, not only as to the specificity of their biological action. The following three criteria were used to divide them into subgroups:
(a) antigenic similarity — detectable by virus-neutralization;
(b) host range — i.e. the ability to infect chicken cells of a certain genotype, possessing receptors for a certain subgroup of leukosis viruses;
(c) interference pattern — i.e. ability to interfere with only related super-infecting viruses.

Thus, if the viruses are antigenically related and have the same host range and interference pattern, they can be assigned to the same subgroup [12,13]. This assignment is based on the similarity in the structures and functions of the viral envelope, because the envelope carries a virus-neutralizing antigen and allows penetration of the virus into the cell probably as a result of interaction with cell receptors. Also, the interference represents a specific block to virus penetration into the cell during which the interfering virus, which is produced by budding through a cell membrane or is firmly bound to it, prevents the passage of the superinfecting virus into the cell [14,15].

Virus penetration

It has been shown in another model already that virus penetration into the cell may take place, even if the corresponding cell receptors are lacking, when the virus is passed over to the cell during cell fusion [16]. Crittenden [17] found that also genetically resistant cells may succesfully be infected with leukosis virus when co-cultivated with cells producing this virus. In this experimental arrangement, cell fusion or formation of intercellular cytoplasmic bridges between the two types of cells might have taken place as a factor permitting the direct transmission of the virus to the cytoplasm of the resistant cell. Similarly, cell fusion may be responsible for overcoming resistance or interference with large doses of virus especially when spontaneous cell fusion was found to take place in mixed cultures of chicken fibroblasts and mammalian cells with a frequency of $10^{-4} - 10^{-5}$ [18,19].

Phenotypic mixing

If a chicken cell is infected with two viruses belonging to different subgroups, their progeny may contain particles carrying coat proteins of the two types of the virus used for infection [20]. This gives rise to phenotypically mixed viruses. The formation of phenotypically mixed virions containing coat proteins of both parental viruses is illustrated in fig. 1. As judged by the criteria of the

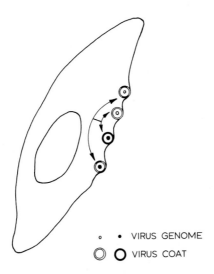

o • VIRUS GENOME

◎ ○ VIRUS COAT

Fig. 1. Illustration of phenotypic mixing.

classification, phenotypically mixed viruses behave in accordance with the nature of their envelope. It stands to reason that if they are cloned at the terminal dilution, they form only the envelope which is coded for by their genome and thus completely lose the alterations caused by phenotypic mixing.

Phenotypic mixing is a common phenomenon in avian leukosis viruses and must be taken into account in their characterization. The mechanism of phenotypic mixing is particularly important in infectivity of the widely studied Bryan strain of RSV. In the case of this strain of RSV, it was found that RSV(O) type α or β', which is not infectious by itself, is responsible for transformation of chicken fibroblasts. However, in the Bryan strain of RSV, Rous-associated virus (RAV) is present in excess [21] which supplies RSV(O) with its coat, permitting in this way the penetration of phenotypically mixed virus into the susceptible cells. As has been found by Weiss [22], RSVβ'(O) is nevertheless able to produce infectious progeny of RSVβ(O) but only in those chicken cells that contain a gs antigen which is an internal component of avian leukosis viruses [23].

RAV(60)

The ability to produce a gs antigen in certain chicken embryos is inherited as a dominant character [24]. According to Hanafusa *et al.* [25] this ability is accompanied by the formation of viral coat antigen but not a virion. These authors were successful in rescuing a new leukosis virus from gs-positive cells by superinfecting them with the known leukosis viruses. The RAV(60) obtained in this way multiplies further alone in avian cells of an appropriate genotype. Vogt and Friis [26] found in certain gs-positive chicken fibroblasts release of the virus designated RAV(O) which has similar properties as RAV(60).

The mechanism of this rescue is independent of phenotypic mixing because RAV(60) forms its own coat. The rescue of RAV(60) may be the result of derepressive action by the superinfecting virus or by some form of interaction of the genomes of both viruses.

All these findings relative to RAV(60) also shed some light on infectivity of RSVβ(O) in chicken gs-positive cells. It was found that RSVβ(O) obtains its coat from RAV(60) which indicates that the infectivity of this RSV is due to phenotypic mixing. This situation is schematically illustrated in fig. 2 which shows the formation of phenotypically mixed RSVβ(O) containing coat protein of RAV(60). This virus is then infectious for certain avian cells. In agreement with this suggestion are experiments in which chicken cells were successfully infected with RSVβ (O), when the penetration of this virus into the cells was facilitated by cell fusion [27].

The RAV(60) represents a very interesting model for studies on the integration and expression of oncogenic viruses. The possibility is not excluded that a systematic study of various genotypes of chicken cells and their individual stages of differentiation will provide evidence on different degrees of expression of the RAV(60) genome.

An earlier finding of Dougherty and Di Stefano [28] that "non-infectious" virus particles, corresponding in their morphology to avian leukosis viruses, are detectable in tissues of chicken embryos derived from a number of flocks of leukosis-free chickens, suggests that viruses of the RAV(60) type may be present as virus-like particles in chicken tissues.

Another type of RSV(O) designated α needs not only a suitable viral coat

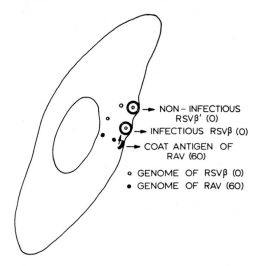

Fig. 2. Chart illustrating phenotypic mixing between RSVβ'(O) and RAV(60).

but also complementation in other functions, probably DNA polymerase, from another leukosis virus in order to become infectious [29].

It should be emphasized that the above relationships hold for the Bryan strain of RSV. Presence of associated viruses is not necessary for the replication and infectivity of many other RSV strains. It is not known whether the co-operation between viruses present in the Bryan strain of RSV reflects the original state of RSV or whether it is the result of selection, as to high virus production. A further strain of chicken sarcoma virus more recently isolated by Thurzo *et al.* [30] also behaves as a virus independent of the associated viruses. Only a detailed analysis of a sufficient number of the primary chicken sarcomas may throw light on these questions.

Transformation of mammalian cells

In the case of infection and transformation of mammalian cells with avian sarcoma viruses, the structure of the viral envelope is probably not a decisive factor.

It should be mentioned that the efficacy of infection and transformation of mammalian cells with RSV is much less than that of chicken cells. The most effective way in this regard is co-cultivation of RSV-producing chicken cells with mammalian cells in which, in addition to a continuous presence of the virus, the direct transfer of the virus or viral genome to mammalian cell thanks to intercellular bridges between both types of cells may play a role [31].

Altaner and Temin [32] showed that the transformation of rat cells with chicken sarcoma virus B77 takes place independently of coat antigen present in this virus. It is therefore likely that the nature of the viral genome or of the functional structures different from the viral coat plays a decisive role in this system. A systematic study of transformation of mammalian cells and other heterologous cells with avian viruses might thus reveal the subtle similarities and differences between these viruses in functions other than those associated with viral envelope and provide a more complete picture of the mutual relationships between these viruses and also of their interaction with the cell, particularly with the cell genome.

Smida and Smidová [33] recently showed that there are significant differences between the strains of sarcoma viruses, even when belonging to the same subgroup, in their affinity to foreign avian hosts.

In some cases, after passage in foreign-species-cells, both in birds [34,35] and in mammals [32,36,37], the oncogenic and transformation activity of avian sarcoma virus on the heterologous host is significantly increased. Experiments performed in mammals suggest that this change is not correlated with changes in viral coat antigens. Furthermore, experiments in which the cloned virus was used [32], thus excluding the possibility that selection of preexisting variants occurred in foreign hosts, may be interpreted by assuming that the change in the affinity of the virus to a foreign cell is the outcome of genetic interaction between the virus genome and the cell.

The persistence of the virus genome and its expression in the cell is directly related to the above questions. An advantageous model for such studies are mammalian cells transformed with RSV (see for references [38]). Such cells are usually virogenic, they contain a complete virus genome but do not form viral particles.

The virus genome is being retained in the population of virogenic cells; for example, in the longest studied rat tumor XC, it has been retained for more than ten years during which time it was continuously passaged *in vivo* or *in vitro*. The virus genome is also present in cells from several tens of the tested clones of virogenic cells [39]. The mechanism of persistence of virus genome in the virogenic cell population has not yet been elucidated. This may be due to a higher numer of free copies of the viral genome in the cell and so there is a high probability that the viral genome will be transmitted to daughter cells during mitosis. Because of long-term stable persistence of RSV genome in the population of different types of mammalian cells it is likely, however, that the virus genome is integrated in the cellular genome as a provirus as proposed by

Svoboda *et al.* [40] or that it is bound to and replicates with some self-replicating cellular structures. The possible ways of integration of RSV genome were recently discussed in detail by Temin [41].

It should be mentioned that in the stable line of hamster BHK cells transformed with RSV the virus genome is lost with a high frequency and this loss is accompanied by loss of the morphological and antigenic properties which are typical for the RSV-transformed cell [42]. It is not known to what extent a quantitatively or qualitatively different type of integration of the virus genome in the cell is involved. It should, however, be mentioned that BHK cells are by themselves a spontaneously transformed cell line, whereas the previously studied virogenic lines were obtained either from tumors induced by RSV or by transformation of primary mammalian cell cultures with RSV.

Rescue of avian tumor viruses from mammalian cells

As has already been stated, the RSV genome persists in virogenic cells but is not fully expressed. However, gs antigen and a tumor specific transplantation antigen (TSTA) are synthesized. A full expression of the virus genome is obtained when the virogenic cell is fused with an indicator cell which is represented by the chicken fibroblast [43,44]. In further experiments, using different indirect methods, it was pointed out that the heterokaryon is the site for synthesis of an infectious virus [18,45]. By studying individual hetero-karyons we have shown that each heterokaryon is a virus producer [19].

The results presented in table 1 are an example of testing the formation of infectious RSV in heterokaryons obtained after fusion of five different lines of virogenic cells with chicken fibroblasts [46]. The table shows that all heterokaryons tested produced the virus. No RSV production was found in heterokaryons formed after fusion of "non-virogenic" mammalian cells with BLEF cells. The non-virogenic cells were originally derived from tumors, which arose after injection of SR-RSV and PR-RSV into mice [52], and were already earlier shown not to give rise to Rous sarcomas after transfer to chickens. Gs avian leukosis antigen was not detected in these tumors which, however, contain tumor specific transplantation antigen (TSTA) as the only characteristics indicating their relation to RSV; the TSTA cross-reacts immunologically with antigens of other RSV-induced virogenic tumors. It was possible that these tumors contain a strongly defective RSV genome which, however, may direct the formation of TSTA and transformation of the cell. On this assumption attempts were made to carry out complementation experiments in which non-virogenic cells were fused with indicator cells pre-infected with avian

Table 1

Rescue of RSV in individual heterokaryons formed by fusion of different types of mammalian virogenic cells with chicken fibroblasts (BLEF) and attempts to rescue RSV by fusion of non-virogenic RSV-transformed mammalian cells and BLEF.

	Origin of cells and transforming virus	Number of mammalian and chicken cells used for heterokaryon formation	Dose of β-PL inactivated RIF-free Sendai virus (HAU)	Incubation of heterokaryons without close contact with indicator BLEF (days)	Incubation of heterokaryons in close contact with indicator BLEF (days)	Titer of rescued infectious RSV (PFU/ml)
Virogenic cells	Chinese hamster cells SR-RSV	1 RSCH × 7 BLEF	400	–	5	50
		4 RSCH × 5 BLEF	500	6	–	642
	Syrian hamster cells SR-RSV	1 RSH × 2 BLEF	400	–	5	82
		1 RSH × 1 BLEF	400	–	5	20
		1 RSH × 1 BLEF	250	5	–	27
	Mouse cells SR-RSV	8 RVA$_2$ × 3 BLEF	400	–	5	25
		1 RVA$_2$ × 3 BLEF	500	–	6	500
		1 RVA$_2$ × 2 BLEF	250	5	–	64
	Rat cells PR-RSV	1 B mix × 8 BLEF	400	–	5	41
		1 B mix × 2 BLEF	250	5	–	48
	Rat cells PR-RSV	1 XC × 2 BLEF	400	–	5	35
		1 XC × 5 BLEF	250	5	–	16
Non-virogenic cells	Mouse cells SR-RSV	1 RVA$_4$ × 5 BLEF	500	–	5	–
		1 RVA$_4$ × 1 BLEF	500	5	–	–
	Mouse cells PR-RSV	1 RVP$_3$ × 5 BLEF	500	–	7	–
		1 RVP$_3$ × 1 BLEF	1 000	5	–	–

leukosis viruses from three different subgroups which synthesize gs antigen but do not transform the chicken fibroblasts (table 2). Although these experiments

Table 2

Tests for RSV production in Sendai virus-treated cultures which arose by mixing non-virogenic RSV-transformed mammalian cells and chicken fibroblasts (BLEF) preinfected with helper virus.

Composition of cell mixture A X B (infected with helper virus)*	Tests for presence of infectious RSV in culture medium (day of collection)		% A cells fused with B cells
	7	14	
RVA_4 X BLEF (RAV(50))	0	0	NT
RVA_4 X BLEF (RAV(49))	0	0	4%
RVA_4 X BLEF (F(42))	0	0	3.2%
RVP_3 X BLEF (RAV(49))	0	0	3.7%
RVP_3 X BLEF (RAV(50))	0	0	NT
RVP_3 X BLEF (F(42))	0	0	NT

* BLEF cells were infected with respective helper virus 3 days before fusion. Multiplicity of infection was equal to 1. The amount of 5×10^6 BLEF was mixed with 5×10^6 non-virogenic cells irradiated with 7,000 R and the mixture was treated with 1,000 HAU Sendai virus. NT = not tested.

were negative in all instances, the possibility cannot be excluded that a portion of RSV genome persists in the non-virogenic cells; such a defective viral genome is not complemented with the helper viruses used.

The molecular mechanism permitting a full expression of RSV genome in a heterokaryon is not yet clear. The most probable explanation seems to be that certain functions, which are necessary for a full expression of RSV genome, are lacking in the virogenic cell. These functions are complemented by fusion of this cell with an indicator cell. The latter cell has a high degree of specificity which is determined by both the species origin and the degree of differentiation. It appeared that the fusion of virogenic cells with mammalian fibroblasts of different mammalian species never give rise to infectious RSV or RSV coat antigen. Similarly, negative results were obtained with fusion of virogenic cells with chicken erythrocytes, macrophages, thymocytes, hepatocytes and cells of the mesonephros.

Our recent observations showed that chicken fibroblasts obtained from the C line embryos and duck fibroblasts from Khaki Campbell embryos are fully effective in RSV rescue after fusion with virogenic cells. Both types of cells were repeatedly tested for the presence of gs antigen during one-month cultivation and this antigen was never detected. This result indicates that endogenous chicken viral genomes of the RAV(60) type, which are manifested by gs antigen formation, are not involved in the mechanism of RSV rescue from mammalian cells.

It should be pointed out that virogenic mammalian cells transformed with RSV represent a unique experimental system for studies of replication, expression and integration of a known tumor virus genome in the cell which does not harbor homologous chicken endogenous viral genomes of RAV(60) type and therefore such genomes cannot phenotypically or genotypically modify the tumor virus genome studied.

Obviously, mammalian cells contain their own endogenous viral genomes and C-type viruses, but, according to the present experience in different laboratories – including ours – they do not interact, even phenotypically, with chicken leukosis viruses.

The development of new models permitting the expression of different functions of the virus genome will undoubtedly contribute to an understanding and determination of these functions. On the other hand, procedures allowing a full functional complementation of the virus genome are very important for a possible rescue of such genomes.

Viral mutants

The question of which functions are available in the virus has been studied by means of viral mutants. Goldé and Latarjet [47] and Goldé [48] found that two types of mutants occur after irradiation of SR-RSV with gamma rays. Mutants of the one type differ from the original virus only in that they are not capable of transforming the chicken cells although they multiply well in the infected cells. Mutants of the other type transform the chicken cells although they do not give rise to an infectious virus. After irradiation of sarcoma virus B77 Toyoshima *et al.* [49] and Graf *et al.* [50] also obtained viral mutants which transformed chicken fibroblasts without producing infectious virus. Transformed cells, however, produced viral particles and these cells regressed after a few passages in vitro.

A series of interesting results were obtained with temperature-sensitive (ts) mutants of avian sarcoma viruses [51]. Temperature-sensitive (ts) mutants include different steps of virus replication, *e.g.* an early or a late step. Moreover, studies of ts mutants showed again that virus replication is independent of its transformation capacity because mutants were obtained which reproduce well ınder non-permissive temperatures but do not transform the cell. Finally, it has)een consistently found by different investigators that the transformation is a ·eversible state so that the temperature shift to a non-permissive temperature is ıccompanied by loss of transformation and vice versa. The present findings on ·s mutants indicate already that the state of transformation includes at least ·wo functional changes in the cell, such as morphological change and ability to ~row in soft agar, which might be defined in greater detail by means of these ınutants and possibly separated, and their relationship to oncogenicity *in vivo* ınight be determined.

All these findings strongly suggest that a certain portion of RSV genome is lirectly responsible for transformation and maintenance of the transformed ·tate of the cell.

Also other functions of the virus genome which are responsible for the ındividual stages of infection and synthesis of the structural components of a irion will probably be elucidated by means of the mutants.

In general, it can be said that the initial scattered information on avian ·eukosis viruses is at present acquiring a more coherent nature and may provide ~ood guidelines for studies of other RNA oncogenic viruses and virus genomes vhich have already been detected or await detection.

References

[1] W.S. Robinson, A. Pitkanen and H. Rubin, Proc. Natl. Acad. Sci. U.S. 54 (1965) 137.
[2] L. Harel, A. Goldé, J. Harel, L. Montagnier and P. Vigier, Compt. Rend. Acad. Sci., Paris 261 (1965) 4559.
[3] W. Levinson, J.M. Bishop, N. Quintrell and J. Jackson, Nature 227 (1970) 1023.
[4] J. Říman and G.S. Beaudreau, Nature 228 (1970) 427.
[5] W. Bernhard, R.A. Bonar, D. Beard and J.W. Beard, Proc. Soc. Exptl. Biol. Med. 97 (1958) 48.
[6] F. Haguenau, A.J. Dalton and J.B. Moloney, J. Natl. Cancer Inst. 20 (1958) 633.
[7] E.A. Eckert, R. Rott and W. Schäfer, Virology 24 (1964) 426.
[8] R.J. Huebner, D. Armstrong, M. Okuyan, P.S. Sarma and H.C. Turner, Proc. Natl. Acad. Sci. U.S. 51 (1964) 742.
[9] H. Bauer and W. Schäfer, Z. Naturforschung 20b (1965) 815.
10] H. Temin and H. Rubin, Virology 6 (1958) 669.
11] H. Temin, Virology 10 (1960) 182.
12] P.K. Vogt and R. Ishizaki, Virology 26 (1965) 664.
13] R.G. Duff and P.K. Vogt, Virology 39 (1969) 18.
14] F.T. Steck and H. Rubin, Virology 29 (1966a) 628.
15] F.T. Steck and H. Rubin, Virology 29 (1966b) 642.
16] J.F. Enders, A. Holloway and E.A. Grogan, Proc. Natl. Acad. Sci. U.S. 57 (1967) 637.
17] L.B. Crittenden, J. Natl. Cancer Inst. 41 (1968) 145.
18] J. Svoboda and R. Dourmashkin, J. Gen. Virol. 4 (1969) 523.

[19] O. Machala, L. Donner and J. Svoboda, J. Gen. Virol. 8 (1970) 219.

[20] P.K. Vogt, Virology 32 (1967) 708.

[21] H. Rubin and P.K. Vogt, Virology 17 (1962) 184.

[22] R.A. Weiss, J. Gen. Virol. 5 (1969) 511.

[23] R.M. Dougherty and H.S. Di Stefano, Virology 29 (1966) 586.

[24] L.N. Payne and R.C. Chubb, J. Gen. Virol. 3 (1969) 379.

[25] T. Hanafusa, H. Hanafusa and T. Miyamoto, Proc. Natl. Acad. Sci. U.S. 67 (1970) 1797.

[26] P.K. Vogt and R.R. Friis, Virology 43 (1971) 223.

[27] T. Hanafusa, T. Miyamoto and H. Hanafusa, Virology 40 (1970) 55.

[28] R.M. Dougherty and H.S. Di Stefano, Proc. Natl. Acad. Sci. 58 (1967) 808.

[29] H. Hanafusa, T. Hanafusa and M. Miyamoto, *In:* L.G. Silvestri (ed.), The Biology of oncogenic viruses, Proceedings of the Second Lepetit Colloquium, Paris 1970 (North-Holland, Amsterdam, 1971) p. 170.

[30] V. Thurzo, M. Slabeciusová, M. Klímek, V. Kovárová-Smidová, Čsl. Onkológia 1 (1954) 230.

[31] J. Svoboda and P. Chýle, Folia Biol. Prague 7 (1963) 46.

[32] C. Altaner and H.M. Temin, Virology 40 (1970) 118.

[33] J. Smida and V. Smidová, Neoplasma 17 (1970) 587.

[34] F. Duran-Reynals, Cancer Res. 2 (1942) 343.

[35] F. Duran-Reynals, Cancer Res. 3 (1943) 569.

[36] T. Kuwata, Cancer Res. 24 (1964) 947.

[37] I.N. Kryukova, I.B. Obuch and T.I. Biryulina, Nature 219 (1968) 174.

[38] J. Svoboda and I. Hložánek, Advan. Cancer Res. 13 (1970) 217.

[39] J. Svoboda and P. Veselý, Experientia 23 (1967) 754.

[40] J. Svoboda, P. Chýle, D. Šimkovič and I. Hilgert, Folia Biol. Prague 9 (1963) 77.

[41] H.M. Temin, *In:* L.G. Silvestri (ed.), The biology of oncogenic viruses, Proceedings of the Second Lepetit Colloquium, Paris 1970 (North-Holland, Amsterdam, 1971), p. 176.

[42] I. Macpherson, Science 148 (1965) 1731.

[43] P. Vigier, Compt. Rend. Hebd. Soc. Sci. 264 (1967) 422.

[44] N. Yamaguchi, M. Takeuchi and T. Yamamoto, Jap. J. Exptl. Med. 37 (1967) 83.

[45] P. Vigier, *In:* Défectivité, démasquage et stimulation des virus oncogènes, Proceedings of the Second International Symposium on Tumor Viruses, Royaumont 3 - 5 June, 1969 (C.N.R.S. Paris, 1970), p. 205.

[46] J. Svoboda, O. Machala, L. Donner and J. Sovová, Int. J. Cancer 8 (1971).

[47] A. Goldé and R. Latarjet, Compt. Rend. Acad. Sci., Paris 262 (1966) 420.

[48] A. Goldé, Virology 40 (1970) 1022.

[49] K. Toyoshima, R.R. Friis and P.K. Vogt, Virology 42 (1970) 163.

[50] T. Graf, H. Bauer, H. Gelderblom and D.P. Bolognesi, Virology 43 (1971) 427.

[51] L.G. Silvestri, ed., The biology of oncogenic viruses, Proceedings of the Second Lepetit Colloquium, Paris 1970 (North-Holland, Amsterdam, 1971).

[52] J. Bubeník, P. Koldovský, J. Svoboda, V. Klement and R. Dvořák, Folia Biol. Prague 13 (1967) 29.

INTERACTIONS BETWEEN HOST GENOME AND AVIAN RNA TUMOR VIRUSES

L.N. PAYNE
*Houghton Poultry Research Station, Houghton
Huntingdon, England*

1. Introduction

Interactions between host genome and avian tumor viruses are of two fundamentally different types: (1) host genes may influence the response of the host to a tumor virus, and determine whether or not its oncogenic potential is expressed, and (2) the tumor virus may modify the genome of the host, possibly in such a way that the modification leads to tumor production. This review is restricted to situations in which the host is the domestic fowl, although it is of course well known that Rous sarcoma virus (RSV) is also oncogenic in other avian species and mammals [1]. There are a number of more or less well characterised examples of the first type of interaction, which are of interest not only to oncologists but also to practical geneticists because of their possible application to the control of avian tumors in the field. Probable interactions of the second type have been recognised recently, and promise to have far-reaching consequences in our understanding of the way in which avian tumor viruses cause tumors. Knowledge of both types of interaction is reviewed in this paper.

2. Influence of host genes on response to tumor viruses

Research on genetic factors affecting response to tumor viruses falls into 3 main areas: (1) identification of genetically controlled differences, (2) discovery of where and how these are mediated, and (3) elucidation of their mode of inheritance. Numerous as yet poorly defined sequential events occur between infection of a bird by a tumor virus and the development of clinical neoplasia, many or all of which will be influenced by genetic factors. Where tumor production in the bird is the variable measured it is to be expected that a number of host genes will affect the final outcome, and the inheritance of different response patterns will appear to be polygenic. In recent years progress has been made in dissecting the polygenic mechanisms by use of assay systems which eliminate some sources of variability such as host immune responses coupled with use of inbred lines of fowl to remove variability at individual genetic loci. In this way simple genetic loci have been identified which control the process of infection of the cell by virus. As Crittenden and Okazaki [2] have pointed out in connection with resistance to leukosis, each component of resistance may have a relatively simple basis when considered alone. Examples have also been discovered in recent years of control of response by single genes in a number of other infectious diseases (see Allison [3]). Single gene inheritance of resistance is of interest because it is easier to fix in a population, and also because it makes investigation of gene action easier.

To provide a framework for this review, three stages in the oncogenic process will be considered: (1) virus infection, (2) neoplastic transformation of the infected cell, and (3) progressive multiplication of the transformed cells to produce a visible tumor. While some of the examples of genetic factors which influence response to avian RNA tumor viruses may be classified with some confidence, the place of others is uncertain.

3. Genetic resistance to virus infection

3.1. Mode of action
Studies on resistance to infection have been greatly facilitated by the ability of certain viruses, notably RSV, to produce tumor pocks on the chorioallantoic membrane (CAM) of the chick embryo, and tumor foci in embryonic cells grown *in vitro*. Long ago, Keogh [4] recognised that some CAMs fail to develop pocks, and Prince [5] presented evidence that genetic factors were responsible for the non-reacting membranes. Genetic differences in the number of pocks which develop on the CAM in response to viruses of different subgroups have been observed between inbred lines of fowl in our laboratory (Payne and Biggs [6-8]) (table 1) and by Crittenden and his colleagues [9,10]. The phenotypic differences are designated by use of the nomenclature proposed by Vogt and Ishizaki [11]. Thus C/O indicates chicken cells resistant to no subgroup tested, C/A indicates resistance to subgroup A virus, etc. (See also Crittenden [12].) It is of interest that whereas the differences observed by Crittenden probably arose from the continued selection for susceptibility or resistance to leukosis (see Waters [13]), those seen in the Reaseheath lines were apparently the result of random genetic drift, since no conscious selection was made for different leukosis responses.

Table 1
Relative sensitivities of chorioallantoic membranes of chicken embryos from different inbred lines in response to avian tumor viruses of different subgroups (data from Payne and Biggs [8]).

Virus subgroup	Strain of virus	Inbred line and phenotype			
		I C/O	C C/A	R C/AC	W C/B
A	BS-RSV	1.00[a]	0.003	NT[bc]	0.23
B	BH-RSV(RAV2)	1.00	1.18	0.76	0.0005
C	RSV(RAV49)	1.00	0.55	NT	0.23
C	MH$_2$	1.00	0.52	0.006	0.30

[a] Sensitivity of C/O membranes = 1.00.
[b] NT = not tested.
[c] Cultured embryo cells are resistant (see [6]).

The inbred lines show differing CAM response patterns to strains of RSV of subgroups A, B and C, and these differences are also expressed by chick embryo cells in tissue culture [6-8,14]. No RSV can be extracted from resistant cultures which fail to produce foci of transformed cells, indicating that resistance is against virus replication as well as transformation [6]. Hanafusa [15] showed that the host range of RSV was determined by its outer coat, and it was therefore suggested by Rubin [16] and Vogt and Ishizaki [11] that genetic susceptibility of the cell is dependent on the presence of specific virus receptors on the cell surface. If the normally excluded virus genome can be introduced into the resistant cell, as by the use of phenotypically mixed virus [17] or by co-cultivation with γ-irradiated infected susceptible cells [18], then the resistant cells can replicate the virus, indicating that resistance is mediated via an early event. Since resistant cells adsorb virus from surrounding medium with an efficiency equal to that of susceptible cells, it appears that the block to infection occurs during virus penetration or uncoating [18,19].

3.2. Mode of inheritance

Investigations by various workers on the mode of inheritance of resistance to viruses of subgroups A, B and C, and to strains of RSV of unspecified subgroup, have shown the major influence on each virus of a single autosomal locus. Various methods were used to determine the phenotype of individuals and for genetic analysis of the results (table 2). In our investigations we found

Table 2
Investigations in which responses to avian tumor viruses of different subgroups were
controlled by genes at single autosomal loci.

Virus subgroup	Strain of virus	Method of pheno-type determination[a]	Method of genetic analysis[b]	Authors
A	BS-RSV	IC	Seg. ratios	[20]
A	BS-RSV	IC, CAM, TC	Seg. ratios	[14]
A	BH-RSV(RAV1)	CAM	Seg. ratios	[10]
B	BH-RSV(RAV2)	TC	Seg. ratios	[16]
B	SR-RSV & H-RSV	CAM	Seg. ratios	[7]
B	BH-RSV(RAV2)	CAM	Seg. ratios	[10]
C	RSV(RAV49) & MH2	CAM	Seg. ratios	[8]
Unclassified	Duran-Reynals RSV	CAM	gene frequency	[5]
Unclassified	Bryan RSV	CAM	Castle's formula	[21]

[a]   IC = intracranial inoculation;
    CAM = inoculation onto chorioallantoic membrane;
    TC = inoculation of tissue cultured cells.
[b]   Seg. ratios = Mendelian segregation ratios.

enumeration of RSV pocks on the CAMs, and determination of segregation ratios of susceptible and resistant individuals, in F_2 and backcross generations between two differing inbred lines, to be a satisfactory method of genetic analysis. The response patterns to viruses of subgroups A, B and C in crosses between two differing lines agree well with expectations from Mendelian theory if resistance to each subgroup is controlled by a single, recessive autosomal gene. An example is shown in fig. 1 and table 3. The presence of 11% resistant embryos in the pure I line was unexpected and is not readily explained (see [7]).

In these studies we found full dominance of susceptibility over resistance, as has Crittenden and his colleagues. Two exceptions to this rule have been reported by Prince [5] and Bower et al. [21,22], who observed intermediate responses in F_1 and F_2 generations between susceptible and resistant lines. They suggested partial dominance of the allele for susceptibility, or differences in gene penetrance or expressivity. However, their parental lines were not completely uniform in response and it seems possible that the presence of

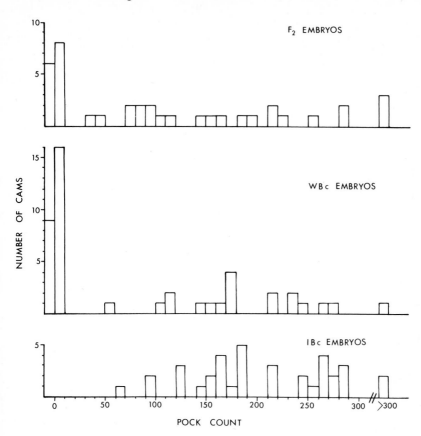

Fig. 1. Distribution of pock counts after inoculation of CAMs of F_2 and first backcross generation embryos with SR-RSV (subgroup B). (Data from Payne and Biggs [7].)

multiple alleles coding for differing response levels could account for the intermediate response. It should be mentioned also that it is not certain that the type of resistance they measured was to virus infection as distinct from neoplastic transformation. Munroe [23] reported non-reactor CAMs from which RSV could be isolated, suggesting resistance to transformation rather than virus infection and replication.

The three genetic loci controlling response to A, B and C subgroup viruses have been designated *tva* (tumor virus a), *tvb* and *tvc* on the basis of the nomenclature proposed by Crittenden *et al.* [10], with susceptibility alleles a^s, b^s, and c^s, and resistance alleles a^r, b^r, and c^r. As discussed above, it seems likely that there are multiple alleles at these loci, which are expressed as

Table 3
Comparison of observed proportions of chicken embryos susceptible to SR-RSV (subgroup B) with those predicted by single autosomal locus hypothesis (data from Payne and Biggs [7]).

Line or cross		Genotype	Phenotype[a]	No. of embryos tested	Susceptible Embryos(%) Expected	Observed	Deviation $\chi^{2\,b}$
I		$b^S b^S$	S	35	100	88.5	–
W		$b^r b^r$	R	37	0	0	–
F_1		$b^S b^r$	S	NT[c]	100	NT	–
F_2	1	$b^S b^S$	S	42	75	73.8	0.03 NS[d]
	2	$b^S b^r$	S				
	1	$b^r b^r$	R				
Back- crosses							
I × F_1	1	$b^S b^S$	S	65	100	100	–
	1	$b^S b^r$	S				
W × F_1	1	$b^r b^r$	R	40	50	47.5	0.03 NS
	1	$b^S b^r$	S				

[a] S = susceptible, R = resistant.
[b] With Yates's correction.
[c] NT = not tested.
[d] NS = not significant.

different levels of susceptibility. Such alleles could explain the different degrees of resistance to subgroup A RSV shown by the C and R lines [6], and the range of intermediate responses observed by Crittenden and Motta [24] in non-inbred commercial heavy-breed stocks.

Tests by Crittenden et al. [10] and ourselves [25] revealed no linkage between the tva and tvb loci, or between the tvb and tvc loci, but there was evidence for linkage between tva and tvc [25]. In the crosses tested, there was a close association between resistance to subgroup A RSV and resistance to subgroup C RSV. Since this association is not invariably found, close linkage rather than control by a single pleiotropic gene appears to be more likely.

The only other linkage relationship known for a tv locus was reported by Crittenden et al. [26] between tvb and the newly discovered R blood group system. Attempts to associate susceptibility to subgroups A and B with alleles of the 11 known blood group systems failed. Search for associations of this type are of interest not only to provide markers for selection of resistance genes, but also for the light they may throw on the nature of virus receptors. The possibility that virus receptors might be antigenically expressed as blood group substances or other antigens is worth pursuing, as is the possibility of common antigens in the virus coat and the cell virus receptor.

Genetic systems other than the single loci described above may influence the CAM response to tumor viruses. Dhaliwal [27] found evidence for dominance of resistance to RSV and MH2 viruses in F_1 crosses between susceptible and resistant lines, and we identified a single cock in a non-inbred flock of Rhode Island Red fowl who conferred resistance on all his progeny (table 4). Extracts

Table 4

Dominance of resistance to BS-RSV (subgroup A) in progeny of Rhode Island Red (RIR) sire no. 206 mated to randomly selected RIR dams.

Sire no.	Dam no.	No. of embryos tested	Pock count range (%) O	1-100	>100
206	36	8	100.0	0.0	0.0
	37	13	61.5	38.5	0.0
	41	10	80.0	20.0	0.0
	42	10	100.0	0.0	0.0
	43	8	100.0	0.0	0.0
	44	9	66.7	33.3	0.0
	46	11	100.0	0.0	0.0
218	51	14	0.0	7.1	92.9
	53	11	9.1	9.1	81.8
	54	9	0.0	11.1	88.9
	55	11	0.0	0.0	100.0
	57	12	8.3	16.7	75.0
	58	7	0.0	28.5	71.5
	59	7	0.0	14.3	85.7
	61	12	0.0	0.0	100.0
	64	13	7.7	15.4	76.9

from resistant CAMs after inoculation of subgroup A RSV contained no virus, which indicates that the dominant resistance trait was against virus infection as well as neoplastic transformation. Crittenden and Motta [24] failed to find the bimodal distribution of pock counts in commercial heavy-breed fowl challenged with subgroups A and C RSV that were expected if single autosomal recessive genes were responsible for resistance, and they suggested instead the operation of a more complex system. Multiple alleles could account for their findings or it is possible that other genetic loci were involved. Bimodal populations suggestive of control by loci similar to *tva* and *tvb* were found when white-egg commercial stock were challenged with subgroups A and B RSV, and when heavy-breed fowl were challenged with subgroup B RSV. The reason for the different types of response pattern between heavy-breed and white-egg stocks is not known.

The nature of genetic resistance to subgroup D viruses [28] has not been elucidated. Subgroup D virus is known to be related to subgroup B viruses in host range, antigenicity and interference patterns [28], and it would be of obvious interest to examine the influence of the *tvb* locus on subgroup D virus.

Genetic resistance to subgroup E viruses, of which the infectious type of RSV(O) is the prototype [29], appears to be of a more complex type than the simple loci which control response to subgroups A, B and C. In collaborative studies with P.K. Pani and R.A. Weiss we have studied the segregation of susceptibility and resistance to $RSV\beta(O)$ in the Reaseheath C and I lines and their crosses. The results, which will be reported in detail elsewhere [30], suggest the presence of a dominant autosomal gene for susceptibility to $RSV\beta(O)$, designated e^s in the I line, and its recessive allele, e^r in the C line. Also present in the I line is a dominant autosomal, epistatic, gene, I^e, which inhibits the expression of e^s, with its recessive allele i^e, present in the C line. The two loci, designated "*tve*" and "Inhibitor ^{e} (I^e)" are unlinked. The results, shown in table 5, are in good agreement with those expected from the hypothesis. Results from second generation backcross embryos to the C line were also consistent with the hypothesis.

4. Relationship between response to RSV and to leukosis virus

Although most studies on the genetic resistance of cells to tumor viruses have been conducted with sarcoma-producing viruses, because of their ability to produce easily recognisable cell transformation within a few days, it is clear that cells resistant to RSV are also resistant to infection by leukosis viruses of the same subgroup [11]. This is because viruses within a subgroup share common coat properties which are necessary for determining host range [1]. Lines of fowl resistant to tumor formation by RSV following challenge as embryos or cultured cells also resist induction by leukosis viruses of leukosis and other tumors. Similarly, RSV-resistant progeny from parents which have been identified genotypically by means of progeny tests with RSV are also found to be resistant to leukosis virus belonging to the same subgroup as the RSV used in the progeny test. In a recent series of experiments, line 15 sires of

Table 5
Comparison of observed proportions of chicken embryos susceptible to $RSV\beta(O)$ (subgroup E) with those predicted by the two locus hypothesis.

Line or cross		genotype	phenotype[a]	No. of embryos tested	Susceptible embryos (%)		Deviation χ^{2b}
					Expected	Observed	
C		$i^e i^e e^r e^r$	R	166	0	0.60	–
I		$I^e I^e e^s e^s$	R	26	0	0	–
F_1		$I^e i^e e^s e^r$	R	8	0	0	–
F_2	9	$I^e\text{-}e^s\text{-}$	R	250	18.75	18.80	0.00 NS[c]
	3	$I^e\text{-}e^r e^r$	R				
	3	$i^e i^e e^s\text{-}$	S				
	1	$i^e i^e e^r e^r$	R				
Back-crosses							
$C \times F_1$	1	$I^e i^e e^s e^r$	R	220	25.00	23.60	0.13 NS
	1	$I^e i^e e^r e^r$	R				
	1	$i^e i^e e^s e^r$	S				
	1	$i^e i^e e^r e^r$	R				
$I \times F_1$	1	$I^e I^e e^s e^s$	R	53	0	0	–
	1	$I^e I^e e^s e^r$	R				
	1	$I^e i^e e^s e^s$	R				
	1	$I^e i^e e^s e^r$	R				

[a] S = susceptible, R = resistant.
[b] With Yates's correction.
[c] NS = not significant.

genotype either $a^s a^s$ or $a^r a^r$, identified in progeny tests with subgroup A RSV, were mated to line 7 dams of genotype $a^r a^r$, to produce susceptible progeny of genotype $a^s a^r$ and resistant progeny of genotype $a^r a^r$, respectively. The two types of progeny were inoculated as embryos or exposed by contact with subgroup A leukosis viruses RPL 12, RPL 28, RPL 29 and RPL 30. The incidences of hemorrhages and the acute neoplasms, erythroblastosis and sarcoma, and of the chronic neoplasm, lymphoid leukosis, were greatly reduced in resistant $a^r a^r$ chickens when compared to susceptible $a^s a^r$ birds [31,32]. The resistance was specifically directed against subgroup A viruses, since RPL 25 leukosis virus and the BAI strain of myeloblastosis virus, both of which contain subgroup B virus, were almost equally oncogenic in $a^r a^r$ and $a^s a^r$ chicks (fig. 2). The a^r gene

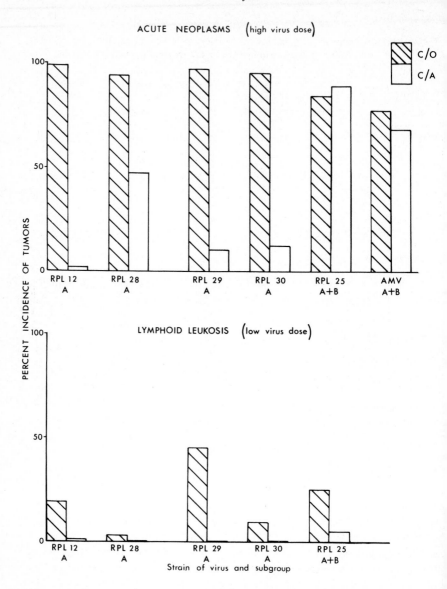

Fig. 2. Incidence of acute and chronic neoplasms in C/O ($a^S a^r$) and C/A ($a^r a^r$) chickens after inoculation with different strains of leukosis virus, showing influence of the *tva* locus on oncogenesis by subgroup A viruses. (Data from Payne *et al.* [31] and Crittenden and Burmester [32].)

influences not only neoplasms but antibody production to subgroup A viruses. Crittenden and Okazaki [2] observed significantly fewer $a^r a^r$ (formerly designated rsrs) birds with antibodies to subgroup A virus than $a^s a^r$ (formerly Rsrs) after RPL 12 inoculation, presumably due to restriction of the antigenic challenge in the resistant birds.

4.1. Commercial application of genetic resistance

The use of homozygous recessive birds, for example of genotype $a^r a^r$, as tester parents for identifying the genotype of birds they are mated to, on the basis of observed segregation ratios in progeny tests with RSV, has been adopted by commercial geneticists as a means of selecting stock genetically resistant to leukosis. This approach should be successful where the simple type of inheritance of resistance operates, as it appears to in white-egg stock [24]. Studies conducted in our laboratory in conjunction with F. & G. Sykes Ltd., showed that it was possible to identify $a^s a^s$, $a^s a^r$, and $a^r a^r$ males of one line with dams of a homozygous recessive line $a^r a^r$, on the basis of the progeny from the 3 types of mating being all susceptible, 1:1 susceptible and resistant, or all resistant [33]. The incidence of lymphoid leukosis and related neoplasms after inoculation of subgroup A lymphoid leukosis virus into progeny from the three types of male mated to recessive females is shown in table 6. The incidence of

Table 6

Influence of a^r gene on incidence of lymphoid leukosis and related neoplasms induced by subgroup A leukosis virus in progeny of Sykes A x B cross (data from Biggs *et al.* [33]).

Genotype of sire (Sykes A)	Genotype of dam (Sykes B)	No. of sire families[a]	No. of progeny	Mean % incidence of leukosis and related neoplasms	Range of mean % incidence per sire family
$a^s a^s$	$a^r a^r$	21	1194	25.1	9.6–45.7
$a^s a^r$	$a^r a^r$	14	801	11.3	5.4–18.4
$a^r a^r$	$a^r a^r$	3	151	0.6	0.0– 1.8

[a] About 20 dams per sire.

leukosis was lowest in families where the sire was homozygous for the a^r gene. In agreement with these findings, Crittenden and Burmester [32] found 7.6% mortality from lymphoid leukosis in $a^s a^r$ chickens exposed to field infection, compared with 0.0% in $a^r a^r$ birds, a significant difference.

Crittenden *et al.* [34] have recently devised a method for identifying the phenotype of adult birds by inoculating cultured pin feather cells with RSV. This technique will simplify selection of genetically resistant fowl for mating.

It is perhaps surprising that while the incidence of subgroup A leukosis viruses is high in commercial chickens [31,35], the incidence of the a^r gene is low [24]. It appears that natural selection against leukosis has operated on genes other than those controlling infection (see later), and that the a^s gene may be of value. Crittenden [36] and Purchase [37] have suggested that there may be a selection pressure against the a^r gene arising through the increased susceptibility to leukosis of $a^s a^r$ progeny without maternal protective antibody obtained when antibody-negative $a^r a^r$ dams are mated to sires carrying the a^s gene. Another possibility, although there is as yet no evidence for it in fowl, is that the susceptibility gene for one virus may be the resistance gene for another, perhaps more virulent, virus. An example of this is the N-B locus in mice, at which there is reciprocal susceptibility and resistance to cell infection by murine leukemia viruses [38]. Both of these possibilities will result in maintenance of a polymorphism which may be valuable, and the introduction of resistance genes on a large scale in commercial poultry should be approached with caution [12]. Further discussions on commercial breeding for resistance are given by Goodwin [39] and Dickerson [40].

5. Genetic resistance to neoplastic transformation

It appears to be generally true that cells or chick embryos that are resistant to RSV are also resistant to tumor formation by leukosis viruses of the same subgroup as the RSV. The converse does not follow. Some strains or individuals which are susceptible to infection by RSV are found to be resistant to tumor induction by leukosis virus, and in this circumstance it has been suggested that the resistance is due to some mechanism other than control of cell infection.

The classical and best documented evidence for this type of resistance are the observations by Crittenden *et al.* [14] on the responses of line 6 and line 15 I chickens to RPL 12 subgroup A leukosis virus. Both lines have cellular susceptibility to the virus, being $a^s a^s$ in genotype. High doses of virus induce a high incidence of erythroblastosis in both lines, but whereas low doses induce a high incidence of lymphoid leukosis in line 15 I, only a low incidence is induced in line 6. These findings suggest that there may be genetically determined resistance to neoplastic transformation of the lymphoid target cell, which is believed to occur in the bursa of Fabricius [41]. The difference may lie in the line 6 target cell itself, or in an interaction of this cell with its environment, investigation of which should be amenable to study of response of bursal cells to virus *in vitro*, or to *in vivo* cell transfer studies. It is possible that the resistance of line 6 to lymphoid leukosis may lie not in resistance to lymphoid transformation *per se*, but to immune rejection of transformed cells at an early stage (see later).

It is of interest that reciprocal F_1 crosses between line 6 $(a^s a^s)$ and line 7 $(a^r a^r)$ had a higher susceptibility to lymphoid leukosis than either parental line. This suggests that line 6 contributed susceptibility to virus infection, and line 7 susceptibility to lymphoid transformation, both traits being a dominant character [14].

6. Genetic resistance to tumor progression

6.1. Mode of action

Tumors induced in chickens with RSV may, after a period of growth, undergo regression and disappear. The onset of regression is coincident with a decrease in virus yield [42-44], which is independent of antibody production to the virus [44] and interferon [45,46]. Studies by Rubin [45] suggest that regression is caused by cell-mediated immunity directed against virus coat antigens. The induction of tumor-specific transplantation antigens has been shown in mice for RSV [47] and leukosis virus [48], and similar antigens could be concerned in tumor rejection in the fowl.

Circumstantial evidence for regression of lymphoid leukosis was found by Cooper *et al.* [41] in a study of the pathogenesis of the disease. This neoplasm arises in a lymphoid follicle of the bursa of Fabricius, where the tumor remains localised for up to 14 weeks before metastasizing to other organs. Some birds appear to be able to regress the localised bursal tumor, because whereas about 70% of birds developed bursal tumors, only 40% of birds developed disseminated leukosis. The mechanism of the regression requires investigation. It is possible that cell-mediated immunity directed against tumor-specific antigen, perhaps to the antigen described by Kakuk and Olson [49], is responsible. Against this possibility perhaps is the observation that thymectomy did not increase the incidence of lymphoid leukosis [50].

6.2. Mode of inheritance

The ability to regress RSV-induced tumors is clearly influenced by genetic factors. Greenwood *et al.* [51] found distinct differences between different lines of Brown Leghorns in the proportion of birds that developed regressive tumors. For example, in the breeding line only 11/333 birds regressed their tumor compared to 14/32 in the non-moult line. By selecting offspring from one particular male they established a "non-susceptible (NS)" line with a high proportion of regressive or small tumors. This type of resistance appeared to be recessive, since it was reduced when NS dams were mated to susceptible (N) cocks.

Quantitative aspects of growth of subcutaneous Rous sarcomas in two pure lines of White Leghorns (WL) and Giant Jungle Fowl (GJF) and their F_1 and F_2 crosses were studied by Gyles *et al.* [52,53]. Highly significant differences in the proportions of negative responses, regressive tumors, and progressive tumors were found between the groups. The WL had significantly more progressive tumors, and fewer regressive tumors and negative responses than did the GJF. In the crosses there was evidence for slight partial dominance for susceptibility. The tumors were also scored for size, appearance and growth rate. WL developed larger tumors, with a higher appearance score, in a shorter time, than did GJF. F_1 crosses tended to have tumors slightly larger than midpoint values between the pure lines, with larger scores but development rates slightly less than the midpoint. Tumor size and score gave the same relative ranking of responses of pure lines and F_1 generation as were observed in CAM inoculation tests on similar lines by Bower *et al.* [22]. This suggests that progression or regression of tumors is related at least in part to the susceptibility of normal cells to infection and transformation. Rous sarcomas are believed to grow partly by recruitment of new transformed cells [54], and the efficiency of host immune responses in causing regression could depend on the rate of virus reinfections. In other words, the effect of genetic factors on regression may be mediated via cell infection rather than through differences in the strength of cell-mediated immunity. In a later study, Gyles *et al.* [55] studied the tumor response of progeny derived from matings of parents from progressive, regressive and negative tumor response classes, and suggested that they were measuring genetic resistance to transformation after virus infection, together with a mechanism causing tumor regression. Without knowledge of the status of their birds at the *tva* locus it is difficult to equate their findings with those of other workers. It is clear that research is needed on the genetics of tumor regression in birds of known genotype at the loci which influence virus infection of cells.

7. Genetic factors with unidentified modes of action

Some of the examples discussed of genetic factors which influence response to tumor viruses have been allocated to the three sections according to their presumptive mode of action. Thus the genetic factors affecting CAM response to RSV studied by Bower *et al.* [21,22], Dhaliwal [27] and Crittenden and Motta [24] have been considered, for convenience of discussion, in the section on resistance to infection although this mode of resistance was not specifically established. A type of genetic resistance for which the mode of action is unknown was described by Waters and Burmester [56,57] for erythroblastosis induced by RPL 12 virus. They found clear evidence for dominance of resistance to erythroblastosis, apparently dependent on a single pair of autosomal genes.

Crittenden *et al.* [58] have recently analysed the results of a series of 7 diallele cross experiments in which lines 6, 7, 9 and 15 I were mated in all combinations and exposed to a number of tumor viruses by a variety of routes. They demonstrated the dominating influence of resistance to cell infection by subgroup A virus contributed by line 7 ($a^r a^r$), which they termed the first line of defence, and of resistance to lymphoid leukosis contributed by line 6, which they termed the second line of defence. In addition there was evidence of other genetic factors involving sex linkage, maternal effects and intermediate resistance of hybrids, which suggests that the second line of defence is genetically complex.

8. Modification of host genome by avian tumor viruses

Although many advances have been made in recent years in knowledge of avian RNA tumor viruses and their replication (see Vogt [1]), the mechanism whereby the virus converts a normal cell into a neoplastic cell remains unknown. Theories of viral carcinogenesis fall in general into two main classes (1) non-cytogenic theories, in which the cell genome is not altered but in which the continued presence of the viral genome changes the cell in some way such that it takes on neoplastic properties, and (2) cytogenetic theories, in which the neoplastic properties arise from an alteration of the host cell genome. There is increasing evidence that a change of the latter type is associated with oncogenesis by RSV.

9. Mutagenic effects of RSV

A change in the host cell genome represents a somatic mutation and may be considered in terms of the possible mutational units. Mutation could arise from duplication of the entire genome (polyploidy), from changes in the numbers of

individual chromosomes (aneuploidy), from structural changes in a chromosome or chromatid (breaks and exchanges), and from changes in individual
genes (point mutation). The mutation may be associated with loss or gain of
host genes, modification of host genes, or acquisition of new genes.

Surprisingly few studies have been made on the effects of avian tumor
viruses on chicken chromosomes, probably partly because of technical
difficulties of working with avian chromosomes. Temin and Rubin [59] found
no significant differences in mode or spread of chromosome counts between
young cultures of RSV-transformed cells and normal cells, but older cultures
of transformed cells contained many polyploid cells. Bayreuther and Thorell
[60,61] reported the largest pairs of chromosomes to be normal in erythroblastosis, and in sarcomas induced by RSV and Fujinami virus. Ponten [62]
found normal karyotypes in 11/12 Rous sarcomas, and hyperdiploidy in 1/12.
Karyotypes from tumor cells from virus induced erythroleukemia were also
normal, whereas cells of the long-transplanted RPL 12 lymphoma were
hyperdiploid. These findings rule out any consistent gross structural or
numerical chromosomal abnormality associated with neoplastic transformation,
(although minor changes amongst the numerous microchromosomes would be
easy to overlook) and suggest that abnormalities in chromosome complement
that are observed in some tumors are secondary changes associated with
continued tumor growth, passage or transplantation. Similar conclusions were
drawn from a study of 91 primary sarcomas induced by RSV in mice by Mark
[63], who suggested virus-induced mitotic lability was responsible for the
appearance of heteroploid lines. The ability of viruses, both oncogenic and
non-oncogenic, to cause chromosomal changes is well known [64]. Sanford [65]
reviewed in general the possible association between malignancy and chromosomal abnormalities in cultured cells, and concluded that the changes were
independent.

Thus, avian tumors and most other malignancies (see Allison [66]) appear to
arise independently of gross chromosomal changes; if genomic change is
involved in neoplastic change in avian cells it would appear to be either
cryptostructural or a point mutation. No mutagenic effects of RSV or other
avian tumor viruses unassociated with neoplasia have been reported in the fowl,
although it is of interest that Burdette and Yoon [67] found an increased
incidence of melanomatous tumors, chromosomal aberrations and visible
mutations in drosophila fed as larvae on RSV. Material from progeny of flies
exposed to RSV failed to produce tumors when inoculated into chicks,
suggesting non-persistence of viral genome.

The effects of RSV described above suggest non-specificity, whereas the
regularity with which RSV induces tumors suggests that any mutagenic effect

must be specific. If the mutation that leads to neoplasia occurs in a pre-existing host gene, then the continued presence of viral genome would be unnecessary for maintenance of neoplastic properties. The fact that in all avian tumors and most mammalian tumors induced by RSV there is evidence of persistence of viral genome [68] suggests that its presence is essential for the malignant character of the cell.

10. Evidence for genetic integration of viral genome

The nature of the persistent viral genome in RSV-transformed cells is largely unknown. A number of workers, notably Temin [69] and Prince [70], have postulated that RSV can exist in the transformed cell in a non-replicating, hidden state, the provirus. The provirus theory is discussed by Temin [71] at this Symposium, but the observations on which it is based may be briefly summarised:

(1) Under certain circumstances non-RSV-producing transformed cells can be obtained from which infectious RSV can later be rescued [1,72,73].

(2) Treatment of cells immediately after RSV-infection with DNA inhibitors, such as actinomycin D, amethopterin, FUDR and cytosine arabinoside, inhibits RSV production [72,74]. This indicates a DNA-dependent step early in the infection cycle, which Temin [72] suggested may be the formation of a DNA provirus.

(3) Hybridization experiments between viral RNA and cell DNA show greater binding with DNA from RSV or AMV-infected cells than from normal cells, consistent with the presence of a provirus DNA copy of RSV or AMV RNA [75,76], although some workers have failed to confirm these findings [see 77].

Recently, integration of viral DNA into the genome of transformed cells has been shown to occur with SV40 and polyomavirus (see Dulbecco [78]). It is logical therefore to consider the possibility that the DNA provirus of RSV might be integrated into the host genome, and inherited as a new gene responsible for the neoplastic properties of the transformed cell. Genetic support for integration of provirus DNA comes from our studies on the inheritance in apparently normal, infection-free chick embryos, of the group-specific (gs) antigen of the avian RNA tumor viruses. The presence of the gs-antigen in leukosis-virus free embryos was first observed by Dougherty *et al.* [79,80], and confirmed as present in inbred I line embryos but absent in C line embryos in our laboratory [81]. From studies on the segregation of the gs-antigen in F_1, F_2 and backcross generations in crosses between the C and I lines we postulated that presence of antigen was controlled by a single,

Table 7

Occurrence of complement-fixing group specific antigen in purebred and crossbred chick embryos from the I and C lines (data from Payne and Chubb [81]).

Line or cross	No. of embryos tested	Embryos with antigen (%)		Deviation $\chi^{2\,a}$
		Expected	Observed	
I	28	100	100	–
C	32	0	0	–
F_1	57	100	100	–
F_2	222	75	74.3	0.02 NS[b]
Back-crosses				
I × F_1	130	100	93.1	–
C × F_1	138	50	41.3	3.83[c]
C × (C × F_1) 11 Homozygous dams	162	0	0	–
9 Heterozygous dams	120	50	48.3	0.08 NS

[a] With Yates's correction.
[b] NS = not significant.
[c] p = 0.05.

dominant autosomal gene [81] (table 7). The deviation of observed gs-antigen-positive embryos from the expected in the C × F_1 cross, which was significant at about the 5% level, may have been due to chance, or to failure to detect antigen present in a few embryos (see [81]). Various hypotheses were considered to account for the presence of a common antigen in tumor viruses and normal embryos [79,81], but the suggestion most consistent with more recent findings is that the embryos contained virus-induced gs-antigen, coded for by tumor virus genome. Since there was no evidence of mature, infectious virus in the gs-antigen-positive cells it appears that the genome is partially repressed. There are at least three simple hypotheses to account for the phenotypic expression of the gs-antigen:

(1) the viral genome may be integrated in the I line and absent in the C line;

(2) the viral genome may be integrated in both the C line and I line, and its expression may be dependent on a segregating regulator gene;

(3) the viral genome may be present in a non-integrated state in both lines, but its expression may be dependent on regulation by a host gene.

A newly discovered biological activity of cells which carry the gs-antigen, which strengthens the identity of natural and viral gs-antigens, has been found in studies with RSV(O). The infectious type of RSV(O) is produced only in cells which possess gs-antigen, and cells from at least some gs-antigen-positive embryos harbor a virus, not belonging to known viral subgroups A, B, C and D, which acts as a helper virus for non-infectious RSV(O), converting it to the infectious variant [29,82-84]. These findings, which are described in detail by Weiss [85] at this Symposium, suggest that many chick embryos carry an unusual type of leukosis virus, possibly genetically integrated into a host chromosome. The concept of integration, which arose by analogy with lysogeny in the phage-bacterium relationship, is made more acceptable by the important discovery by Temin and Mizutani [86], Baltimore [87], and others [88], of an RNA-dependent DNA-polymerase which catalyses the synthesis of a DNA copy of viral RNA, together with DNA-dependent DNA polymerase necessary to convert the RNA-DNA hybrid into a double-stranded DNA molecule [89,90].

11. Some implications of genetic integration

The conventional view of infection by avian leukosis virus as consisting of horizontally and congenitally transmitted infectious virus will need to be broadened if the evidence for genetic transmission of viral genome is validated. The concept of the leukosis-free flock and the methods for the development of such a flock will have to be greatly modified. Indeed, the existence of any chickens free from integrated viral genome may be questioned.

Extensive investigations by Huebner and Sarma and their colleagues [91-96] notably in mice and chickens indicate that antigenic and viral expression of covert viral genome may not be seen until late in life or until stimulated by "derepressors" such as X-rays or chemical carcinogens. The time of first appearance of an expression of the genome varies between strains of animal, and systematic study will be required in attempts to exclude the occurrence of viral genome.

The question of the relationship between the leukosis virus rescuable from gs-antigen positive cells and field isolates of leukosis virus needs elucidating. On the basis of the helper activity of rescued virus for RSV(O) it appears that the helper virus belongs to a new subgroup, E. Is all integrated virus a subgroup E virus, and has the widespread occurrence of the epistatic dominant resistance gene already mentioned resulted in selection of a variant virus for which transmission by the ordinary process of cell infection has been largely by-passed?

Products of the viral genome may have immunological significance. Huebner and colleagues [95,96] have commented on the absence of gs-antibodies to homologous tumor viruses in chickens, mice and other species, which may be due to induction of immunological tolerance. If so, gs-antibodies should be produced in chickens lacking gs-antigen, such as C line. Whether tolerance is an advantage or disadvantage in responding to later, active virus infections remains to be determined.

More generally, the evidence for genetic integration of leukosis virus genome in the chicken provides support for the "oncogene" theory of neoplasia propounded by Huebner and his colleagues [91-93], which seeks to explain the generality of tumors in terms of infection by RNA tumor viruses.

12. Summary

Host genes may influence the response of the chicken to avian tumor viruses, and tumor viruses may modify the genome of the host. Host genetic factors have been identified which affect virus infection, neoplastic transformation of the infected cell, and progressive growth of the transformed cell. Genes controlling cell infection are the best studied, and single genetic loci have been identified which control infection by viruses of subgroups A, B and C. Infection by RSV(O), placed in subgroup E, appears to be controlled by genes at two loci.

Evidence for integration of viral genetic material with the genome of the host is reviewed.

References

[1] P.K. Vogt, Adv. Virus Res. 11 (1965) 293.
[2] L.B. Crittenden and W. Okazaki, J. Natl. Cancer Inst. 36 (1966) 299.
[3] A.C. Allison, Arch. Gesamte Virusforsch. 17 (1965) 280.
[4] E.V. Keogh, Brit. J. Exptl. Pathol. 19 (1938) 1.
[5] A.M. Prince, J. Natl. Cancer Inst. 20 (1958) 843.
[6] L.N. Payne and P.M. Biggs, Virology 24 (1964) 610.
[7] L.N. Payne and P.M. Biggs, Virology 29 (1966) 190.
[8] L.N. Payne and P.M. Biggs, J. Gen. Virol. 7 (1970) 177.
[9] L.B. Crittenden and W. Okazaki, J. Natl. Cancer Inst. 35 (1965) 857.
[10] L.B. Crittenden, H.A. Stone, R.H. Reamer and W. Okazaki, J. Virol. 1 (1967) 898.
[11] P.K. Vogt and R. Ishizaki, Virology 26 (1965) 664.
[12] L.B. Crittenden, World's Poult. Sci. J. 24 (1968) 18.
[13] N.F. Waters, Poult. Sci. 30 (1951) 531.

[14] L.B. Crittenden, W. Okazaki and R.H. Reamer, Natl. Cancer Inst. Monograph 17 (1964) 161.

[15] H. Hanafusa, Virology 25 (1965) 248.

[16] H. Rubin, Virology 26 (1965) 270.

[17] P.K. Vogt, Virology 32 (1967) 708.

[18] L.B. Crittenden, J. Natl. Cancer Inst. 41 (1968) 145.

[19] F. Piraino, Virology 32 (1967) 700.

[20] N.F. Waters and B.R. Burmester. J. Natl. Cancer Inst. 27 (1961) 655.

[21] R.K. Bower, N.R. Gyles and C.J. Brown. Genetics 51 (1965) 739.

[22] R.K. Bower, N.R. Gyles and C.J. Brown, Virology 24 (1964) 47.

[23] J.S. Munroe, Natl. Cancer Inst. Monograph 17 (1964) 177 (Discussion).

[24] L.B. Crittenden and J.V. Motta, Poult. Sci. 48 (1969) 1751.

[25] L.N. Payne and P.K. Pani, J. Gen. Virol. 13 (1971) 253.

[26] L.B. Crittenden, W.E. Briles and H.A. Stone, Science (N.Y.) 169 (1970) 1324.

[27] S.S. Dhaliwal, J. Natl. Cancer Inst. 30 (1963) 323.

[28] R.G. Duff and P.K. Vogt, Virology 39 (1969) 18.

[29] T. Hanafusa, H. Hanafusa and T. Miyamoto, Proc. Natl. Acad. Sci. U.S. 67 (1970) 1797.

[30] L.N. Payne, P.K. Pani and R.A. Weiss, J. Gen. Virol. in press.

[31] L.N. Payne, L.B. Crittenden and W. Okazaki, J. Natl. Cancer Inst. 40 (1968) 907.

[32] L.B. Crittenden and B.R. Burmester, Poult. Sci. 48 (1969) 196.

[33] P.M. Biggs, R.J. Thorpe and R.T. Hodges, unpublished results.

[34] L.B. Crittenden, E.J. Wendel and D. Ratzsch, Avian Dis. in press.

[35] B.W. Calnek, Avian Dis. 12 (1968) 104.

[36] L.B. Crittenden, Genetics 52 (1965) 438 (Abstract).

[37] H.G. Purchase, J. S. Afr. Vet. Med. Assoc. 40 (1969) 25.

[38] T. Pincus, J.W. Hartley and W.P. Rowe, J. Exptl. Med. 133 (1971) 219.

[39] K. Goodwin, World's Poult. Sci. J. 22 (1966) 299.

[40] G.E. Dickerson, World's Poult. Sci. J. 24 (1968) 107.

[41] M.D. Cooper, L.N. Payne, P.B. Dent, B.R. Burmester and R.A. Good, J. Natl. Cancer Inst. 41 (1968) 373.

[42] A.M. Prince, J. Natl. Cancer Inst. 23 (1959) 1361.

[43] B. Stenkvist and J. Ponten, Acta Pathol. Microbiol. Scand. 58 (1963) 273.

[44] T. Shimizu and H. Rubin, J. Natl. Cancer Inst. 33 (1964) 79.

[45] H. Rubin, Cold Spring Harbor Symp. Quant. Biol. 27 (1962) 441.

[46] M. Dinowitz and H. Rabin, J. Natl. Cancer Inst. 36 (1966) 189.

[47] N. Jonsson, Acta Pathol. Microbiol. Scand. 67 (1966) 339.

[48] H. Bauer, J. Buběnik, T. Graf and C. Allgaier, Virology 39 (1969) 482.

[49] T.J. Kakuk and C. Olson, Amer. J. Vet. Res. 28 (1967) 1491.

[50] R.D.A. Peterson, B.R. Burmester, T.N. Frederickson, H.G. Purchase and R.A. Good, J. Natl. Cancer Inst. 32 (1964) 1343.

[51] A.W. Greenwood, J.S.S. Blyth and J.G. Carr, Brit. J. Cancer 2 (1948) 135.

[52] N.R. Gyles, J.L. Miley and C.J. Brown, Poult. Sci. 46 (1967) 465.

[53] N.R. Gyles, J.L. Miley and C.J. Brown, Poult. Sci. 46 (1967) 789.

[54] J. Ponten, J. Natl. Cancer Inst. 29 (1962) 1147.

[55] N.R. Gyles, B.R. Stewart and C.J. Brown, Poult. Sci. 47 (1968) 430.

[56] N.F. Waters, B.R. Burmester and W.G. Walter, J. Natl. Cancer Inst. 20 (1958) 1245.

[57] N.F. Waters and B.R. Burmester, Poult. Sci. 42 (1963) 95.
[58] L.B. Crittenden, H.G. Purchase, J.J. Solomon, W. Okazaki and B.R. Burmester, in preparation.
[59] H.M. Temin and H. Rubin, Virology 6 (1958) 669.
[60] K. Bayreuther and B. Thorell, Exptl. Cell Res. 18 (1959) 370.
[61] K. Bayreuther, Nature (London) 186 (1960) 6.
[62] J. Ponten, J. Natl. Cancer Inst. 30 (1963) 897.
[63] J. Mark, Hereditas 57 (1967) 23.
[64] W.W. Nichols, Hereditas 55 (1966) 1.
[65] K.K. Sanford, Int. Rev. Cytol. 18 (1965) 249.
[66] A.C. Allison, Proc. Roy. Soc. B. 177 (1971) 23.
[67] W.J. Burdette and J.S. Yoon, Science (N.Y.) 155 (1967) 340.
[68] J. Svoboda and I. Hložánek, Adv. Cancer Res. 13 (1970) 217.
[69] H.M. Temin, Cancer Res. 26 (1966) 212.
[70] A.M. Prince, Neoplasma 13 (1966) 13.
[71] H.M. Temin (this Symposium).
[72] H.M. Temin, Cold Spring Harb. Symp. Quant. Biol. 27 (1962) 407.
[73] H. Hanafusa, T. Hanafusa and H. Rubin. Proc. Natl. Acad. Sci. U.S. 49 (1963) 572.
[74] J.P. Bader and A.V. Bader, Proc. Natl. Acad. Sci. U.S. 67 (1970) 843.
[75] H.M. Temin, Proc. Natl. Acad. Sci., U.S. 52 (1964) 323.
[76] M.A. Baluda and D.P. Nayak, Proc. Natl. Acad. Sci. U.S. 66 (1970) 329.
[77] T. Kušanová, Folia Biol. (Prague) 15 (1969) 96.
[78] R. Dulbecco, Science (N.Y.) 166 (1969) 962.
[79] R.M. Dougherty and H.S. Di Stefano, Virology 29 (1966) 586.
[80] R.M. Dougherty, H.S. Di Stefano and F.K. Roth, Proc. Natl. Acad. Sci. U.S. 58 (1967) 808.
[81] L.N. Payne and R.C. Chubb, J. Gen. Virol. 3 (1968) 379.
[82] R.A. Weiss, J. Gen. Virol. 5 (1969) 511.
[83] P.K. Vogt and R.R. Friis, Virology 43 (1971) 223.
[84] R.A. Weiss and L.N. Payne, Virology 45 (1971) 508.
[85] R.A. Weiss (this Symposium).
[86] H.M. Temin and S. Mizutani, Nature (London) 226 (1970) 1211.
[87] D. Baltimore, Nature (London) 226 (1970) 1209.
[88] S. Spiegelman, A. Burny, M.R. Das, J. Keydar, J. Schlom, M. Travnicek and K. Watson. Nature (London) 227 (1970) 563.
[89] S. Mizutani, D. Boettiger and H.M. Temin, Nature (London) 228 (1970) 424.
[90] J. Riman and G.S. Beaudreau, Nature (London) 228 (1970) 427.
[91] R.J. Huebner and G.J. Todaro, Proc. Natl. Acad. Sci. U.S. 64 (1969) 1087.
[92] R.J. Huebner, G.J. Todaro, P. Sarma, J.W. Hartley, A.E. Freeman, R.L. Peters, C.E. Whitmire, H. Meier and R.V. Gilden. Second Intern. Symp. on Tumor Viruses. Editions du Centre national de la Recherche Scientifique, Paris, p. 33.
[93] R.J. Huebner, In: R.M. Dutcher, Comparative leukemia research, Proceedings of the IVth International Symposium on Comparative Leukemia Research, Cherry Hill, N.J., 1969. (S. Karger, Basel, München, Paris, New York, 1970) p. 22.

[94] P.S. Sarma, F. Edwards, R.J. Huebner, H.C. Turner and L. Vernon, *In:* R.M. Dutcher, Comparative leukemia research, 1969, Proceedings of the IVth International Symposium on Comparative Leukemia Research, Cherry Hill, N.J. 1969 (S. Karger, Basel, München, Paris, New York, 1970) p. 168.

[95] R.J. Huebner, G.J. Kelloff, P.S. Sarma, W.T. Lane, H.C. Turner, R.V. Gilden, S. Oroszlan, H. Meier, D.D. Myers and R.L. Peters. Proc. Natl. Acad. Sci. U.S. 67 (1970) 366.

[96] R.J. Huebner, P.S. Sarma, G.J. Kelloff, R.V. Gilden, H. Meier, D.D. Myers and R.L. Peters, Ann. N.Y. Acad. Sci. 181 (1971) 246.

HELPER VIRUSES AND HELPER CELLS*

R.A. WEISS**
Department of Microbiology,
University of Washington School of Medicine,
Seattle, Wash. 98105, U.S.A.

This article is concerned with avian tumor viruses that exist in latent form in normal cells. Evidence for endogenous viruses has been sought by four approaches: homology between cellular and viral nucleic acids; presence of virus specific proteins, such as antigens, in "uninfected" cells; complementation of defective viruses by the endogenous virus; and rescue of the latent virus in infectious form. The latter two provide the most convincing evidence, and in order to understand them it is useful to review the interactions that occur between known avian tumor viruses, particularly between defective viruses and "helper" viruses.

Avian tumor viruses are broadly classified as sarcoma and leukosis viruses. Sarcoma viruses "convert" or "transform" fibroblasts in culture (fig. 1a). This property is used in the focus assay of sarcoma viruses [1]. Leukosis viruses do not transform fibroblasts and are therefore called non-transforming (NT) viruses (fig. 1b). NT viruses may, however, transform other cell types, such as lymphopoietic or haemopoietic cells, and some are leukemogenic *in vivo*. Thus the transforming property of the virus may depend on the epigenetic state of the cell, though there is evidence [2] that NT viruses lack a nucleic acid component which is present in sarcoma viruses. Non-transforming viruses are called "helper" viruses when they complement functions of transforming viruses which are defective for virus replication but not for cell transformation.

*I am most grateful to Drs. P.K. Vogt, R.R. Friis and E. Katz for many discussions concerning the work and the manuscript, and to Dr. P.K. Vogt for providing facilities for this work to be carried out.

The original work presented here was undertaken during the tenure of an American Cancer Society – Eleanor Roosevelt – International Cancer Fellowship awarded by the International Union Against Cancer, and it was supported by the American Cancer Society Institutional Grant IN-26L to the University of Washington and by U.S. Public Health Service Grant no. CA 10569 from the National Cancer Institute.

**Current address: Imperial Cancer Research Fund, Lincoln's Inn Fields, London W.C.2, U.K.

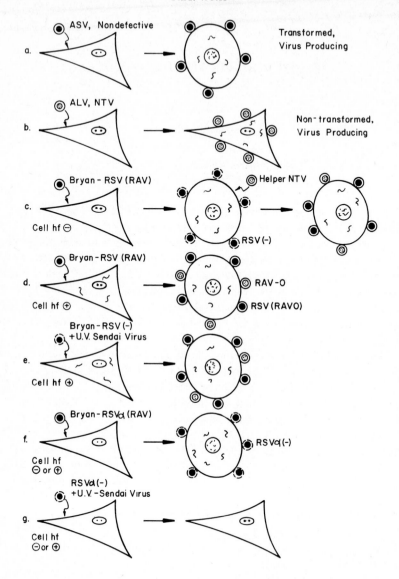

Fig. 1. Defectiveness and rescue of avian RNA tumor viruses. Triangles depict non-transformed cells and circles transformed cells. Particles at the cell surface depict virus progeny. ASV, avian sarcoma virus; ALV, avian leukosis virus; NTV, non-transforming virus; hf, helper factor.

1. Defectiveness of Bryan strain Rous sarcoma virus

In 1962 two reports suggested that the replication of Bryan strain Rous sarcoma virus (BH-RSV) was complex and might require more than one infecting virus particle. Rubin and Vogt [3] found that Bryan RSV was a mixed stock of transforming RSV and a non-transforming leukosis virus, which they named Rous associated virus (RAV). Temin [4] meanwhile observed that chicken cells infected by solitary particles of BH-RSV failed to replicate progeny virus, although the cells became transformed. By isolating and subcultivating single Rous foci from plates infected with high dilution of RSV, it was shown that these transformed cells from solitary infection did not produce infectious RSV. The cells contained the viral genome which could be rescued by superinfection with an avian leukosis "helper" virus to release infectious RSV (fig. 1c). This finding was confirmed by H. Hanafusa and his colleagues [5] who suggested that the transforming capacity of BH-RSV might be related to its inability to reproduce. However, it was later shown that other strains of RSV were not defective in virus replication [6-8] yet could transform cells as efficiently as the Bryan strain.

Hanafusa *et al.* [9,10] and Vogt [11] demonstrated that the envelope of re-activated BH-RSV possessed the same properties as the helper virus used for rescue, i.e. the RSV was neutralized by antiserum specific to the helper virus and possessed the same host range and interference pattern. Repeated solitary infections with the rescued RSV yielded non-producer cells once more [5], indicating that rescue of RSV was not due to genetic recombination between RSV and helper virus. These findings showed that phenotypic mixing, first described in bacteriophages [12], occurred among avian tumor viruses. Following mixed infection by two viruses, the progeny virus contains genomes of either type with mixed coat components coded by both genomes. In the case of defective RSV, the envelope components were provided by the helper virus and it was assumed that no RSV particles were produced without the helper virus. RSV particles which have the same genomes but different coats are referred to as pseudotypes [13] and the origin of the coat is written in parentheses, e.g. RSV(RAV-1). These "wolves in sheeps' clothing" have proved extremely useful in the classification of avian tumor viruses into subgroups on the basis of host range, interference patterns and antigenicity [14]. Phenotypic mixing was subsequently demonstrated amongst non-defective avian tumor viruses also [15,16].

The first indication that Bryan RSV was not defective in the original sense of being unable to replicate, came from electron microscopic studies of Dougherty and Di Stefano [17] which showed that virus particles morphologically indistinguishable from avian tumor viruses budded from the surface of "non-producing" BH-RSV transformed cells. These particles were apparently not infectious. Robinson [18] demonstrated that the particles had similar physical and chemical properties to RSV and showed [19] that if they were introduced into cells by means of inactivated Sendai virus, the cells became transformed and RSV pseudotypes could be subsequently rescued by helper viruses. About the same time, however, Vogt [20] and Weiss [21] discovered that the particles released by "non-producer" cells were, after all, infectious, but they possessed a different host range from that of the A, B, C and D subgroups of avian tumor viruses. The virus was named RSV(0) due to its apparent lack of helper specified envelope.

RSV(0) is commonly said to have a narrow host range on account of its restriction in chickens [20-22]. Actually the narrow host range appears to be more in our way of thinking than in the virus, since RSV(0) is infectious for a wide variety of other fowl than the domestic fowl, including Red jungle fowl, Japanese quail, certain pheasants, partridges, guinea fowl and turkeys [14,23, unpublished observations]. The susceptibility of chickens to the A, B and C subgroups of avian tumor viruses is genetically controlled by single, independent autosomal loci [24,25]. In each case, a dominant allele determines the presence of receptors on the cell surface which are required for viral penetration. The genetic control of susceptibility to RSV(0) in chickens is more complex and appears to depend on two genes, one, a dominant, autosomal gene for susceptibility which presumably codes for a cell surface receptor, the other, an epistatic, dominant, autosomal gene which inhibits the expression of the first gene [26].

2. A helper factor in normal chicken cells

The first hint that there might be viral information expressed in normal cells came from the observations of Dougherty and his colleagues [27,28] that apparently leukosis-free chick embryos contained an antigen which reacted in the complement fixation for avian leukosis (COFAL) test. The antigen was indistinguishable from the group-specific (gs) antigen of avian tumor viruses. Payne and Chubb [29] showed that the presence of this antigen in inbred Reaseheath chickens was controlled by a single autosomal locus with dominance for expression. Using the same chickens, I observed that synthesis of infectious RSV(0) following solitary infection only occurred in cells derived from gs positive embryos [23]. When RSV was cloned in gs negative cells no infectious virus was released. Host dependent formation of infectious RSV(0) was also observed by the Hanafusas [30] who did not at that stage search for *gs* antigens or other viral markers in the permissive cells.

These findings suggested that Bryan RSV was "conditionally" defective according to the type of chick cell in which it was cloned. Wise by now to the pitfalls of interpreting viral defectiveness merely on the basis of limited infectivity, both Hanafusa [30] and I [23] checked whether "non-infectious" virus might be synthesized by the non-permissive cells and we found that virus particles were, indeed, released (fig. 1c, d). Host range studies on bantam, quail and pheasant in addition to all known chicken phenotypes failed to reveal a host cell naturally susceptible to this virus [23]. However, the particles were active for transformation and replication if introduced into cells with the aid of inactivated Sendai virus [23,30] (fig. 1e).

Thus it was shown that particles with biologically active and apparently identical genomes were released by *gs* positive and *gs* negative cells. The difference between infectious and non-infectious RSV particles resided in their envelope properties, and it appeared that *gs* positive cells contained some factor or information which acted like a helper virus in complementing a biological deficiency in the envelope and in determining its host range and antigenicity [23,31,32]. The agent was named chick helper factor (*chf*) [32]. RSV(0) was not deficient in *gs* antigen itself, and both chicken and quail cells which released non-infectious RSV, though lacking the "natural" *gs* antigen before infection, reacted positively in the COFAL test [23]. There was no evidence, biological or physical [23,29,32], that cultures carrying the helper factor released mature virus particles prior to infection with RSV, hence the term "helper cells" in the title of this article.

3. Rescue of chick helper factor

My studies in 1969 [23] also demonstrated that the infectious RSV(0) released from *gs*[+] cells could be indefinitely propagated in infectious form in *gs*[−] cells, provided that the cells were infected with relatively high titres (1000 f.f.u. or more per 10^6 cells). In contrast, on solitary infection of *gs*[−] cells, progeny RSV(0) reverted to the non-infectious form. These observations indicated that the helper factor genome could be rescued and transmitted to cells lacking the factor. This was subsequently confirmed by Hanafusa *et al.* [32], who also showed that the factor could be rescued by non-transforming viruses, such as RAV-2.

The continued propagation of infectious RSV(0) in factor-negative cells following mass infection led to two related hypotheses: that factor positive cells contained a latent helper virus which was "activated" to infectious form by infection with RSV [23] or that a minority of the RSV(0) particles themselves incorporated the additional genetic information of the helper factor [32]. Hanafusa et al. [33] then demonstrated that the helper factor could be isolated as an independently replicating virus from stocks of RAV-2 grown in gs^+ cells. The virus, named RAV-60, was a typical RNA containing avian leukosis virus bearing the same envelope properties as RSV(0), and Hanafusa et al. [33] suggested that RAV-60 might be a genetic recombinant between RAV-2 and helper factor.

The rescue of helper factor [23,32,33] demonstrates that apparently normal chick embryo cells contain at least partial genetic information for an RNA tumor virus. This information is not normally expressed by release of mature virus particles. However, Vogt and Friis [34] recently demonstrated that occasional embryos of line 7 chickens spontaneously release a non-transforming virus which they named RAV-0. This virus was detected in sonicated embryonic tissues and in the medium of fibroblast cultures. Like RAV-60, it is a typical C-type particle with indistinguishable envelope properties from RSV(0), though unlike RAV-60, RAV-0 appears to be inefficient for independent infection of quail fibroblasts. About 12% line 7 embryos spontaneously release RAV-0. As line 7 cells are susceptible to RSV(0), a spontaneous activation of helper factor could establish itself as a RAV-0 viraemia. Gs^+ line 7 cultures which do not spontaneously release RAV-0 are activable by RSV(0) in the same way as other gs^+ cultures [34].

It is evident that the envelope properties of infectious particles of RSV(0) are conferred on the RSV by phenotypic mixing with helper factor and it is therefore logical to refer to RSV(0) as the pseudotype RSV(RAV-0). The non-infectious particles released by cells lacking helper factors may be designated RSV(-).

4. Association between natural gs antigen and helper factor

The dependence of chick helper factor (chf) on the presence of natural gs antigen noted by Weiss [23] was confirmed by Hanafusa et al. [32] and Vogt and Friis [34]. Further studies by Weiss and Payne [35] showed that the helper factor was closely linked with presence of gs antigen in Reaseheath I- and C-line chickens and their hybrids (table 1). The synthesis of gs antigen in Reaseheath chickens is determined by a single, dominant, autosomal allele, designated gs^+ [29,35], and the segregation of helper factor with gs antigen suggests that both are controlled at the same locus, and that this might represent the site of

Table 1
Association of *gs* antigen and helper factor.

Fowl	*gs* antigen	No. of embryos with helper factor
Reaseheath C-line	–	0/10
Reaseheath I-line	+	12/12
C ♂♂ × (I × C) ♀♀	–	0/11
	+	9/9
Brown Leghorn	–	2/14
	+	24/24
White Leghorn C/B	–	1/18
	+	33/33
White Leghorn C/O	–	7/16
	+	19/19
Ring-necked pheasant	–	0/9
	+	0/25
Japanese quail	–	0/46

integration of an avian tumor virus genome. Alternatively, this locus might act as a regulatory gene.

Further studies in this laboratory have revealed that not all chicken strains show a perfect association between presence of helper factor and the natural *gs* antigen detectable in the COFAL test (table 1). We found that several C/O White Leghorns and one C/B White Leghorn, which were negative in a COFAL test of embryonic viscera and muscle, carried helper factor in a majority of the fibroblasts later cultivated. COFAL tests were made on fibroblast cultures of some of these embryos after two weeks *in vitro,* at which time they were *gs* positive. The COFAL test is relatively insensitive and the *gs* antigen comprises more than one polypeptide (36-38). A given preparation of antiserum may react preferentially with one component [39] and it is not yet known whether all the components are present in the "natural" *gs* antigen of embryonic tissues. Payne [personal communication] has noted that while many Brown Leghorn embryos are *gs* negative at 11 days incubation, most become *gs* positive at hatching. Such embryos may contain active helper factor before they reveal titratable *gs* antigen. Dougherty *et al.* [27,28] observed C-type virus particles in the liver and pancreas of *gs* negative chicken embryos. It is possible that these "non-infectious" particles, and those of Sarma *et al.* [40] are related to RAV-0.

Amongst chickens, however, no embryos or cultures which lacked active helper factor contained detectable *gs* antigen. Thus 4 classes of chick embryos were recorded:

(1) gs^-; chf^-
(2) gs^-; chf^+
(3) gs^+; chf^+
(4) gs^+; RAV-0 producing

In contrast to chickens, helper factor was not unequivocally detected in ring-necked pheasants, although a majority of the embryos contained gs antigen which reacted in the COFAL test. The presence of infectious RSV in sonicated foci or X-irradiated infective centres, was tested on pheasant, quail, C/O or C/B assay cells with negative results (table 1). However, prolonged culture of 25 initially non-infectious RSV foci picked from gs^+ or gs^- pheasant cultures gradually revealed increasing titres of infectious RSV(RAV-0). A similar complication has been found with several lines of gs^- Japanese quail cells transformed by RSV(RAV-0) in this laboratory and previously [35]. It is not yet understood whether this is due to residual, slow growing RAV-0 introduced at original infection with RSV(RAV-0) or whether it represents the conversion of cells from a state where helper factor is present but not functioning, to a state where it is active.

5. A common helper factor among different strains of fowl

The envelope specificity of rescued virus was examined by studying the RSV pseudotype in six distinct breeds of gs positive fowl, originating in three continents (table 2). All varieties released RSV with the same host range and all

Table 2
RSV (RAV-0) rescued from different strains of fowl.

Type of fowl			Host range			Neutralization by RSV(RAV-0) anti-serum
Strain	Location	Phenotype*	Quail	C/O	C/E	
Brown Leghorn	U.K.	C/O, C/E	+	+	−	+
Reaseheath I-Line	U.K.	C/E	+	+	−	+
Reaseheath W-Line	U.K.	C/BE	+	+	−	+
Line 7	U.S.A.	C/A	+	+	−	+
White Leghorn	U.S.A.	C/O, C/E, C/BE	+	+	−	+
Red Jungle Fowl	Malaysia	C/O, C/E	+	+	−	+

*The C/O phenotype is susceptible to all subgroups; C/A, C/B and C/E are resistant to subgroup A, B and RSV(RAV-0) respectively.

were neutralized by anti-serum to RSV(RAV-0) prepared in pheasants. This is particularly significant for Red jungle fowl embryos obtained in the Tasek Bera region of Malaya. These fowl have no history of contact with domestic breeds of chicken [41]. It therefore seems that the endogenous helper factors resembling RAV-0, classified as subgroup E, [33] represent the natural C-type virus of this species. Since this virus may not be readily obtained from *gs* positive ring-necked pheasants, further species of Galliformes are currently under examination for the presence of *gs* antigens and rescuable helper factors. Perhaps the "avian" tumor virus group would be more aptly named the chicken tumor virus group.

The widespread genetic resistance to subgroup "E" viruses among chickens, in contrast to the susceptibility of other species of fowl, may be related to the presence of subgroup E helper factors in chickens. Cellular resistance to infection with RSV(RAV-0) is due either to the absence of the susceptibility allele, e^s, of the receptor gene or to the presence of the epistatic inhibitor gene, I^e which prevents expression of e^s [26]. Thus selection of resistant phenotypes can operate on two independent loci. However, it is possible that the inhibitor gene itself represents another expression of the *gs* locus, which controls the presence of helper factor.

6. Infective centre test for helper factor

Because a negative COFAL test for *gs* antigen was unreliable as an indicator of the absence of functional helper factor in White Leghorns, *gs* negative embryos are now additionally tested for presence of helper factor as a routine measure in this laboratory. In fig. 2 a scheme is illustrated for the detection of spontaneous RAV-0 release and presence of latent helper factor. Both tests are based on the infective centre technique for the detection of virus-producing cells [42]. Spontaneous production of RAV-0 is detected by taking a sample of medium from the cell culture in question and after removing viable cells by sonication or centrifugation, the medium is plated onto Japanese quail cells concurrently with 100 focus forming units (f.f.u.) of RSV(RAV-0). Two similar quail cultures are infected with RSV(RAV-0) alone. After 24 hours to allow for the eclipse period of RSV, one culture, infected with RSV alone, is overlaid with agar medium as a control focus assay, while the remaining two are X-irradiated with 5000 R at which no further cell division takes place but virus release is not inhibited. Following irradiation, non-irradiated quail indicator cells are added and cultures are overlaid with agar 6-8 hours later for focus assay. Only those cells which have been doubly infected with RSV(RAV-0) and RAV-0 will

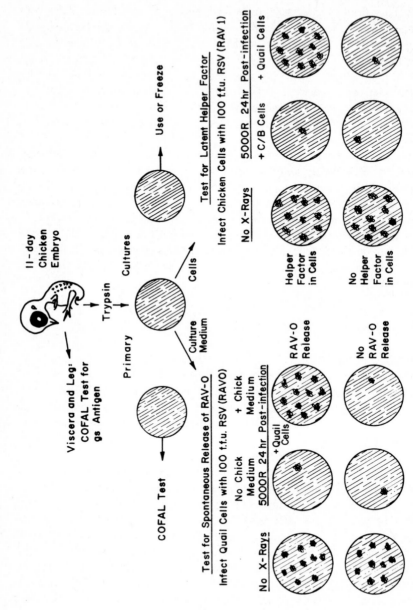

Fig. 2. Characterization of congenital tumor viruses in chicken embryos. Shaded discs depict fibroblast cultures and clusters of dots within them depict Rous cell foci.

register as infective centres. The irradiated culture which was infected with RSV(RAV-0) alone serves as a control plate for the number of double infections due to the presence of RAV-0 in the RSV(RAV-0) stock. RAV-0 will not be detected unless there are sufficient infectious particles to infect a majority of cells in the culture.

The detection of helper factor is based on the same principle; in this case the chick cells themselves are infected with RSV(RAV-1) and two plates are X-irradiated 24 hours later. Unirradiated C/B cells are added to one plate which registers only the number of infective centres doubly infected with RSV-(RAV-1) and RAV-1, as C/B cells are insusceptible to RSV(RAV-0). Quail cells are added to the other irradiated plate which registers the number of infective centres due to both RSV(RAV-1) and RSV(RAV-0) released as a result of helper factor pre-existing in the chicken cells. Table 3 shows the result of such

Table 3

Infective centre test for helper factor. C/B cultures were infected with 300 f.f.u. RSV(RAV-1), and irradiated with 5000 R 24 hours later. Addition of quail (Q) cells reveals infective centres releasing RSV(RAV-0) or RSV(RAV-1) while C/B cells reveal only RSV(RAV-1).

		Foci		
Embryo	COFAL titre	No X-rays	X-rays + C/B cells	X-rays + Q cells
1	1:2	360	13	360
2	1:8	310	9	260
3	1:4	260	15	250
4	1:8	240	15	240
5	0	320	16	18
6	0	280	18	21
7	0	310	12	15
8	1:8	320	16	270

an assay for eight C/B chicken embryos. In this case the presence of helper factor correlated well with the COFAL test. If the cells to be tested are susceptible to subgroup B viruses, RSV(RAV-2) or non-defective SR-RSV-B may be conveniently used since quail cells are insusceptible to subgroup B and will therefore reveal the RAV-0 pseudotype only.

An experiment on the timing of release of the pseudotype SR-RSV(RAV-0), determined by the endogenous helper factor, showed that it is detectable as soon as SR-RSV itself begins to be released. For this study, chf^+ C/E cells were infected with SR-RSV-B which had been recloned twice in chf^- cells. The infective centre technique was used to demonstrate the release of SR-RSV-

(RAV-0) (fig. 3). The greater number of infective centres releasing SR-RSV-B compared to SR-RSV(RAV-0) 24 hours or more after infection may be due to dominance of the B subgroup envelope component in phenotypic mixing.

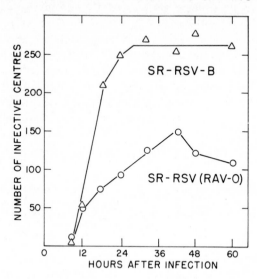

Fig. 3. Release of SR-RSV(RAV-0) pseudotype following infection of $gs+$ cells with SR-RSV-B. Cultures were infected with 250 f.f.u. SR-RSV-B and at different times after infection four plates were X-irradiated with 5000 R. Two plates were then seeded with C/E cells and two with quail cells as indicator cells for infective centres releasing SR-RSV-B and SR-RSV(RAV-0) respectively. Agar overlay medium was substituted six hours after adding the indicator cells, and foci were counted six days later.

7. Complementation between helper factor and RSV mutants

The defectiveness of the envelope of BH-RSV played an important role in the discovery of chick helper factor [23,32]. In 1968, Hanafusa and Hanafusa [22] described a variant of BH-RSV named α, which appears to be genetically distinct from RSV(0). RSVα is non-infectious, even when released from cells carrying the helper factor, and inactivated Sendai virus does not facilitate its infection [30] (fig. 1f, g). RSVα can nevertheless be rescued as an infectious pseudotype, RSVα(RAV), on superinfection of RSVα producing cells with RAV. Hanafusa and Hanafusa [43] recently made the important discovery that RSVα did not possess functional RNA dependent DNA polymerase (reverse transcriptase), common to RNA tumor viruses [44,45]. Of several avian tumor viruses tested, only RSVα(RAV) failed to activate the production of RAV-60 from cells carrying the helper factor [33]. The failure to obtain complementation between helper factor and RSVα indicates that helper factor does not possess functional reverse transcriptase either [43]. Other helper viruses complement RSVα not only by phenotypic mixing of envelope components but of the enzyme too. After rescue of RSVα as a pseudotype by RAV-1, about 15% of re-isolated clones behave as the common, or β form of RSV(0) [22]. The Hanafusas suggested that this is due to genetic recombination with RAV-1, and further suggested [33] that the rescue of RAV-60, which possesses functional reverse transcriptase, might involve recombination with the virus used for activation. However, genetic recombination among avian tumor viruses remains to be proved.

Other RSV mutants, which are defective for different functions involved in viral replication, will be useful for the characterization of helper factors in normal cells. Defective mutants of the Schmidt-Ruppin strain RSV (SR-RSV) have been described by Goldé [46] and by Kawai and Yamamoto [47]. Using Prague strain RSV of subgroup A mutagenized with 5-aza-cytidine, we have recently isolated mutants which are defective for replication of infectious RSV (Weiss and Vogt, unpublished results). Preliminary investigations show that these mutants fall into three classes: (1) mutants that are not complemented by RAV-7 or by chick helper factor; (2) mutants that are complemented by RAV-7 but not by chick helper factor, a similar situation to that of RSVα(0); (3) mutants that are complemented both by RAV-7 and by chick helper factor. Two mutants release particles with subgroup A properties following complementation by chick helper factor. It remains to be seen whether a virus similar to RAV-60 is also released. Mutants of avian tumor viruses which are temperature sensitive for viral replication [48] promise to be a powerful tool for investigating the control of helper factor activity in normal cells.

8. Implications of helper cells for RSV genetics

A majority of eggs, even from "leukosis free" flocks, carry helper factor and much of the experimental work of avian tumor virologists has unwittingly been carried out using cells which perform viral functions and from which a virus may be isolated. It is, therefore, necessary to re-apparaise what we know concerning avian tumor virus functions. It is possible that well known "non-defective strains" of virus might be defective after all, but complemented by helper factor for structural or non-structural cistrons which do not show up as host range differences. In this laboratory repeated cloning of Schmidt-

Ruppin and Prague RSV and of B77 in chick cells lacking helper factor did not reveal any dysfunction. Surprisingly, cloning in Japanese quail did so. The replication of Prague RSV-C in quail cells is severely reduced and that of B77 sarcoma virus undetectable, although the cells became transformed [Friis, unpublished observations]. Superinfection with RAV-0 or RAV-1 failed to rescue the sarcoma virus. The significance of these findings is not yet clear, but we should keep an open mind whether these and other [49] host-dependent modifications of viral performance might be related to endogenous viral functions within the natural host cell.

Where cells carrying active helper factors are used as assay cells one might also expect complications in interpreting, for example, the inactivation of virus treated with ultra-violet (UV) or ionizing radiations [46,50,51]. The estimation of target size for replication may be spuriously small since the endogenous virus will complement defects in many replicative functions.

9. Induction of virus with physical and chemical carcinogens

The failure to rescue helper factor with RSVα(RAV) [33] suggested that helper factor does not have functional reverse transcriptase and therefore should not be inducible by non-viral carcinogens. However, the occurrence of spontaneous release of RAV-0, which possesses reverse transcriptase [52], in line 7 embryos suggested that the helper factor may not be deficient in the enzyme in non-producing cultures of this line. We have also noticed new appearance of RAV-0 in a few long term cultures, though it is possible that it was released in lower titres before it became detectable.

Several laboratories have reported the induction of murine RNA tumor viruses following *in vivo* treatment with ionizing radiations [53-55] or long term cultivation *in vitro* [56]. The chick helper factor system is particularly suitable for induction experiments of this type because the whole process may be initiated in culture, starting with normal, early passage cells, and because there is, in addition to careful negative controls, a good positive control, namely, activation by RSV. Therefore, several embryo cultures bearing rescuable helper factor, and others which did not possess helper factor, were treated with X-irradiation, UV-irradiation, 20-methylcholanthrene, urethan, and mitomycin C [52]. Following treatment, gs^- pheasant cells were seeded onto the treated cultures and were passaged twice a week in order to promote the reproduction of induced viruses. The results of induction in gs^+ Reaseheath I-line cells is shown in table 4. Induced leukosis viruses (ILV) became detectable after 2 to 3 weeks co-cultivation of carcinogen-treated cells with pheasant cells. Pheasant

Table 4
Induction of RAV-0 in I-line cells by carcinogens.

Treatment*	Co-cultivation with pheasant	Detection of RAV-0**
None	21 days	−
DMSO 1%, 8 days†	14 days	−
X-rays 1000 R, 50 kV, 20 mA no filter	21 days	+
UV-light 2.5 seconds germicidal lamp, 40 cm distance	21 days	+
20-Methylcholanthrene 0.5 µg/ml, 8 days	14 days	+
Urethan 100 µg/ml, 21 days	14 days	+
RSV(RAV-1) solitary infection, 7 days	−	+

* Several cultures of I-line fibroblasts were treated by each of the methods listed; after which gs^- pheasant cells were added to the cultures.
** RAV-0 was assayed by its helper activity for BH-RSV on co-infection of quail cells (see fig. 2).
† Dimethylsulphoxide, which was used as a solvent for 20-methylcholanthrene.

cells alone did not release ILV. ILV was also found in cultures of gs^+ line 7 embryos after treatment with carcinogens or mitomycin C. Between 10^{-5} and 10^{-6} cells were induced to release virus. These new findings will require considerable analysis before we can begin to understand the complexities of this system, but it is clear that cells bearing latent helper factor may be converted to overt virus producers and that the probability of this event taking place is considerably increased by suitable treatment with chemical or physical carcinogens. The induced viruses of the I-line and line 7 chickens represent typical avian leukosis virus particles. They possess the same buoyant density, RNA characteristics, reverse transcriptase, and envelope characteristics as spontaneously released RAV-0. Induction experiments with gs^- cells lacking active helper factor were also successful. Moreover, the majority of cells treated with carcinogen were converted from gs^- chf^- to gs^+ chf^+ [52].

10. The virogene and protovirus hypotheses

The idea that information for RNA tumor viruses might exist as part of the normal cell genome was suggested by Payne and Chubb [29] and by Bentvelzen [57]. It has received strong advocacy from Huebner and his associates [58-60] and from Temin [61,62]. The data reviewed here show that an endogenous viral genome does exist in many chicken embryos, and that it may be activated to form infectious virus particles by infection with other chicken RNA tumor viruses or by treatment of cells with non-viral carcinogens. The activated viruses have similar envelope specificities to RAV-0, and, as rescued from fibroblasts or Rous transformed cells, behave as non-transforming viruses. It is not yet known whether RAV-0 or the induced viruses are leukemogenic *in vivo*. In most strains of chicken the presence of the virus in latent but activable form is associated with the "natural" *gs* antigen, which is controlled by a chromosomal locus. This locus could represent the site of an integrated DNA copy of the viral genome, but it probably represents a regulatory gene for the partial expression of latent RNA tumor virus present in all chickens. In the latter case, positive control is indicated since *gs* antigens and rescuable helper factor are expressed in heterozygous embryos [29,35], and there is no genetic evidence for supposing that the viral genome itself is associated with the host genome. Either model is compatible with Huebner and Todaro's oncogene and virogene hypothesis [58] or Temin's protovirus hypothesis [61,62].

One approach to this question is to study the homology of cellular DNA to viral nucleic acid. This was first undertaken by Temin [63] in an attempt to detect the DNA provirus in cells infected with RSV. It later became apparent [64-66] that DNA of normal, uninfected cells showed a degree of homology to viral RNA which obscured the significance of virus-like DNA in infected cells. In spite of Dougherty and Di Stefano's [27] discovery of *gs* antigen in normal cells and Payne and Chubb's [29] demonstration of its genetic control, molecular biologists until recently ignored the existence of these two classes of embryos when comparing the homology of viral RNA to "uninfected" cellular DNA. In collaboration with H. Varmus, W. Levinson and J.M. Bishop, we have examined this point [67]. C/B embryos were classified as *gs⁻ chf⁻* and *gs⁺ chf⁺* by the techniques described above, using a small amount of tissue for COFAL tests and for culture. The remaining parts of the embryos were grouped into the two classes and DNA was extracted from them. DNA was also prepared from *gs⁻* Japanese quail. RAV-0 was harvested from line 7 cells spontaneously releasing the virus. Double-stranded ^{3}H-DNA product was prepared from RAV-0 using its own reverse transcriptase and template. The reassociation kinetics of rapidly annealing viral DNA strands were examined in the presence of excess DNA from chf^+ and chf^- embryos. Homologous sequences were found in both classes and there was no significant difference in the amount of virus-like DNA between the two classes of embryo. No homology was observed between the viral DNA product and HeLa cell DNA or salmon sperm DNA. These results suggest that equivalent sets of virogenes may exist in the genome of both chf^+ and chf^- cells. Further characterization of cellular DNA and of cellular RNA from chf^+ and chf^- embryos is in progress.

11. Conclusion

Normal chicken cells contain viral genomes which may be activated to form infectious C-type virus particles by infection with other avian tumor viruses or by treatment with non-viral carcinogens. Viruses induced in a wide variety of chicken strains all resemble RAV-0 in their biological and biochemical properties. A chromosomal locus controls the partial expression of the endogenous virus. These observations may be pertinent to the origin of RNA tumor viruses and to carcinogenesis.

References

[1] P.K. Vogt, *In:* K. Habel and N.P. Salzman, Fundamental techniques in virology (Academic Press, New York, 1969) p. 198.
[2] P. Duesberg and P.K. Vogt, Proc. Natl. Acad. Sci. U.S. 67 (1970) 1673.
[3] H. Rubin and P.K. Vogt, Virology 17 (1962) 184.
[4] H.M. Temin, Cold Spring Harbor Symp. Quant. Biol. 27 (1962) 407.
[5] H. Hanafusa, T. Hanafusa and H. Rubin, Proc. Natl. Acad. Sci. U.S. 49 (1963) 572.
[6] R.M. Dougherty and R. Rasmussen, Natl. Cancer Inst. Monograph 17 (1964) 337.
[7] H. Hanafusa, Natl. Cancer Inst. Monograph 17 (1964) 543.
[8] A. Goldé and P. Vigier, Compt. Rend. Acad. Sci. 262 (1966) 2973.
[9] H. Hanafusa, T. Hanafusa and H. Rubin, Proc. Natl. Acad. Sci. U.S. 51 (1964) 41.
[10] H. Hanafusa, Virology 25 (1965) 248.
[11] P.K. Vogt, Virology 25 (1965) 237.
[12] A. Novick and L. Szilard, Science 113 (1951) 34.
[13] H. Rubin, Virology 26 (1965) 270.
[14] P.K. Vogt, Comparative leukemia research 1969, Bibl. Haemat. 36 (Karger, Basel, 1970) p. 153.
[15] H. Hanafusa and T. Hanafusa, Proc. Natl. Acad. Sci. U.S. 55 (1966) 532.
[16] P.K. Vogt, Virology 32 (1967) 708.
[17] R.M. Dougherty and H.S. Di Stefano, Virology 27 (1965) 351.
[18] H.L. Robinson, Proc. Natl. Acad. Sci. U.S. 57 (1967) 1655.
[19] W.S. Robinson, H.L. Robinson and P.H. Duesberg, Proc. Natl. Acad. Sci. U.S. 58 (1967) 825.
[20] P.K. Vogt, Proc. Natl. Acad. Sci. U.S. 58 (1967) 805.

[21] R.A. Weiss, Virology 32 (1967) 719.
[22] H. Hanafusa and T. Hanafusa, Virology 34 (1968) 630.
[23] R.A. Weiss, J. Gen. Virol. 5 (1969) 511.
[24] L.B. Crittenden, H.A. Stone, R.H. Reamer and W. Okazaki, J. Virol. 1 (1967) 898.
[25] L.N. Payne, This symposium.
[26] L.N. Payne, P.K. Pani and R.A. Weiss, J. Gen. Virol. in press.
[27] R.M. Dougherty and H.S. Di Stefano, Virology 29 (1966) 586.
[28] R.M. Dougherty, H.S. Di Stefano and F.K. Roth, Proc. Natl. Acad. Sci. U.S. 58 (1967) 808.
[29] L.N. Payne and R.C. Chubb, J. Gen. Virol. 3 (1968) 379.
[30] T. Hanafusa, T. Miyamoto and H Hanafusa, Virology 40 (1970) 55.
[31] R.A. Weiss, J. Gen. Virol. 5 (1969) 529.
[32] H. Hanafusa, T. Miyamoto and T. Hanafusa, Proc. Natl. Acad. Sci. U.S. 66 (1970) 314
[33] T. Hanafusa, H. Hanafusa and T. Miyamoto, Proc. Natl. Acad. Sci. U.S. 67 (1970) 1797.
[34] P.K. Vogt and R.R. Friis, Virology 43 (1971) 223.
[35] R.A. Weiss and L.N. Payne, Virology 45 (1971) 508.
[36] F.K. Roth and R.M. Dougherty, Virology 38 (1969) 278.
[37] D. Armstrong, J. Virol. 3 (1969) 133.
[38] D.W. Allen, P.S. Sarma, H.D. Niall and R. Saur, Proc. Natl. Acad. Sci. U.S. 67 (1970) 837.
[39] H. Bauer and D.P. Bolognesi, Virology 42 (1970) 1113.
[40] P.S. Sarma, F. Edwards, R.J. Huebner, H.C. Turner and L. Vernon, In: Comparative leukemia research 1969, Bibl. Haemat. 36 (Karger, Basel, 1970) p. 168.
[41] R.A. Weiss and P.M. Biggs, J. Natl. Cancer Inst. (1972) in press.
[42] H. Rubin, Virology 10 (1960) 29.
[43] H. Hanafusa and T. Hanafusa, Virology 43 (1971) 313.
[44] H.M. Temin and S. Mizutani, Nature 226 (1970) 1211.
[45] D. Baltimore, Nature 226 (1970) 1209.
[46] A. Goldé, Virology 40 (1970) 1022.
[47] S. Kawai and T. Yamamoto, Japan. J. Exptl. Med. 40 (1970) 243.
[48] R.R. Friis, K. Toyoshima and P.K. Vogt, Virology 43 (1971) 375.
[49] C. Altaner and H.M. Temin, Virology 40 (1970) 118.
[50] K. Toyoshima, R.R. Friis and P.K. Vogt, Virology 42 (1970) 163.
[51] T. Graf, H. Bauer, H. Gelderblom and D.P. Bolognesi, Virology 43 (1971) 427.
[52] R.A. Weiss, R.R. Friis, E. Katz and P.K. Vogt, Virology 46 (1971) 918.
[53] L. Gross, Acta Haematol. 19 (1958) 353.
[54] M. Lieberman and H.S. Kaplan, Science 130 (1959) 387.
[55] A. Timmermans, P. Bentvelzen, P.C. Hageman and J. Calafat. J. Gen. Virol. 4 (1969) 619.
[56] S.A. Aaronson, J. Hartley and G.J. Todaro, Proc. Natl. Acad. Sci. U.S. 64 (1969) 87.
[57] P. Bentvelzen, Genetical control of the vertical transmission of the Mühlbock mammary tumor virus in the GR mouse strain (Hollandia, Amsterdam, 1968).
[58] R.J. Huebner and G.J. Todaro, Proc. Natl. Acad. Sci. U.S. 64 (1969) 1087.
[59] R.J. Huebner, G.J. Kelloff, P.S. Sarma, W.T. Love, H.C. Turner, R.V. Gilden, S. Orozlan, H. Meier, D.D. Myers and R.O. Peters, Proc. Natl. Acad. Sci. U.S. 67 (1970) 366.

[60] R.J. Huebner, This Symposium.
[61] H.M. Temin, J. Natl. Cancer Inst. 46 (1971) III.
[62] H.M. Temin, This Symposium.
[63] H.M. Temin, Proc. Natl. Acad. Sci. U.S. 52 (1964) 323.
[64] J. Harel, L. Harel and A. Goldé, Compt. Rend. Acad. Sci. D. 263 (1966) 745.
[65] M.A. Baluda and D.P. Nayak, Proc. Natl. Acad. Sci. U.S. 66 (1970) 329.
[66] M. Yoshikawa-Fukada and J.D. Ebert, Proc. Natl. Acad. Sci. U.S. 68 (1971) 743.
[67] H. Varmus, R.A. Weiss, R.R. Friis, W. Levinson and J.M. Bishop, Proc. Natl. Acad. Sci. U.S. 69 (1972).

A COMMENT ON THE EXISTENCE OF
TUMOR VIRUS GENES IN CHICKEN CELLS*

H. HANAFUSA
The Public Health Research Institute of the
City of New York, Inc., 455 First Avenue,
New York, N.Y. 10016, U.S.A.

Recent studies on the mechanism of virus reproduction of functionally defective Rous sarcoma virus (RSV) have given a new insight into the viral genes present in "normal" chicken cells. The first notion on the presence of such viral genetic elements was obtained from the finding of virus specific group-specific antigen in certain chickens [1,2]. Second, it was discovered that there are two classes of chicken embryos among the populations which are uniform in their full susceptibility to known avian leukosis-sarcoma viruses [3,4]: upon infection with a single particle of Bryan RSV, one class of cells gives rise to the formation of infectious RSV originally called RSV(0) and another class produces only non-infectious RSV. Analysis of the basis of these differences in two types of embryos led to a demonstration in the former type cells of a genetic element similar to avian tumor virus in its functions [5]. Since this genetic factor is acting as an agent like helper virus for formation of infectious RSV, it was called chick cell-associated helper factor (chf). Although no complete virus is formed from them, the chf-containing cells carry two viral functions: the formation of gs-antigen and the formation of viral coat antigen of a certain specificity. This latter function allows these cells to complement a defective function of the Bryan RSV.

The clearest evidence for the presence of chf in some chicken cells was that infection by RSV or avian leukosis virus (ALV) that had been grown in chf-positive cells carry a new agent which converts chf negative cells to producers of infectious RSV(0). In later studies, this transmissible agent was isolated as a new Rous associated virus, RAV-60 [6]. Thus, chf can be defined as a precursor of RAV-60 present in certain chicken cells. It could be a defective genome of ALV or a complete genome, some functions of which are somehow suppressed in these cells.

*This work was supported by U.S. Public Health Service research grant CA 08747 and CA 12177 from the National Cancer Institute.

137

In 1968, Payne and Chubb [2] described the fact that the presence of gs-antigen in some chickens is a characteristic which is inheritable to offspring by an autosomal gene. The character of gs-antigen positive was found to be dominant over gs-negative. Weiss [3] has shown that chick embryos derived from a gs-positive line have a capacity to produce RSV(0) but those from a gs-negative line produce non-infectious RSV following Bryan RSV infection. Studies on chf positive C/O and chf-positive C/O′ embryos confirmed this finding. Therefore, the possibility was raised that either the structural gene for chf itself is located on chromosomes, or that the expression of chf itself or chf-provirus is determined by another internal gene, or both.

Recently, we have obtained evidence suggesting that all chick embryos, including those of gs-antigen negative, have the genetic information of chf. Thus the difference of chick embryos in chf-functions should be controlled by a regulatory gene [7].

Presence of gs-negative chick cells which induce low titer of infectious RSV

C/O and C/O′ cells were classified by the capacity to produce infectious RSV [RSV(f)]* following Bryan RSV infection. The detailed description was given in a recent paper [7]. The two methods employed differ in the infecting viruses, one with non-infectious virus, RSV(−)* together with UV-Sendai virus and another with RSV(RAV-2). In both cases, infected cultures produce RSV(f) only when the cultures contain chf. By these tests, typical C/O produced high titers of RSV(f), more than 1 FFU RSV(f) per transformed cell and C/O′ produced no detectable RSV(f). However, with more than 400 individual embryos tested, we found some embryos behave intermediate between typical C/O and C/O′. These embryos, termed C/O′-L (low titer RSV(f)-producing C/O′), produced less than 10^{-3} FFU RSV(f) per transformed cell (table 1). These embryos were always gs-negative as shown in table 2.

The yield of RSV(f) following infection of C/O′-L type cultures with RSV was variable, sometimes less than 10^{-5} FFU per transformed cell, but was consistent with a particular single embryo even after many subcultures. It was also shown that transformed cell lines derived from many foci induced in C/O′-L cells of a single embryo produced equal amounts of infectious virus. The

*Since we know now RSV(0) is formed by the assistance of chf, it will be termed RSV(f). Non-infectious RSV formed in chf-negative cells will be called RSV(−). The subscript β will be omitted from β type RSV because this type appears to be the wild type of Bryan RSV.

Table 1
RSV(f) production from C/O, C/O ′and C/O ′-L type chick embryo cells.

Method A

Embryo no.	Cell type	No. of foci formed	RSV(f) produced (FFU/ml)		
			Day 2	Day 5	Day 7
931	C/O′	420	0	0	0
934	C/O′	386	0	0	0
932	C/O	218	139	5000	>10⁵
936	C/O	342	218	5000	>10⁵
901	C/O′-L	476	0	5	2
930	C/O′-L	380	0	33	200

Method B

931	C/O′	0	1	0
934	C/O′	0	0	0
932	C/O	2660	2730	572
936	C/O	5110	960	2660
901	C/O′-L	2	1	2
930	C/O′-L	9	10	20

Cells of individual chick embryos were infected with either RSV(−) plus UV-inactivated Sendai virus (method A) or RSV(RAV-2) (method B), and the titer of RSV(f) produced from the infected cultures was assayed in quail embryo cell cultures.

Table 2
Correlation between the presence of gs-antigen and helper function in individual embryos.

Type of embryo	Titer of RSV(f) produced by RSV-infection		No. of embryos with gs-titer	
			<2	≧4
C/O	high	(h_H)	8 ($h_H gs^-$)	161 ($h_H gs^+$)
C/O′	undetectable	(h^-)	58 ($h^- gs^-$)	0
C/O′-L	low	(h_L)	48 ($h_L gs^-$)	0

The amount of gs-antigen of each embryo was determined by the complement fixation test [2,9,10] using the viscera which were removed when the primary cultures were prepared.

possibility that production of RSV(f) by C/O´-L cells is due to trivial reasons inherent in the techniques used has been examined and ruled out. Cross breeding experiments have shown that C/O´-L type embryos have recessive alleles as C/O′ type for the expression of chf. Thus, the presence of such embryos suggests that the genetic information of chf is not limited to C/O type but in C/O′ or C/O´-L type it is suppressed under internal and quantitative control.

Recovery of RAV-60 from C/O′-L and C/O′ cells

Previously, we have shown that RAV-60 can be isolated from C/O cells following infection with ALV [6]. RAV-60 can also be isolated from RSV(f) stocks obtained from C/O type cells following selective growth in quail cells (unpublished observation), indicating that RSV (β type) is also capable to activate RAV-60 from chf.

Since chf seems to exist in C/O´-L cells, an attempt was made to isolate RAV-60 from these cells and also from C/O′ cells. However, the expected amounts of RAV-60 in ALV stocks obtained from C/O′ cells are exceedingly small (it should be less than 1 infectious unit per 10^6 infectious units of ALV). In order to detect such a small amount of virus, C/O´-L or C/O′ cells infected with ALV were co cultured with quail cells which are susceptible to RAV-60. Thus, if RAV-60 is activated from these chicken cells by ALV, this particle would have an immediate chance of infecting and replicating in the neighboring quail cells. The mixed cultures were serially transferred and challenged by RSV(f) to detect RAV-60 growth by interference. Results are shown in table 3. It can be seen that the susceptibility of control quail cells to RSV(f) did not alter after many subcultures regardless of their infection with RAV-1. The ratio of quail and chick cells was carefully kept constant in all mixed cultures during transfers so that simple cocultivation did not reduce susceptibility to RSV(f). Only cocultures infected with RAV-1 did eventually develop resistance to RSV(f) infection at various transfers depending on the type of cells. The establishment of resistance to RSV(f) indicates the recovery of RAV-60 from even C/O´-L or C/O′ cells and in faet a virus indistinguishable from RAV-60 was isolated from culture fluid of the cells which manifested resistance to RSV(f) by the same technique used for the recovery of RAV-60 from C/O cells, previously described [6].

These findings suggest that the genetic information. of chf is present almost ubiquitously in chicken cells. The difference between C/O and C/O′ cells is therefore not due to the presence or absence of the structural genes of chf, but

Table 3
Recovery of RAV-60 from chicken cells.

Culture	No. of embryos tested	No. of embryos which developed resistance to RSV(f) after 9 transfers	No. of transfers required to induce resistance
Quail	5	0	
Quail + RAV-1	5	0	
Quail + C/O	3	0	
Quail + C/O + RAV-1	3	3	2-3
Quail + C/O′-L	6	0	
Quail + C/O′-L + RAV-1	6	6	6-7
Quail + C/O′	5	0	
Quail + C/O′ + RAV-1	5	5	7-9

Quail cells were mixed with chick derived from various types of embryos and a half of each set was infected with RAV-1. The cultures were serially transferred and at every transfer they were challenged by RSV(f).

rather due to their expression. Since the allele for positive chf functions is dominant in heterozygotes [2], the expression of the chf or chf-provirus may be activated by some internal product. Or C/O cells may have a mutation in the operator gene which becomes insensitive to a repressor as suggested in mouse mammary tumor virus system by Bentvelzen and Daams [8]. The mechanism of control would be assessed better when we know the nature and products of chf in the cells. At the moment, there is no proof for the genetic information for chf being in DNA.

Recently, Rosenthal *et al.* [11] demonstrated that C/O and C/O′ cells contain an equal amount of DNA that is complementary to RNA of ALV including RAV-60. If one assumes that this DNA represents the provirus of chf, the results would at least be consistent with the view of the existence of such chf-provirus in both types of cells.

Finally, Vogt and Friis [12] have found that a leukosis-like virus is spontaneously produced from gs-positive C/A cells, which are susceptible to subgroup E virus, and they have designated it RAV-0. RAV-0 is similar to RAV-60 in its antigenic relatedness to RSV(f) but differs from RAV-60 in its inability to propagate in infected cells by itself [12]. No RAV-0 like virus has been found in C/O type cells used in this study. It is conceivable, however, that RAV-0 is a precursor of RAV-60 which acquires self-replicating ability through interaction with ALV used for RAV-60 induction.

H. Hanafusa

The function of chf-genes in tumor virus production or in viral carcinogenesis is unknown, but it could be equivalent to the oncogene [13] or to the protovirus [14] proposed as an integrated form of RNA tumor viruses.

References

[1] R.M. Dougherty and H.S. Di Stefano, Virology 29 (1965) 586.

[2] L.N. Payne and R.C. Chubb, J. Gen. Virol. 3 (1968) 379.

[3] R.A. Weiss, J. Gen. Virol. 5 (1969) 511.

[4] T. Hanafusa, T. Miyamoto and H. Hanafusa, Virology 40 (1970) 55.

[5] H. Hanafusa, T. Miyamoto and T. Hanafusa, Proc. Natl. Acad. Sci. U.S. 66 (1970) 314.

[6] T. Hanafusa, H. Hanafusa and T. Miyamoto, Proc. Natl. Acad. Sci. U.S. 67 (1970) 1797.

[7] T. Hanafusa, H. Hanafusa, T. Miyamoto and E. Fleissner, in preparation.

[8] P. Bentvelzen and J.H. Daams, J. Natl. Cancer Inst. 43 (1969) 1025

[9] R.J. Huebner, D. Armstrong, M. Okuyan, P.S. Sarma and H.C. Turner, Proc. Natl. Acad. Sci. U.S. 51 (1964) 742.

[10] E. Fleissner, J. Virol. 5 (1970) 14.

[11] P.N. Rosenthal, H.L. Robinson, W.S. Robinson, T. Hanafusa and H. Hanafusa, Proc. Natl. Acad. Sci. U.S. in press.

[12] P.K. Vogt and R.R. Friis, Virology 43 (1971) 223.

[13] R.J. Huebner and G.J. Todaro, Proc. Natl. Acad. Sci. U.S. 64 (1969) 1087.

[14] H.M. Temin, J. Natl. Cancer Inst. 46 (1971) III-VII.

Part 4

MOUSE LEUKEMIA VIRUSES

MOUSE LEUKEMIA: INTERACTION OF MULTIPLE COMPONENTS IN A COMPLEX ONCOGENIC SYSTEM*

Henry S. KAPLAN
Department of Radiology,
Stanford University School of Medicine,
Stanford, Calif., U.S.A.

1. Introduction

That the mechanisms of action of the RNA tumor viruses are now being pursued with increasing sophistication at the cellular and even the molecular level is amply documented in several other papers at this Symposium. In opening this session on the murine leukemia viruses, I felt that it would be desirable to present a panoramic view of the evolution of this field of investigation at the *in vivo* level, to emphasize the complexity of the natural system within which these tumors develop.

The term "mouse leukemia" has been rather loosely used to refer to a variety of neoplasms of the lymphatic and hematopoietic systems. The neoplasm most intensively studied, to which I shall confine my presentation, is more appropriately designated as a diffuse, poorly-differentiated lymphocytic lymphosarcoma, which occurs in virtually all strains of mice and, in almost all of them, tends to arise in the thymus gland and to disseminate secondarily to the other lymphatic tissues, to major viscera, and to the bone marrow, with the late occurrence of a frank lymphatic leukemia in those animals which survive sufficiently long. In some high-leukemia strains, notably AKR and C58, these tumors arise "spontaneously", whereas most other strains exhibit a very low spontaneous incidence but may develop an equally high incidence after exposure to ionizing radiations or a variety of chemical agents, including the carcinogenic hydrocarbons, urethane, certain alkylating agents, the nitroquinoline oxides, and estrogen [1].

This work was supported by grant CA 03352 from the National Cancer Institute, National Institutes of Health, U.S. Public Health Service, Bethesda, Md., U.S.A.

143

2. Viral etiology of the mouse leukemias

2.1. "Spontaneous" leukemias

Gross [2] first succeeded in demonstrating the presence of a viral agent in the spontaneous lymphomas of the high-leukemia AKR and C58 strains. Cell-free extracts prepared from these tumors, inoculated into newborn C_3H mice, induced a high incidence of identical tumors in this normally low-leukemia strain, and the agent could be propagated from one tumor generation to the next by serial passage, with progressive increase in tumor incidence and reduction in latent period. In time, the agent was purified, identified as a type C virus by electron microscopy, and extensively characterized biophysically and immunologically.

2.2. Radiation-induced lymphomas

The demonstration by our group [3-5] that thymic grafts restore the incidence of lymphomas in thymectomized, irradiated C57BL mice and in their F_1 hybrids, that the tumors thus induced originate in the unirradiated thymus grafts, and that most of the tumors can be shown to be of donor genotype provided conclusive proof of the existence of a completely indirect induction mechanism and led to a search, which soon proved successful [6-8], for the presence of leukemogenic viruses in extracts of radiation-induced lymphomas. The agent thus recovered was again concentrated by serial passage, purified, and demonstrated by electron microscopy to have the morphology of a type C virus [9], essentially indistinguishable from that of the Gross virus, and was named the radiation leukemia virus (RadLV). It is now evident that this was a misnomer, since the virus extracted from chemically-induced lymphomas of strain C57BL [10] is almost certainly the same virus; perhaps a new system of nomenclature for the murine leukemia viruses is now needed.

2.3. Chemically-induced lymphomas

Leukemogenic agents, again presumably viral in nature, have now been extracted from lymphomas induced by virtually all of the known chemical leukemogens, including the hydrocarbons [10-12], urethane [11], and nitro-quinoline oxide [13]. Moreover, the group-specific antigen characteristic of the murine leukemia viruses has been detected in chemically-induced lymphomas [14]. Thus, viruses appear to be associated with all of the murine lymphomas and lymphatic leukemias, whether "spontaneous" or induced by external physical or chemical agents.

3. The multiple components of this oncogenic system and their interactions

It is now well-established that there are at least five major components of this oncogenic system: (1) the virus; (2) the thymus; (3) the bone marrow; (4) constitutional and environmental factors affecting the host; and (5) external physical or chemical inducing agents. The complex interactions of these components have now been partially elucidated *in vivo* [1].

3.1. The radiation leukemia virus (RadLV)

Advantage has been taken of the discovery that the virus is most efficiently propagated by direct intrathymic inoculation [15] to study its intrathymic replication by electron microscopy [16] and to obtain consistently high titer preparations for both *in vivo* and *in vitro* studies. It is a spherical type C virus, with a diameter of approximately 110 mμ and with a relatively thick lamellated outer layer, a dense inner membrane, and a nucleoid of relatively low density [16]. It has been purified from mouse lymphoma tissue and from rat plasma on sucrose gradients, in which it has a buoyant density of approximately 1.16, identical with that of the other known murine leukemia viruses. It appears to be a single-stranded RNA-containing virus, on the basis of its ribonuclease-sensitive red fluorescence with acridine orange and *in vitro* labeling with tritiated uridine, and its RNA has a sedimentation rate of 71S, like that of RSV (RAV$_1$), with an associated molecular weight of about 1.0-1.2 x 10^7 daltons [17].

Although the neo-antigens which it induces on lymphoid tumor cells are indistinguishable from those induced by the Gross virus [18], the host range (strain specificity patterns) of the two viruses are strikingly different [1]. "Wild-type" RadLV, freshly extracted from a newly-induced lymphoma, is active in strain C57BL, BALB/c, and their hybrids and relatively inert in strain C$_3$H, CBA, and AKR; conversely, the Gross virus is active in the latter strains and inert in the former.

Like the Gross virus, RadLV is vertically transmitted through the embryo in its strain of origin, C57BL. Unlike the Gross virus, however, it is not extractable in active form from C57BL embryo or neonatal tissues, though virus particles of similar morphology have been observed by electron microscopy in the fetal C57BL thymus [19]. Although the virus ultimately emerges spontaneously in the tissues of extremely old C57BL mice [20,21], it appears to require the action of external physical or chemical agents for its activation and release from the tissues of younger animals [22-24].

The host range of RadLV appears to undergo modulation after serial passage, perhaps as a result of phenotypic mixing. After serial passage in

C57BL, it becomes active in the AKR strain, from which it can again be recovered in a form which remains active in strain C57BL; conversely, after adaptation to and serial passage in the SJL/J strain, it acquires sustained activity in the latter strain but loses activity in its strain of origin, C57BL [1].

Although RadLV is appreciably more difficult than most of the other murine viruses to propagate *in vitro*, it has been shown to have the capacity to rescue defective murine sarcoma virus from hamster tumor cell cultures [25], and this property has been made the basis of an *in vitro* assay for RadLV [26,27]. The pseudotype of MSV resulting from the helper action of RadLV appears to be specific, since it shares the host-range preference of RadLV for strains C57BL and BALB/c.

Recently, we have demonstrated that the prior inoculation into young C57BL mice of certain other closely related viruses can strikingly inhibit the leukemogenic activity of RadLV inoculated some weeks later [28]. To date, such inhibitory action has been demonstrated with wild-type Gross/AKR virus, with SJL-adapted RadLV, and with the RadLV pseudotype of MSV (table 1).

Table 1

Inhibition of RadLV leukemogenesis in C57BL mice by prior inoculation of other, related viruses. *

| | Lymphoma incidence | | | |
| | Exp. 1 | | Exp. 2 | |
Virus pre-inoculated	No.	%	No.	%
Gross/AKR ("wild type")	14/35	40	5/37	14
Control; none	41/45	91	33/42	79
SJL-adapted RadLV	11/43	26	–	
Control; none	37/45	82	–	
Gross/AKR, heated	15/20	75	–	
Gross/AKR, unheated	2/20	10	–	
Control; none	15/23	65		
MSV (RadLV)	12/39	31	–	
Control; none	29/48	61	–	
C57BL thymocytes incubated *in vitro* with virus, then injected: Gross/AKR first, then RadLV	15/24	63	–	
RadLV only	16/24	67	–	

* Data of M. Lieberman and H.S. Kaplan; manuscript in preparation.

Heat inactivation of Gross virus abolished its inhibitory activity. Incubation of thymus lymphoid target cells with Gross virus *in vitro,* prior to their incubation with RadLV, yielded the same tumor incidence as control cell preparations incubated with RadLV alone, suggesting that viral interference by competition for specific sites on the target cell membrane is not a tenable explanation. The alternative hypothesis that the mechanism responsible for such inhibition is immunologic in nature has now received direct support from the observation that antisera from C57BL mice previously inoculated with MSV-(RadLV) exhibit virus-neutralizing activity against appropriate dilutions of RadLV (table 2). From the fact that earlier attempts to immunize mice against their own

Table 2

RadLV leukemogenesis in C57BL mice injected with serum and spleen cells from syngeneic donors with regressed MSV (RadLV)-induced sarcomas.*

Material	RadlV	Lymphomas	
injected	dilution	Number	Percent
None	10^{-1}	16/16	100
Normal cells		20/21	95
Experimental cells		18/18	100
Normal serum		19/21	91
Experimental serum		14/18	78
None	10^{-3}	10/18	56
Normal cells		10/19	53
Experimental cells		18/26	69
Normal serum		9/24	38
Experimental serum		0/14	0**

     *   Data of M. Lieberman and H.S. Kaplan; manuscript in preparation.
     ** X^2 of this group vs. sum of other groups = 8.8; $p < 0.01$

viruses have failed, it has been presumed that they are tolerant to these vertically transmitted agents. If so, then perhaps we have found a way to break tolerance by the inoculation of other, very closely related viruses.

3.2. The thymus

In most strains of mice, the thymus is essential for the induction of lymphomas, the development of which is virtually abolished by thymectomy and restored by the implantation, either subcutaneously or intrarenally, of thymic grafts [3,15]. It is also well established that the thymus is the locus of genetic susceptibility [5] and of the direct oncogenic action of the virus [15]. There is now abundant evidence that the thymus provides at least two quite different components to this tumor-induction system: (1) the lymphoid target cells, which undergo neoplastic transformation as a consequence of the action of RadLV; and (2) the epithelial-reticular stroma, which provides an environment essential for the progression of preneoplastic target cells to an autonomous, fully neoplastic state.

3.2.1. The target cells.   The immature lymphoblastic cells of the outer cortex of the neonatal thymus are the most abundant known sources of target cells [29]. The relative abundance and susceptibility of target cells in the thymus are strongly influenced by their state of differentiation, as well as by the age and genetic constitution of the host animal [29-31]. When parental strain thymus grafts are implanted intrarenally in thymectomized, irradiated F_1 hybrid host animals and the subsequent direct intrathymic injection of RadLV is delayed for different intervals of time, the genotype of the resulting tumors has been shown to correspond closely to the time course of the shift from donor- to host-type cells in such grafts [1,32], suggesting that the virus must act very rapidly to alter the reproductive behavior of the lymphoid cells that it infects at the time of injection.

3.2.2. The epithelial-reticular thymic stroma.   Susceptible thymic target cells infected with active preparations of RadLV and injected intrasplenically into thymectomized, histocompatible hosts yield no lymphomas unless susceptibility is restored to the host animals by the implantation of thymic grafts. That the intrasplenically-inoculated target cells migrate to the intrarenal thymic grafts is strongly suggested by the observation that the thymic grafts, when re-excised and reimplanted into secondary, intact hosts 15 to 60 days later, give rise to a high incidence of lymphomas. In contrast, the animals from which the thymic grafts were removed, even as late as 60 days after initial injection of infected target cells, fail to develop lymphomas unless they receive a new thymus graft. It appears that the infected target cells must remain for a surprisingly long period of time in intimate proximity to the epithelial-reticular cells of the thymus in order to undergo progression to an autonomous, fully neoplastic state. The nature of this transition is as yet unknown, but it is well established that thymuses of certain genetic constitution provide a significantly more favorable environment than others for this sequence of events [29].

3.3. The bone marrow

It is known that the bone marrow is a principal site for storage of the RadLV in its oncogenically inert state. In addition, intact bone marrow appears to exert a strong inhibitory influence on the development of lymphomas in mice treated with partial-body X-irradiation [33] or with hydrocarbon carcinogens [34]. This antileukemogenic action of the bone marrow may be inactivated by irradiation [33] or by chemical agents such as urethane [35].

The mechanism of this protective effect appears to be related, in part, to the migration of stem cells from the bone marrow through the blood stream to the thymus [36,37], where they undergo metaplasia to become thymus cells, thus promoting the accelerated regeneration of the radiation-injured thymus [33]. Another mechanism of action involves the preferential reabsorption by intact bone marrow of RadLV particles in the peripheral blood. The plasma clearance rates of RadLV were estimated at serial intervals after the intravenous injection of RadLV into mice that had been pretreated with whole-body or with thigh-shielded irradiation [38]. The plasma samples were inoculated intrathymically into intact baby C57BL test mice to ascertain the leukemogenic activity remaining in the plasma. The data indicate that RadLV is cleared much more rapidly from the blood stream of the thigh-shielded-irradiated animals than from the whole-body-irradiated animals (table 3), suggesting that intact, unirradiated bone marrow has the capacity to quench RadLV viremias by readsorption.

Table 3
Effect of whole-body *vs.* thigh-shielded irradiation on the plasma clearance rate of RadLV.*

Time of sampling after i.v. virus inoc.	Whole-body irradiation		Thigh-shielded irradiation	
Minutes	Lymphomas no.	%	Lymphomas no.	%
15	55/62	89	15/38	39
30	14/52	27	4/52	7.7
45	15/60	25	1/60	1.7
60	5/59	8.5	1/75	1.3,

* Data of H.S. Kaplan and M. Lieberman; manuscript in preparation.

3.4. Constitutional and environmental factors affecting the host
It has been shown that age, sex, genetic constitution, nutritional state, and endocrine factors within the host can all exert a strong influence on

susceptibility to lymphoma development [1]. A particularly striking example of the influence of genetic factors was observed in an experiment involving two different F_1 hybrids of strain C57BL with strains C_3H and BALB/c, respectively, in both of which C57BL thymus grafts, C57BL target cells, and the same RadLV preparation were utilized [29]. The lymphoma incidence in the (C57BL x BALB/c) F_1 mice was 89%, whereas that in the (C57BL x C_3H) F_1 mice was only 33%, with an appreciably longer mean latent period. Pincus *et al.* [39] have recently demonstrated by elegant *in vitro* techniques that the murine leukemia viruses tend to fall into two broad classes, with respect to genetic susceptibility patterns: the *N-tropic* viruses, of which the Gross virus is the prototype, which are propagated in all H-2^k and certain other strains, and the *B-tropic* viruses, of which RadLV may be considered the prototype, which are propagated in H-2^b and H-2^d strains, such as C57BL and BALB/c.

3.5. External physical and chemical agents

Careful analysis of the mode of action of X-irradiation in inducing lymphomas in strain C57BL mice indicates that at least four different effects are involved, and that their simultaneous occurrence may explain why X-irradiation is such a powerful leukemogenic agent in this system. The actions identified to date are: (a) "activation" and release of RadLV; (b) thymic injury and regeneration; (c) injury to the bone marrow; and (d) immunosuppression.

3.5.1. "Activation" and release of RadLV. The release of leukemogenically active virus from C57BL bone marrow within several days after exposure to X-irradiation [23,24] or to certain chemical leukemogens [12] is now well established. Although the phenomenon has obvious analogies to the induction of temperate bacteriophage in lysogenic hosts exposed to the same types of agents, the details of the mechanism are not yet known. However, radiation must have other actions as well, since it also potentiates the response to RadLV in C57BL mice [40].

3.5.2. Thymic injury and regeneration. It has long been known that radiation injures the thymus and that the phase of injury is followed by one of regeneration during which the thymus is abundantly repopulated by immature lymphoblastic target cells, recapitulating the situation which exists in the unirradiated neonatal thymus. Direct evidence that small, subleukemogenic doses of X-rays restore susceptibility of the adult thymus to intrathymically inoculated RadLV has now been obtained [41]. It has also been shown that at least two classes of chemical leukemogenic agents, urethane and the hydrocarbons, share the property of producing thymic injury, followed by a phase of regeneration [35,42].

3.5.3. Bone marrow injury. X-rays kill bone marrow stem cells and thus reduce the number available for migration to the radiation-injured thymus, delaying its regeneration and prolonging the phase of maturation arrest of the lymphoid target cells within the thymus [43]. The hydrocarbons and urethane also appear to have the capacity to destroy bone marrow stem cells [34,35]. The data cited above suggest that X-rays are capable of injuring the capacity of the bone marrow to readsorb RadLV from the blood stream after its injection and presumably would also influence the capacity of bone marrow to quench viremias developing after radiation-induced virus release.

3.5.4. Immunosuppression. The immunosuppressive effects of X-irradiation, methylcholanthrene, 6-mercaptopurine, and alkylating agents such as thio-TEPA are well known [44,45]. Haran-Ghera [46] has presented evidence indicating that the immunosuppressive effect of irradiation plays a significant role in its leukemogenic activity in strain C57BL mice. It is postulated that the immune surveillance mechanisms are normally capable of detecting the neo-antigens induced on the surfaces of lymphoid tumor cells by RadLV and of destroying such cells before they can give rise to tumors. By transiently suppressing these immune mechanisms, X-rays and the various chemical agents provide an opportunity for clones of lymphoid tumor cells to gain reproductive momentum and to outgrow the immune response after it recovers.

4. The problem of causality

Is RadLV the true cause of the thymic lymphomas from which it is extracted, or is it merely a secondary "passenger" in tumors induced by irradiation or chemical agents? This interesting question has been discussed in earlier communications [1], and a number of lines of evidence have been presented which favor the view that the virus is the actual causative agent. Strong further support for this view comes from recent studies in which multiple injections of interferon were administered to groups of mice treated respectively with leukemogenic doses of X-irradiation or with RadLV. At appropriately chosen X-ray doses, or of RadLV concentrations, it was possible to demonstrate a very significant decrease in lymphoma incidence and a marked prolongation of latent period in animals serially injected with interferon preparations from cell cultures infected with Newcastle disease virus, as compared with animals injected either with saline or with supernatants from control cultures [47]. Control experiments failed to reveal any evidence of inhibition by interferon of "takes" and growth of transplanted lymphoid tumor cells. In view of the specificity of the antiviral action of interferon, this evidence strongly suggests that RadLV plays an essential role in the induction of lymphomas in X-irradiated C57BL mice.

5. Summary and conclusion

Thus, a coherent theory of murine leukemogenesis emerges from the available evidence concerning this complex system (fig. 1). A family of closely related

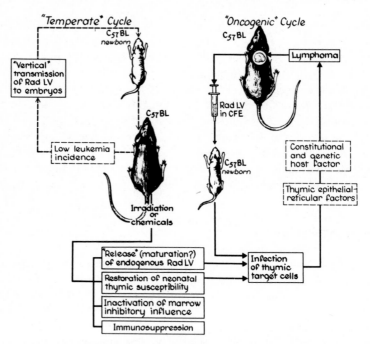

Fig. 1. Virus-mediated radiation leukemogenesis in strain C57BL mice.

RNA viruses, of which the Gross/AKR and the RadLV viruses are the major prototypes in nature, appear to be the universal murine leukemogenic agents. They are apparently ubiquitous in virtually all strains of mice and probably exist in latent form in other animal species as well [48]. In analogy with the temperate viruses of lysogenic bacteria, they are propagated vertically from one generation to the next, but usually remain latent and innocuous throughout the entire life span of the host unless the host-virus relationship is disturbed. The nature of this disturbance has not yet been identified in the high-leukemia strains; in the low-leukemia strains, "activation" of these viruses requires exposure of the host to certain physical or chemical agents which simultaneously restore susceptibility to the thymus, injure certain protective mechanisms in the bone marrow, and impair immune surveillance mechanisms of the host, permitting the neoplastic transformation of thymic lymphoid target cells by the activated virus, and the replication and progression of clones of such altered cells to an autonomous, fully neoplastic state. Once they have been activated, these latent leukemogenic viruses are capable of inducing neoplastic conversion in susceptible lymphoid target cells without the further mediation of external agents and continue indefinitely thereafter to be propagated by, and extractable in active form from, the lymphoid tumors which they induce. It is to be hoped that recently developed *in vitro* techniques will now permit us to pursue the intimate details of these complex cell-virus interactions at the molecular level.

References

[1] H.S. Kaplan, Cancer Res. 27 (1967) 1325.
[2] L. Gross, Proc. Soc. Exptl. Biol. Med. 76 (1951) 27.
[3] H.S. Kaplan and M.B. Brown, Science 119 (1954) 439.
[4] H.S. Kaplan, W.H. Carnes, M.B. Brown and B. B. Hirsch, Cancer Res. 16 (1956) 422.
[5] H.S. Kaplan, B.B. Hirsch and M.B. Brown, Cancer Res. 16 (1956) 434.
[6] H.S. Kaplan, *In:* R.W. Begg, Proceedings Second Canadian Cancer Conference (Academic Press, New York, 1957) p. 127.
[7] L. Gross, Acta Haematol. 19 (1958) 353.
[8] M. Lieberman and H.S. Kaplan, Science 130 (1959) 387.
[9] W. Bernhard, Cancer Res. 20 (1960) 712.
[10] N. Haran-Ghera, Proc. Soc. Exptl. Biol. Med. 124 (1967) 697.
[11] R. Ribacchi and G. Giraldo, Natl. Cancer Inst. Monograph 22 (1966) 701.
[12] J.K. Ball and J.A. McCarter, J. Natl. Cancer Inst. 46 (1971) 751.
[13] R. Kinosita and T. Tanaka, *In:* Viruses, nucleic acids, and cancer (Williams and Wilkins, Baltimore, 1963) p. 571.
[14] H.J. Igel, R.J. Huebner, H.C. Turner, P. Kotin and H.L. Falk, Science 166 (1969) 1624.
[15] N. Haran-Ghera, M. Lieberman and H.S. Kaplan, Cancer Res. 26 (1966) 438.
[16] W.H. Carnes, M. Lieberman, M. Marchildon and H.S. Kaplan, Cancer Res. 28 (1968) 98.
[17] E.F. Walker and H.S. Kaplan, manuscript in preparation.
[18] J.F. Ferrer and H.S. Kaplan, Cancer Res. 28 (1968) 2522.
[19] W.H. Carnes, Fred. Proc. 26 (1967) 748.
[20] G. Rudali and C. Silberman, Nouv. Rev. Franc. Hématol. 5 (1965) 63.
[21] J.F. Duplan, Bull. Cancer 52 (1965) 117.
[22] H.S. Kaplan, Natl. Cancer Inst. Monograph 14 (1964) 207.

[23] N. Haran-Ghera, Intern. J. Cancer 1 (1966) 81.
[24] L. Gross and D.G. Feldman, Cancer Res. 28 (1968) 1677.
[25] H. Igel, R.J. Huebner, B. Deppa, and S. Buhgarner, Proc. Natl. Acad. Sci. U.S. 58 (1967) 1870.
[26] G.M. Hahn, A. Declève, M. Lieberman and H.S. Kaplan, J. Virol. 5 (1970) 432.
[27] A. Declève, M. Lieberman, G.M. Hahn and H.S. Kaplan, J. Virol. 5 (1970) 437.
[28] M. Lieberman and H.S. Kaplan, Proc. Am. Assoc: Cancer Res. 9 (1968) 42.
[29] M. Lieberman and H.S. Kaplan, Natl. Cancer Inst. Monograph 22 (1966) 549.
[30] H.S. Kaplan, Cancer Res. 21 (1961) 981.
[31] A.A. Axelrad and H. van der Gaag, J. Natl. Cancer Inst. 28 (1962) 1065.
[32] M. Lieberman and H.S. Kaplan, Proc. Am. Assoc. Cancer Res. 7 (1966) 43.
[33] H.S. Kaplan, M.B. Brown and J. Paull, J. Natl. Cancer Inst., 14 (1953) 303.
[34] J.K. Ball, J. Natl. Cancer Inst. 44 (1970) 439.
[35] N. Haran-Ghera and H.S. Kaplan, Cancer Res. 24 (1964) 1926.
[36] V. Wallis, A.J.S. Davies and P.C. Koller, Nature 210 (1966) 500.
[37] P.L.T. Ilbery and C.A. Barnes, Intern. J. Cancer 5 (1970) 124.
[38] H.S. Kaplan and M. Lieberman, manuscript in preparation.
[39] T. Pincus, J.W. Hartley and W.P. Rowe, J. Exptl. Med. 133 (1971) 1219.
[40] M. Lieberman, N. Haran-Ghera and H.S. Kaplan, Nature 203 (1964) 420.
[41] M. Lieberman and H.S. Kaplan, manuscript in preparation.
[42] K. Yasuhira, Cancer Res. 24 (1964) 558.
[43] H.S. Kaplan and M.B. Brown, In: J.W. Rebuck, F.H. Bethell and R.W. Monto, The leukemias: etiology, pathophysiology, and treatment (Academic Press, New York, 1957) p. 163.
[44] R.G. Doell, C. de Vaux St. Cyr and P. Grabar, Intern. J. Cancer 2 (1967) 103.
[45] J.R. Eltringham and I. Weissman, Radiology 94 (1970) 438.
[46] N. Haran-Ghera, Brit. J. Cancer 21 (1967) 739.
[47] M. Lieberman, T.C. Merigan and H.S. Kaplan, Proc. Am. Assoc. Cancer Res. 12 (1971) 61; Proc. Soc. Exptl. Biol. Med., in press.
[48] R.J. Huebner, G.J. Kelloff, P.S. Sarma, W.T. Lane, H.C. Turner, R.V. Gilden, S. Oroszlan, H. Meier, D.D. Myers and R.L. Peters, Proc. Natl. Acad. Sci. U.S. 67 (1970) 366.

ANTIGENIC CONVERSION BY LEUKEMIA VIRUSES[1]

G. PASTERNAK, L. PASTERNAK, and B. MICHEEL[2]

German Academy of Sciences,
Research Center of Molecular Biology and Medicine,
Department of Immunobiology, 1115 Berlin-Buch, GDR

1. Introduction

Viruses may exert different effects on susceptible cells. Depending on viral as well as cellular qualities they produce cytopathic effects, including chromosomal aberrations, malignant transformation, or antigenic conversion. Whereas cytopathogenicity and cell transformation by viruses are well-defined events which are generally known, the phenomenon of antigenic conversion is not precisely characterized and experimentally less elaborated.

In tumor research the term "antigenic conversion" was introduced by Stück *et al.* [1]. These authors have shown that established transplanted leukemias acquire a new specific cellular antigen after infection with an unrelated leukemogenic virus. The surface localization of the new antigen is evident from the cells' sensitivity to cytotoxic antibodies directed against the unrelated viral leukemia. Antigenic conversion appeared to be a stable change since passaging of the cells *in vivo* did not alter their sensitivity to cytotoxic antibodies.

The appearance of virus-induced membrane-associated antigens characteristic of the infecting agent has also been observed by others in various malignant and non-malignant tissues. Sjögren [2] was able to show that methylcholanthrene-induced sarcomas of mice contain the polyoma-specific transplantation antigen provided that the tumors had been infected with that virus. Transplantation techniques were also used by Svet-Moldavsky and Hamburg [3], and Hamburg and Svet-Moldavsky [4] in order to show that herpes simplex-, Sendai-, SV40-, or polyoma virus-infected tumors of chemical origin acquire sensitivity to the specific rejection response of virus-immunized animals. Svet-Moldavsky introduced the term "artificial heterogenization" for this phenomenon. Further-

[1] The work by the authors was supported by the Ministry of Health of the GDR.
[2] The technical assistance of Mrs. Johanna Rosin is gratefully acknowledged.

more, non-malignant cells may contain a specific membrane-associated antigen as a consequence of a virus infection. Thus, lymphoid tissues of AKR mice carry the specific surface antigen of Gross leukemia from the time of birth [5], and normal spleen cells of 14-day-old mice carried the Graffi-specific antigen when they had been infected as newborns [6]. Even skin from animals with viral leukemia is antigenically converted since the grafts are rejected after transplantation to genetically compatible hosts [7].

On the basis of these findings, antigenic conversion is the acquisition of new membrane-associated antigen(s) by tumor or normal cells as a consequence of infection with tumor as well as non-tumor viruses. Antigenic conversion may be connected with, but is not dependent on malignant transformation. It may appear spontaneously when cells pick up a virus during natural infection or it can be induced experimentally by either infection of tissue culture cells or by infection *in vivo* of transplanted grafts.

Little is known about the antigens involved in antigenic conversion, especially in the mouse leukemia system. Release of the viruses from the cell membrane and, consequently, presence of viral antigen as an integral part of the membrane could fully explain the acquisition of a new antigen. This is certainly the case in some latent infections with non-oncogenic viruses. However, tumor viruses generally induce the formation of a membrane-associated antigen which is unrelated to the virion antigen. Hence, antigenic conversion may be due to the presence in the membrane of (a) a virion antigen, (b) a membrane-associated new cellular antigen, or (c) both kinds of antigens [8]. Murine leukemia viruses display type-specific antigenic differences not only in the virions, but also in the membrane-associated antigens [8]. It is therefore possible to study certain virus-cell interactions such as the mechanism of antigenic expression or antigen disappearance as well as problems of viral and antigenic interference. The following experiments were directed towards obtaining more information about the role of the viral and the host-cell genome in malignant transformation and antigenic expression.

2. Viral and virus-induced antigens of murine leukemia

Before discussing our experiments on antigenic conversion, a brief summary of present knowledge about the classification of specific antigens of viral leukemia and their distribution may be of help. There are two possibilities of presenting the data. One is based solely on the grouping or typing of the antigens concerned, corresponding to the presence or absence of cross-reactions with immune sera of homologous or heterologous origin. The other considers the nature of the antigens in relation to viral or cellular structures. The second approach is certainly the more difficult one.

Tables 1 and 2 list the antigens of murine leukemia viruses and membrane-associated antigens of viral leukemia as detected by homologous and hetero-logous sera. One of the group-specific antigens of the viral nucleoid is shared by rat, hamster and cat leukemia (table 3) [9-12]. It is of interest that the mouse is apparently unable to produce antibodies to the group-specific antigens of the viral nucleoid. The non-reactivity of the mouse indicates the structural identity of the group-specific antigen with molecular configurations of this species, or a state of immunological tolerance to this viral antigen.

In table 4, the localization of viral and virus-induced antigens is summarized in respect of virus, cell and host. It is known that the virion may also contain host-cell components. T. Aoki[3] reported the presence of H-2^k antigen in 28,6% of the virions released from cells of this genotype, and the absence of H-2^b when released from the H-2^b genotype. Virions of H-2^b origin, however, have the Θ antigen. Whether or not the host-cell antigens of the leukemia viruses play a role in the process of infection, is not yet clear.

Among the cell-bound antigens, the virus-induced new cellular antigen has attracted wide interest. Until now there are only some indirect data suggesting the existence of this type of antigen in viral leukemia (table 5). Distinction between viral envelope antigen and the new cell-antigen, that should be also type-specific, is extremely difficult since no cells containing the new cell-antigen are guaranteed virus free. Although the mere presence of viral antigen as an integral part of the cell membrane could explain the antigenicity and immunosensitivity of leukemia cells, this would be an exception among the viral tumors which are known to contain a virus-induced new cell-antigen. The problem of distinction between viral and virus-induced new cellular antigen also holds true for the soluble antigens which appear in the plasma of infected animals [19]. Two antigens have been identified, the group-specific antigen of the viral nucleoid and the type-specific (ts) antigen of the viral envelope. After adsorption onto ts-negative cells, the ts antigen is capable of eliminating the virus-neutralizing activity from immune sera [20]. It cannot be excluded, however, that a third antigen, the virus-induced new cellular antigen, is also present in the serum of infected animals. Now, if a given leukemia indeed contains two distinct type-specific antigens, *viz.* a viral and a new cellular one, then a doubly infected cell should theoretically have four different antigens. To test this possibility we performed conversion experiments in which cells doubly infected with unrelated leukemogenic viruses, were analyzed.

[3] Presented at the "International Symposium on Relationships between Tumor Antigens and Histocompatibility Systems", Paris, 26-28 February 1971.

G. Pasternak et al.

Table 1
Antigens of murine leukemia viruses.

Localization of antigen	Origin of typing sera	Cross-reactions between G and FMRGr	Designation of antigen	Method of detection
Envelope	Mouse	Absent	Type-specific (ts) a. of viral envelope	Neutralization
	Rat or rabbit	Present	Group-specific (gs) a. of viral envelope	Immunoelectron microscopy
Nucleoid	Mouse	No immune response		Complement fixation
	Rat or rabbit	Present	Group-specific (gs) a. of viral nucleoid	Immunoprecipitation

Table 2
Membrane-associated antigens of murine viral leukemia.

Localization of antigen	Origin of typing sera	Cross-reactions between G and FMRGr	Designation of antigen	Method of detection
Cell surface	Mouse	Absent	Type-specific (ts) membrane-associated a.	Immunofluorescence Immunoelectrŏn microscopy
	Rat	Present	Group-specific (gs) membrane-associated a.	Cytotoxicity Absorption

Table 3
Group-specific (gs) antigens of MuLV in different species as detected by immunoprecipitation with Gross rat serum.

	mouse	rat	hamster	cat
gs 1	+	−	−	−
gs 2	+	−	−	−
gs 3	+	+	+	+

Table 4
Viral and virus-induced antigens of murine leukemia.

I. Antigens of the virion
  1. Viral envelope
     viral antigen (ts)
     components of host cell membrane

  2. Viral nucleoid
     viral antigen (gs)
     host cell components?

II. Cell-bound antigens of viral origin
  1. Membrane-associated antigens
     viral envelope
     virus-induced new cellular antigen

  2. Intracellularly localized antigens
     viral envelope?
     viral nucleoid (gs)
     virus induced new cellular antigen?

III. Soluble antigens in the plasma of infected animals
     gs antigen of viral nucleoid
     ts antigen of viral envelope
     virus-induced new cellular antigen?

Table 5

Criteria for the existence of virus-induced new cellular antigens in murine leukemia	Critical points of argumentation against applicability of statements
1. Independence of immunosensitivity of leukemia cells and virus release [13]	There must be no correlation between virus release and viral antigen present on the membrane
2. Certain virus-infected cell lines absorb predominantly virus-neutralizing antibodies from mouse immune sera and do not alter the anticellular antibodies [14]	Incomplete absorption and higher sensitivity of the anticellular (immunofluorescence) than of the virusneutralizing test
3. Absorption of mouse immune serum with virus removes virus-neutralizing but not cytotoxic activity [15]	Same as 2
4. Immunization of mice with virus-free leukemia cells produces resistance to virus infection [16]	"Virus-free" leukemia cells may produce the virus after inoculation into mice
5. A non-releaser MSV (MLV) tumor was found to be both immunogenic and immunosensitive [17]	The situation is different from leukemia and the antigen is due to MSV and not to MuLV
6. There are Gross mouse immune sera which react with the cell membrane of leukemia cells but not with the virus [18]	Non-labelled virions may have been produced after antibody binding to the cell surface

3. Antigenic conversion by artificial infection

3.1. AKR Gross leukemia

When testing the antigenic conversion by Rauscher virus, Stück *et al.* [1] observed that a BALB/c but not an AKR Gross leukemia acquired Rauscher specificity when passaged in Rauscher-infected animals. Their finding that conversion apparently did not occur in all cases of Gross leukemia motivated our research. One of the main questions was whether the non-converted tumors had picked up the second virus and produced it in spite of the absence of antigenic conversion. Therefore a number of AKR Gross leukemias was infected with Graffi virus by passaging the cells one to five times in Graffi virus-infected mice. Virus release was measured by the mouse antibody production (MAP) test. At the same time we tested the sensitivity of the cells to Graffi-specific immunity *in vivo*, and cytotoxic antibodies *in vitro*, and applied the indirect

Table 6
Antigenic conversion by Graffi virus of AKR Gross leukemia. Search for Graffi virus production and Graffi virus-induced membrane-associated antigens.

Type of leukemia	Release of Graffi virus	Number of positive cases		
		Total number of leukemias investigated		
		Antigens detectable by		
		transplantation-techniques	MIF	cytotoxic test
AKR Gross	0/10	0/5	0/9	0/7
AKR Gross infected with Graffi virus	10/10	1/12	8/11	0/8

membrane immunofluorescence with Graffi-specific antibodies (table 6). Only one of 12 Graffi-virus-superinfected Gross leukemias was sensitive *in vivo* as shown by its rejection in Graffi-immunized animals. The membrane immuno-fluorescene test was also strongly positive. Although the cytotoxic test could not be evaluated for technical reasons, one may assume that this leukemia was antigenically converted by infection with Graffi virus.

Surprisingly all other Gross leukemias passaged in Graffi virus-infected animals permanently produced the Graffi virus at the same rate. Their membrane immunofluorescence was slightly positive; however, the cells were not sensitive to cytotoxic antibodies and to rejection response *in vivo*.

According to the data of Stück *et al.* [1] and our own experience, one should distinguish between complete and incomplete antigenic conversion (table 7). Complete and incomplete conversion could, however, represent quantitative rather than qualitative differences, but even a quantitative difference in antigenic expression would be of interest. The problem is even more complicated in that cloning of cells from one of the incompletely converted tumors has shown that some cells do not contain the Graffi virus [21]. Accordingly, incomplete antigenic conversion could depend on the proportion of infected to non-infected cells. However, since those non-infected cells, which are moreover not resistant to Graffi virus infection, apparently represent only a minor fraction of the tumor-cell population, incomplete antigenic conversion cannot be explained by the presence of a small number of completely converted cells only. The presence of a Graffi antigen on the majority of cells as detected by the indirect membrane immunofluorescence test, furnished another argument against the aforementioned hypothesis. There

Table 7

Criteria of complete and incomplete antigenic conversion of AKR Gross leukemia after infection with Graffi virus.

Activities measured	Complete antigenic conversion	Incomplete antigenic conversion
Virus release	+++	+++
Membrane fluorescence	+++	+
Sensitivity of the cells to cytotoxic antibodies	+++	–
Sensitivity of the cells to the specific rejection response of Graffi virus-immunized mice	+++	–

are some indications that this Graffi antigen is the type-specific antigen of the viral envelope. Such cells eliminate virus-neutralizing antibodies from Graffi immune sera [22]. The Gross-specific antigens seem to be present on Graffi virus-producing cells.

Let us assume that the presence of the Gross type of new cellular antigen in the cell membrane is incompatible with the expression of the Graffi virus-induced new cellular antigen, because they occupy the same sites or interfere at some other step of antigenic expression. Then complete antigenic conversion of Gross leukemia is only possible to occur in cases where the new cellular antigen is absent. Unfortunately our completely converted Gross leukemia was lost and we were not able as yet to select another tumor to be analyzed for the Graffi-specific new cellular antigen.

3.2. Methylnitrosourea-induced leukemia

Table 8 shows the results of a similar conversion experiment with N-methyl-N-nitrosourea (MNU)-induced leukemia of mice. Contrary to the findings with AKR Gross leukemia, the cells of the chemically induced leukemias acquired sensitivity to the specific rejection response of Graff-immunized animals and thus appear to be completely converted. At the time of the experiments we did not have any data on the presence of Gross virus and Gross antigens in this type of leukemia. Type C particles, however, were frequently seen in the majority of cases.[4]

[4] A. Graffi and D. Bierwolf, personal communication

Table 8

Antigenic conversion by Graffi virus of MNU-induced leukemia. Search for Graffi virus production and Graffi virus-induced membrane-associated antigens.

Type of leukemia	Release of Graffi virus	Number of positive cases / Total number of leukemias investigated / Antigens detectable by transplantation techniques	MIF
MNU-induced leukemia of XVII	0/4	0/3	0/33
MNU-induced leukemia infected with Graffi virus	4/4	3/4	7/7

The appearance of complete antigenic conversion shows that MNU leukemia of XVII mice generally behaves different from AKR Gross leukemia. The results suggest that either Gross virus-induced antigens are absent in this chemically induced leukemia, or the host genotype, by controlling the expression of virus-induced membrane-associated antigens, allows the presence of both Graffi and Gross new cellular antigens in XVII but only that of Gross new cellular antigen in AKR.

Before discussing natural infection with Gross virus, another example of antigenic conversion by artificial infection may be mentioned.

3.3. Graffi leukemia SOV 16

Graffi leukemia SOV 16 had lost infectivity and did not contain significant concentrations of membrane-associated antigens any longer. Only intensive immunizations of mice with SOV 16 produced some Graffi virus-neutralizing antibodies. As detected by immunoprecipitation, the group-specific antigen of the viral nucleoid was present in high amounts. Apparently there was a defect in the process of enveloping the viral nucleoid as a result of either the low concentration of envelope antigen or some other inhibitory mechanism. Also any virus-induced new cellular antigen must have been lost during the transplantation passages. Reinfection of SOV 16 with Graffi virus converted the cells to virus producers and led to the expression of membrane-associated antigens (table 9). There was no change in malignancy after reinfection. The regain of virus production is in line with the hypothesis that SOV 16 had lost some viral genes.

Table 9
Antigenic conversion by Graffi virus of the non-specific transplantation leukemia SOV 16.

	Concentration of		
	membrane-associated Graffi antigens as measured by MIF	group-specific antigen of viral nucleoid as measured by immuno-precipitation	Virus release
SOV 16 original line	Extremely low	High	Negative
SOV Gr 16 Graffi virus-infected	High	High	Positive

SOV 16 which was induced by Graffi virus about 15 years ago had lost the virus during cellular passages in genotypically different hosts.

4. Antigenic conversion by natural infection

Tumors as well as normal tissues may pick up viruses and become antigenically converted. Some confusion in definition may arise in this context when taking into consideration the hypothesis of Huebner and Todaro [22] that the cells of many, if not all vertebrates carry vertically transmitted (inherited) RNA tumor virus information, and that besides tumor formation, phenotypic expression of viral information such as membrane-associated antigens may also occur. According to this view, antigenic conversion is not necessarily the outcome of natural infection with Gross-type viruses, but may also be due to virogene derepression. In this context the MNU-induced leukemias were analyzed, also with the hope of learning the possible causes of different conversion behavior after infection with Graffi virus.

4.1. MNU-induced leukemia

The first experiments concerned the immunogenicity of MNU leukemia. Immunization *in vivo* failed if pretreatment of the mice consisted of 2-3 inoculations with X-ray killed tumor-cell suspensions, a technique which is sufficient to produce transplantation resistance against Graffi leukemia. Only after 5-6 inoculations a slight degree of transplantation resistance was demonstrable. Resistance was directed against the homologous leukemia; cross-resistance among MNU leukemias could not be detected so far (table 10). This result indicates the presence of individually distinct antigens in MNU leukemia. In one case a MNU leukemia produced resistance to Gross leukemia cells. Information on the immunological behavior of seven different MNU-leukemias is summarized in table 11. Most of these tumors have TSTA but do

Table 10
Results of immunization and cross immunization with MNU leukemia of XVII mice.

Challenge leukemia	Presence of TSTA as detected by immunization of mice with leukemia				
	MNU 3	MNU 8	MNU 9	MNU 12	Gross
MNU 3	+	−	−	−	−
MNU 8	−	+	−	−	−
MNU 9	−	−	(+)	−	−
MNU 12	−	−	−	+	−
Gross	−	+	n.t.	n.t.	+

n.t. = not tested.

Table 11
Summary of information on the immunological behavior of 7 different MNU-induced leukemias of mice.

MNU leukemia (strain of origin)	Immunogenicity and immuno-sensitivity *in vivo* (immunization and challenge inoculation with same tumors)	Sensitivity to Gross-specific immune response *in vivo*	Reaction with Gross-specific antibodies *in vitro* (MIF-test)	Group-specific antigen of viral nucleoid (immuno-precipitation)
MNU 3 (XVII)	+	−	+	+
MNU 8 (XVII)	+	−	+	(+)
MNU 9 (XVII)	(+)	−	+	+
MNU 12 (XVII)	+	−	+	−
MNU 131 (CBA)	−	n.t.	+	−
MNU 135 (CBA)	+	n.t.	+	−
MNU 122 (CBA)	n.t.	n.t.	−	−

not show sensitivity to the Gross-specific immune response *in vivo*. Transplanted MNU-leukemic cells are not rejected despite the presence of Gross virus-induced membrane-associated antigens as detected by the membrane immunofluorescence test. The presence or absence of the group-specific viral antigen was not correlated with that of the membrane-associated antigens investigated.

Table 12

Summary of information on the presence of viral or virus-induced antigens in primary MNU-induced leukemia.

Strain of origin	Indirect membrane immunofluorescence test*			Group-specific* antigen of viral nucleoid
	Graffi mouse im- mune serum	Gross mouse im- mune serum	Graffi rat immune serum	
XVII	0/15	10/15	3/4	11/14
(XVII × AKR)F$_1$	0/6	5/8	n.t.	4/8
AKR	0/8	10/10	2/2	7/10
CBA	0/4	2/5	n.t.	0/5

*Number of positive leukemias over total number tested. n.t. = not tested.

Table 12 shows that the majority of MNU leukemias of different mouse strains has viral or virus-induced antigens of the Gross type. Membrane-associated antigens of this type are also present in leukemias which have been induced in strains with a low incidence of spontaneous leukemia, such as XVII and CBA. Although in two of five CBA leukemias a membrane-associated Gross antigen was detectable we failed to show the group-specific viral antigen in the five MNU-induced CBA leukemias. Some data on the presence of the group-specific antigen in different tissues are presented in table 13. Finally, table 14 gives a brief description of the four immunologically different types of leukemia which may arise after injection of MNU into newborn mice. From these results the conclusion can be drawn, in correspondence with Huebner and Todaro [23], that the membrane-associated antigens, group-specific viral antigens and oncogenicity are expressed as independent entities.

The presence of individually distinct antigens in MNU leukemia as shown by transplantation tests needs further attention. It is not excluded that the carcinogen is directly producing the disease and that the antigens thus correspond to those of chemically induced sarcomas. On the basis of this hypothesis, virus-induced antigens are only accidentally present. Activation of virus by action of MNU is conceivable because this nitrosamide compound is strongly immunosuppressive [24]. However, in contrast to chemically induced sarcomas, the immunogenicity of MNU leukemia is low and there are even some

Table 13
Summary of information on the presence of group-specific (gs) antigen of viral nucleoid in different tumorous and non-tumorous mouse tissues (detection by immunoprecipitation).

	Number of positive cases — Total number tested
Primary Graffi leukemia of mouse or rat origin	8/8
Primary Gross leukemia of AKR origin	12/14
Primary methyl nitrosourea-induced mouse leukemia	22/37
Normal tissue (spleen, liver, lymph nodes) of adult XVII	0/7
Normal tissue (spleen, liver, lymph nodes) of adult (XVII × AKR)F$_1$	2/11

We are greatly indebted to Dr.L.J. Old who kindly provided us with the serum.

Table 14
Pattern of immunological reactivity *in vitro* of MNU leukemia.

Type of MNU leukemia	Virus-induced membrane antigens detectable by			Group-specific viral antigen as detected by gel diffusion with rat serum
	Graffi mouse immune serum (type-specific)	Gross mouse immune serum (type-specific)	Graffi rat immune serum (group-specific)	
I	−	+	+	+
II	−	−	−	+
III	−	+	+	−
IV	−	−	−	−

tumors which do not produce any immune response in syngeneic mice. Individually distinct antigens are now known to exist in virus-induced mammary tumors of mice [25,26], and recently have also been found in reticulum cell tumors of SJL/J mice [27] and in plasma cell tumors of BALB/c mice [28]. Hence, the presence of individually distinct antigens in MNU leukemias does not necessarily indicate the chemical origin of the tumors.

Another interesting finding is that, although the leukemias did not show cross-resistance *in vivo*, they were positive for the Gross antigen *in vitro*. Apparently this antigen plays only a minor role in the immunosensitivity of the cells *in vivo*. Unfortunately we have as yet no data on the immunosensitivity *in vitro*. Most probably the humoral immune response alone is not sufficient to kill the cell. For that the simultaneous action of immune cells predominantly directed against the individually distinct antigens, may be required.

The differences observed in antigenic conversion by leukemia viruses are still another subject of speculation. Although antigenic conversion by artificial or natural infection of tumor and normal tissues is well defined as regards the way of infection and the materials involved, the phenomena of complete and incomplete antigenic conversions are not yet understood. The definition is solely based on the different immunosensitivity *in vivo* and *in vitro* of converted cells. Either quantitative or qualitative differences in antigenic expression may cause the different behavior of the cells and this might be controlled by the viral as well as by the host genome. That the XVII genotype does not inhibit the full expression of the Gross-type of antigens follows from the finding that two Gross leukemias of the XVII strain show immunosensitivity *in vivo*.

The action of some of the viral genes in a cell does not prevent complete antigenic conversion by an unrelated leukemia virus. This conclusion can be drawn from the experiments with MNU-induced leukemias where Gross-type antigens are present. However, the general impression from these experiments is that complete conversion of cells occurs only if the surface concentration of virus-induced antigens in the original leukemia is low. Evidence of qualitative differences between the two conversion types can only be obtained by separate measurements of viral and virus-induced new cellular antigens. Hopefully, immunoelectronmicroscopic methods will help to solve this problem. As yet, however, there are more open questions in this field than ready answers.

5. Summary

Antigenic conversion by leukemia viruses is the acquisition of a new membrane-associated antigen by tumor or normal cells. It may happen spontaneously by natural infection as well as artificially under laboratory conditions. During the process the cells acquire antigens characteristic of the infecting agent. Experiments are described in which AKR Gross leukemias, methylnitrosourea(MNU)-induced leukemia of XVII mice, and the non-infectious Graffi leukemia SOV 16 were antigenically converted by infection with Graffi virus and immunologically analyzed for the presence of virus-induced antigens. To further understanding of the antigens involved, a summary of information is given on the present knowledge about viral and virus-induced antigens of murine leukemia. Finally, data on the immunological behaviour of

MNU-induced leukemias are presented. It was shown that these leukemias contain cross-reacting antigens of the Gross leukemia type although they show also individually distinct TSTA. The significance of the findings is discussed. Special attention is drawn to the finding that Graffi virus-converted cells may or may not acquire immunosensitivity *in vivo* and *in vitro* to the Graffi-specific immune response. To distinguish between the two phenomena we have introduced the terms complete and incomplete antigenic conversion.

References

[1] B. Stück, L.J. Old and E.A. Boyse, Nature 202 (1964) 1016.

[2] H.O. Sjögren, J. Natl. Cancer Inst. 32 (1964) 361.

[3] G.J. Svet-Moldavsky and V.P. Hamburg, Nature 202 (1964) 303.

[4] V.P. Hamburg and G.J. Svet-Moldavsky, Nature 203 (1964) 772.

[5] L.J. Old, E.A. Boyse and E. Stockert, Cancer Res. 25 (1965) 813.

[6] G. Pasternak and L. Pasternak, J. Natl. Cancer Inst. 38 (1967) 157.

[7] E.J. Breyere and L.B. Williams, Science 146 (1964) 1055.

[8] G. Pasternak, Adv. Cancer Res. 12 (1969) 1.

[9] G. Geering, W.D. Hardy, jr., L.J. Old, E. de Harven and R.S. Brodey, Virology 36 (1968) 678.

[10] W.D. Hardy, jr., G. Geering, L.J. Old, E. de Harven and S. McDonough, Science 166 (1969) 1019.

[11] G. Geering, T. Aoki and L.J. Old, Nature 226 (1970) 265.

[12] L.R. Sibal, M.A. Fink, E.J. Plata, B.E. Kohler, F. Noronha and K.M. Lee, J. Natl. Cancer Inst. 45 (1970) 607.

[13] G. Klein and E. Klein, Science 145 (1964) 1316.

[14] G. Pasternak, Nature 214 (1967) 1364.

[15] R.A. Steeves, Cancer Res. 28 (1968) 338.

[16] S. Oboshi, K. Itakura and K. Maruyama, Gann 58 (1967) 367.

[17] L.W. Law and R.C. Ting, J. Natl. Cancer Inst. 44 (1970) 615.

[18] T. Aoki, E.A. Boyse, L.J. Old, E. de Harven, U. Hämmerling and H.A. Wood, Proc. Natl. Acad. Sci. U.S. 65 (1970) 569.

[19] B. Stück, L.J. Old and E.A. Boyse, Proc. Natl. Acad. Sci. U.S. 52 (1964) 950.

[20] G. Pasternak, L. Pasternak and B. Micheel, *In:* L. Severi, Immunity and tolerance in oncogenesis, Proceedings of the Fourth Quadrennial Conference on Cancer, University of Perugia, 1969 (The Division of Cancer Research, Perugia, 1970).

[21] G. Pasternak and L. Pasternak, Folia Biol. 14 (1968) 43.

[22] B. Micheel and G. Pasternak, Intern J. Cancer 3 (1968) 603.

[23] R.J. Huebner and G.J. Todaro, Proc. Natl. Acad. Sci. U.S. 64 (1969) 1087.

[24] G. Gryschek and G. Pasternak, Acta Biol. Med. Ger. 27 (1971) 195.

[25] J. Vaage, Nature 218 (1968) 101.

[26] J. Vaage, T. Kalinovsky and R. Olson, Cancer Res., 29 (1969) 1452.

[27] E.A. Carswell, H.J. Wanebo, L.J. Old and E.A. Boyse, J. Natl. Cancer Inst. 44 (1970) 1281.

[28] G. Lespinats, J. Natl. Cancer Inst. 45 (1970) 845.

THE RELATION OF LINKAGE GROUP IX TO
LEUKEMOGENESIS IN THE MOUSE[1]

Edward A. BOYSE, Lloyd J. OLD and Elisabeth STOCKERT[2]
Division of Immunology,
Sloan-Kettering Institute for Cancer Research,
New York, N.Y. 10021, U.S.A.

Three loci in linkage group IX of the mouse, − H-2 (histocompatibility-2, [1]), Tla (thymus leukemia antigen, [2,3]) and G_{IX} (Gross IX, [4]), − are defined by serological test that identify antigens on the cell-surface (fig. 1).

The genes of the H-2 locus are expressed in most if not all mouse cells. Tla genes, on the other hand, are expressed (in normal mice) only in thymocytes, and G_{IX} genes only in thymocytes and other lymphoid cells; serological demonstration of the TL and G_{IX} antigens identified at the cell surface is the only criterion by which these two loci and their products can be recognized at the present time.

All three loci have some connection with leukemogenesis in the mouse. H-2 can be dealt with very briefly. The other two loci require more detailed consideration.

1. H-2 and leukemogenesis

The connection between H-2 and leukemia is that alleles at or near the K pole of this compound locus influence susceptibility to the induction of leukemia by inoculated Passage A Gross virus [5,6]. There is also an influence of these alleles on the spontaneous occurrence of leukemia in mice that are natural overt carriers of murine leukemia virus (MuLV) (Gross). As fig. 2 shows, the onset of leukemia is considerably delayed in a congenic strain of AKR mice into which the allele $H\text{-}2^b$, derived from C57BL/6 (B6) (which is highly resistant to

[1] This work was supported in part by NCI grant CA 08748 and a grant from the John A. Hartford Foundation, Inc.
[2] The authors are indebted to Gloria Alexander and Chika Iritani for expert participation in some of these experiments.

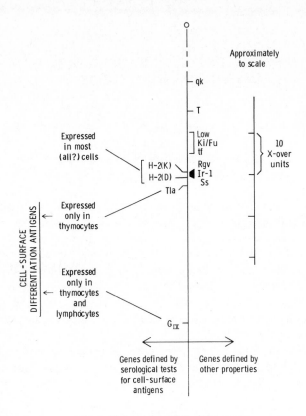

Fig. 1. Linkage group IX of the mouse.

MuLV), has been introduced by serial backcrossing, replacing the native AKR allele H-2^k. It is not certain whether the alleles responsible are actually genes of the H-2 locus itself, defined as the set of genes which specify the H-2 antigens of the cell-surface [6], nor whether the property of resistance *versus* sensitivity to MuLV (Gross) is in fact mediated via components of the cell surface [6].

2. Tla and leukemogenesis

Table 1 gives the essentials of the Tla locus and the TL antigens which it specifies. This unique genetic system has been thoroughly reviewed elsewhere [2,3] and the following brief account is intended only to provide a background

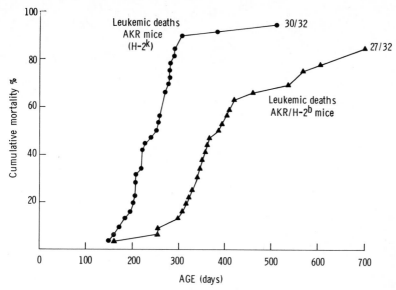

Fig. 2. Influence of H-2 on the incidence of spontaneous leukemia in AKR mice. Mortality from spontaneous leukemia among a group of 32 AKR mice (H-2^k) and 32 AKR/H-2^b congenic mice (females only).

for comparison with the newly recognized locus G$_{IX}$ which shares with Tla a feature unknown so far in any other system of cell-surface antigens. This special feature is that certain strains of mice carry genes at these loci that they normally do not express, but which frequently are expressed in leukemia cells of these strains.

The Tla locus specifies four antigens, TL.1, 2, 3 and 4, and these occur only on thymocytes and leukemia cells.

2.1. TL antigens of normal mice (table 1; columns 1-3)

Antigens 1, 2 and 3 occur on the thymocytes of normal mice. Some strains of mice express all three of them, others only antigen 2, and some none at all (column 3). This defines 3 categories of normal mice: TL$^-$, TL.2, and TL.1, 2, 3 (column 2). Mice can form TL antibody to any TL antigen that they do not express on their thymocytes, and this is how the various TL antisera are prepared. Segregation data from crosses between TL$^+$ and TL$^-$ mice place the alleles responsible for these thymocyte phenotypes in group IX at about 2 units from the D end of H-2 (fig. 1). Crossing-over has not been observed within Tla.

The position of the TL-bearing elements of the thymocyte surface has been

Table 1
The three TL phenotypes of mice.

1	2	3				4				5
Mouse strain	Phenotype	TL antigens								Inferred Tla genotype of strain
		1	2	3	4	1	2	3	4	
		on thymocytes				on leukemic cells				
AKR, B6, A/TL⁻	TL⁻	−	−	−	−	+	+	−	+	Structural genes for TL. 1, 2 and 4 plus respective expression-negative alleles
BALB/c, DBA/2	TL. 2	−	+	−	−	+ or +	+ +	− −	−* +	As above, with substitution of an expression-positive allele for TL. 2
A, B6/TL⁺, AKR. K, C58, SJL, PL	TL. 1, 2, 3	+	+	+	−	+	+	+	−	Structural genes for TL. 1, 2 and 3, plus respective expression-positive alleles

+ = antigen present.
− = antigen absent.

*It has recently been observed that TL.4 is not invariably expressed on leukemia cells carrying other TL components. This complicates the assignment of genotypes in some instances; e.g. in A.BY (TL⁻) mice we have observed three leukemias of phenotype TL.1⁺2⁺4⁻, but this is too few to be *sure* that the A.BY strain lacks the structural gene for TL.4 and so has a distinctive (fourth) genotype.

Note: Mice can make antibodies to those TL antigens that they do not express on their thymocytes; this includes antibodies to TL antigens expressed on their own leukemia cells.

established in relation to other thymocyte surface antigens. They lie adjacent to the H-2(D)-bearing elements [7]. This reflects the genetic linkage of Tla and H-2(D) and provides a so-far-unique example of an association between genetic linkage and proximity of the gene-products on the cell surface. It seems that this spatial orientation should be viewed on a supramolecular scale, for chromatography of soluble membrane products separates H-2 and TL antigens into different fractions of around 50,000 molecular weight [8].

Not only are the TL and H-2(D) antigens situated close to one another on the cell-surface, but they have a reciprocal quantitative relationship to one another. Thus the thymocytes of TL$^-$ mice express more H-2(D) antigens than the thymocytes of TL$^+$ mice [9]. This influence of TL on the representation of H-2(D) is seen in both *cis* and *trans* positions [9] and therefore appears to depend not on coordinate gene activity on a chromosomal scale but on later events in the fabrication of the cell surface.

2.2. TL antigens on leukemia cells (table 1; column 4)

Some leukemias of every mouse strain are TL$^+$, regardless of whether the affected mouse comes from a TL$^+$ or TL$^-$ strain. Antigens 1 and 2 are invariably expressed on all TL$^+$ leukemias. Antigen 3 occurs only on leukemia cells of TL.1, 2, 3 mice. Antigen 4 is found on leukemia cells only, never on thymocytes. Antigens 3 and 4 have so far appeared to be mutually exclusive, so they may be specified by alleles.

2.3. Genetics of TL antigen expression

To simplify discussion, the term "structural gene" (str) will be used to refer to a gene that specifies an antigen directly, if the antigen is a protein and therefore a direct gene product, or indirectly if the antigen is not protein, (the latter being exemplified by the AB blood group genes of man, which code for transferases that specify the AB antigens by attaching the pertinent sugars to an antecedent molecule [10]). Additional (or epistatic) genes, involved in regulating the presence *versus* absence of antigen, will be called "expression genes" (exp), but this is not intended to convey any implication as to what mechanism of control is involved.

The phenotypes of leukemia cells (column 4) reveal that str genes for antigens 1 and 2 are present in all mice, including TL$^-$ which are capable of forming the respective antibodies and so provide the antiserum with which the system is analyzed. Therefore the alleles at the Tla locus in group IX which govern the presence of TL antigen on thymocytes in segregating crosses are not str genes but exp genes.

Thus the segregation data do not reveal where the str TL genes are. There is however some indirect evidence [11] that the str and exp genes for TL are linked and therefore are both at the Tla locus in group IX. The arguments are complicated and here it must suffice simply to indicate that they depend on: a) the half-expression of TL in (TL$^-$ x TL$^+$) heterozygotes, and (b) the finding that TL.3 and 4, which unlike TL.1 and TL.2 do not appear to have *str* genes that are common throughout the species, invariably follow linkage group IX in a variety of genetic tests, including the use of leukemia-cell variants in which part or all of linkage group IX has been selectively deleted. This evidence makes it probable the str and exp genes for TL antigens are all at the Tla locus.

In normal cells, three conditions must be fulfilled before a TL antigen is expressed: (a) the relevant str gene must be present, (b) the relevant exp allele must be present at the Tla locus, and (c) the cell, which originates from bone marrow, must be undergoing differentiation to a thymocyte, under the influence of the thymus. This differentiation process in the thymus activates not only Tla genes but also a cluster of other loci for thymocyte-surface differentiation antigens: θ, Ly-A, Ly-B.C, G_{IX} and others [3,4]. Tla and G_{IX} are the only two of these loci that exhibit aberrant expression in leukemia cells.

The thymocyte is destined to mature to a lymphocyte and will in the process undergo major rearrangements of its coat of antigens, including the complete loss of TL. The TL^+ leukemia cell evidently is arrested at a phase of differentiation preceding this metamorphosis and so is continuing to make its surface under the dictation of the pattern of gene action which was in effect at that time.

2.4. Are the Tla genes viral or cellular?

The suggestion that Tla may be a viral genome has been raised more than once [3,12], mainly on the somewhat flimsy grounds that aberrant expression of TL antigens was seen to be a common feature of leukemogenesis in the mouse, and that since no such phenomenon was known to occur with any other systems of antigen, this might imply an exceptional origin for the Tla genes. Again, a high proportion of mouse leukemias that show no evidence of induction by MuLV are TL^+ [2], so Tla might possibly be viewed as a second leukemogenic viral genome.

But these were only tenuous suggestions, and there the matter rested for lack of evidence connecting the TL antigens with any virion that could be retrieved and studied. The points of resemblance now established between the Tla and G_{IX} loci add some credibility to the hypothesis that Tla is a viral genome.

3. G_{IX} and leukemogenesis

This system [4] is defined by the standard MuLV (Gross) antiserum prepared in rats (fig. 3) [13]. W/Fu inbred rats are extremely susceptible to leukemogenesis by wild-type Gross virus; when approximately 5×10^7 thymocytes from AKR

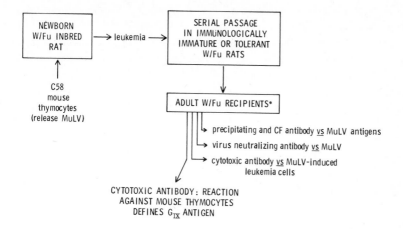

or C58 mice are inoculated at birth, the released MuLV induces leukemia in virtually all recipients. The leukemias can be transplanted into adult W/Fu recipients only with difficulty, because they are highly antigenic. For maintenance in serial passage, immunologically immature or tolerant hosts are used. Transplantation into adult W/Fu rats yields potent antiserum against MuLV-associated antigens. These antibodies neutralize MuLV, react in various serological tests with MuLV antigens, and are cytotoxic for leukemia cells. Because the immunizing leukemia and the immunized rats are syngeneic, all antibodies formed must be directed to MuLV-associated antigens. This antiserum is cytotoxic not only for rat and mouse leukemia cells induced by MuLV, which is not unexpected, but also for the thymocytes of non-leukemic mice of some but not all strains of mice. This antigen recognized on mouse thymocytes by the cytotoxicity test is called G_{IX}.

The G_{IX} system has been serologically analyzed by the same methods that have been applied to the TL system, with the following results [4]:

3.1. G_{IX} antigen of normal mice
Typing of thymocytes by the cytotoxicity test with this standard W/Fu

antiserum categorizes mouse strains as $G_{IX}{}^+$ or $G_{IX}{}^-$. Thymocytes of $G_{IX}{}^-$ mice have no G_{IX} antigen.

Absorption analysis shows that G_{IX} antigen is expressed only on thymocytes and lymphocytes, indicating that the determinant gene or genes are geared to the program of gene action, mentioned in connection with TL, according to which a cluster of genes, including Tla, specifies a unique spectrum of surface components for thymocytes. In other words, the TL and G_{IX} antigens of normal mice belong to the category of "thymocyte surface differentiation antigens".

To study the genetics of G_{IX} expression in normal mice we selected strain 129 as the prototype $G_{IX}{}^+$ strain and B6 as the prototype $G_{IX}{}^-$ strain. Segregation ratios were determined for a variety of crosses involving these two strains. The data, outlined in fig. 4, reveal that two unlinked genes are required

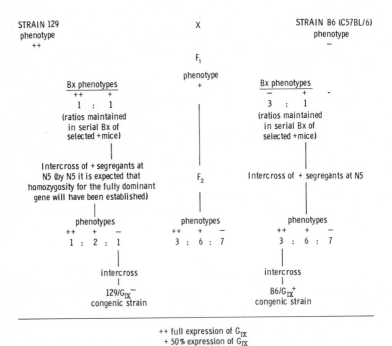

Fig. 4. Segregation ratios expected for an antigen whose expression depends on one fully dominant and one semi-dominant gene. The phenotypes and ratios observed for G_{IX} antigen [data in ref. 4] conform to this scheme for all the populations shown.

for expression of G_{IX} on normal thymocytes. One of them is fully dominant, there being only 2 classes of segregants, in the ratio 1:1, in the positive backcross. The second gene is semi-dominant, which is revealed by the hemi-expression of G_{IX} in heterozygotes.

The linkage group of the semi-dominant gene is IX, at some 35 map units from Tla (fig. 1).

3.2. G_{IX} antigen on leukemia cells

Leukemia cells, like thymocytes, can be typed G_{IX}^+ or G_{IX}^-. The results reveal that G_{IX}^+ leukemias occur not only in G_{IX}^+ mouse strains but also in G_{IX}^- strains. This parallels the occurrence of TL^+ leukemias in both TL^+ and TL^- mice, and is the most striking point of resemblance between the two systems.

3.3. Relation of G_{IX} antigen to MuLV

Within a few days after inoculation of MuLV-carrying C58 or AKR thymocytes, or of Gross Passage A virus, the thymocytes and other lymphoid cells of newborn W/Fu rats become G_{IX}^+. Thus MuLV induces in rat lymphoid cells a surface antigen that in normal mice shows Mendelian inheritance, as described above. Only cells exhibiting productive MuLV infection induce G_{IX} antigen in rats; cells that are G_{IX}^+ but are not producing MuLV do not do so.

It is unlikely that G_{IX} is a structural component of the virion, because the thymocytes of some strains of mice (*e.g.* strain 129, see above) are G_{IX}^+ but contain no other MuLV antigens or demonstrable virions, and on the other hand some mouse leukemias and other tumors produce MuLV and all other MuLV antigens, but not G_{IX} (see below). Furthermore, a series of monospecific antisera prepared against purified structural proteins of MuLV (Gross) did not react with strain 129 thymocytes (Nowinski, personal communication). This evidence is not entirely conclusive and it is desirable that the location of G_{IX} antigen should be established by immuno-electronmicroscopy on cells that are producing MuLV.

Assuming then, as seems likely on the evidence available, that G_{IX} is a non-virion cell-surface antigen, the question arises, "Is it coded by MuLV or by a cellular gene activated by MuLV?" The latter would require that the rat genome must carry the same str gene for G_{IX} antigen that is present in the mouse genome, but there is no compelling reason to rule this out, particularly as there are G_{IX}^- strains of mice that carry the str gene but do not normally express it, as would have to be postulated for the rat. In short, we cannot be sure that MuLV itself codes for G_{IX} antigen, which would constitute the best evidence that MuLV genes are integrated in the genome of the mouse strains in which G_{IX} antigen exhibits Mendelian inheritance.

E.A. Boyse

In the rat, G_{IX} and MuLV are invariably associated with one another. In the mouse, where G_{IX} is inherited by normal mice as an allo-antigen, the situation is more complex, and the association of G_{IX} with MuLV is not invariable. To test for concordance between G_{IX} and MuLV on a large enough scale requires a simple way of testing cells for productive infection with MuLV. This is provided by the standard method of typing cells for GCSA (Gross cell-surface antigen) (fig. 5) [14].

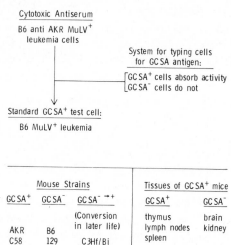

Fig. 5. Standard method of typing cells for presence or absence of GCSA (Gross cell surface antigen); the GCSA$^+$ phenotype signifies productive infection with MuLV. (We have not found any anti-G_{IX} activity in mouse antisera.)

GCSA, which mouse antiserum recognizes, is also a non-virion cell-surface antigen [15], and its presence or absence on cells is determined by the presence or absence of MuLV (Gross). The lymphoid cells of mouse strains that are life-long overt carriers of MuLV, like AKR and C58, are GCSA$^+$, whereas other mouse strains are GCSA$^-$ (table 2) [14]. C3Hf/Bi mice do not belong to either category but may be called a "conversion strain", for in this strain overt MuLV infection appears spontaneously late in life and when this happens their lymphoid cells are converted from GCSA$^-$ to GCSA$^+$ [16, and see 17]. In all mouse strains the expression of GCSA entails the expression of G_{IX} (table 2) [4] and reflects productive infection with MuLV (Gross). The association is especially obvious in C3Hf/Bi mice, whose lymphoid cells undergo spontaneous conversion from MuLV$^-$GCSA$^-$G_{IX}$^-$ to MuLV$^+$GCSA$^+$G_{IX}$^+$ in later life. Thus in normal mice G_{IX} is always expressed if MuLV and GCSA are expressed.

Table 2
G_{IX} and GCSA phenotypes of normal cells.

Strain	Lymphoid cell phenotypes	
	G_{IX}	GCSA
AKR, C58	+	+
B6	−	−
129	+	−
C3Hf/Bi (young)	−	−
C3Hf/Bi (old)	+	+

But the reverse is not true, for G_{IX} expression is dissociated from MuLV and GCSA in the thymocytes of 129 mice and of several other mouse strains whose normal phenotype is MuLV$^-$GCSA$^-$G$_{IX}^+$. Thus with regard to the antigens GCSA and G_{IX} there are three phenotypes of normal mice, GCSA$^+$G$_{IX}^+$, GCSA$^-$G$_{IX}^+$, and GCSA$^-$G$_{IX}^-$. The fourth possible phenotype GCSA$^+$G$_{IX}^-$ has not been observed in normal mice, but it does occur in malignant cells. In fact all four phenotypes have been found in malignant cells of both G_{IX}^+ and G_{IX}^- strains (table 3).

Table 3
G_{IX} and GCSA phenotypes of malignant cells.

A. in GCSA$^-$G$_{IX}^+$ mouse strains

GCSA	G_{IX}	
+	+	6 leukemias
+	−	2 leukemias, 1 sarcoma
−	+	7 leukemias
−	−	2 leukemias

B. in GCSA$^-$G$_{IX}^-$ mouse strains

GCSA	G_{IX}	
+	+	5 leukemias, 1 myeloma
+	−	8 Moloney and 2 Friend leukemias, 1 myeloma, 2 sarcomas, 1 melanoma
−	+	3 myelomas
−	−	8 leukemias, 1 myeloma, 1 sarcoma

C. in GCSA$^+$G$_{IX}^+$ mouse strains (AKR and C58)

All spontaneous leukemias examined were GCSA$^+$G$_{IX}^+$

3.4. Genetics of G_{IX} expression; comparison with TL

The provocative similarity between the two systems, one that is shared by no other known system of cell-surface antigens specified by Mendelian genes, that in both cases there are strains of mice that show no evidence of carrying the relevant str gene unless malignant transformation, (in the case of TL) or productive infection with MuLV (in the case of G_{IX}), takes place. The phenotype of the affected cell then changes from $-$ to $+$. The task of accounting for the Mendelian segregation data in normal mice is the same in both cases, except that the frequent involvement of MuLV in $G_{IX}^- \rightarrow G_{IX}^+$ conversion introduces some special considerations that apparently do not apply in the case of TL; these arise especially from the fact that we cannot be sure that G_{IX}, despite its induction in the rat by MuLV, is specified by the MuLV genome itself rather than by a cellular gene activated by MuLV. Therefore each of these alternatives must be considered separately:

(a) If G_{IX} is a cellular gene not belonging to the MuLV genome then neither of the two chromosomal genes identified can be the str gene for G_{IX}, they must both be exp genes. The argument is the same as that applied to the TL system, namely that since every mouse has the ability to express G_{IX} in malignant lymphoid cells, the presence or absence of the antigen in normal mice cannot be ascribed to presence or absence of the str gene, but must be due to another gene which has alleles for expression *versus* non-expression. In the TL system the segregation data requires one such exp locus (accommodating more than one exp gene), and in the G_{IX} system two are required. In the case of TL there is evidence that the str and exp genes are linked, but no such evidence yet exists in the case of G_{IX}.

(b) Alternatively, if the str gene for G_{IX} belongs to MuLV, then it might itself be one of the two chromosomal genes identified. For in this case the expression *versus* non-expression of G_{IX} might depend upon alternative states or locations of the MuLV genome in G_{IX}^+ or G_{IX}^- mice. Clearly if the str gene for G_{IX} antigen belongs to the MuLV genome it need not be integrated in all strains as it is in the 129 strain which provided the segregation data; it might have a different chromosomal site or a non-chromosomal site in other strains, and this might be the circumstance which determines non-expression.

In short, the uncertainty as to whether the str gene for G_{IX} is cellular or viral necessarily entails uncertainty as to whether either of the chromosomal genes identified in segregation tests is the str gene coding for G_{IX}. This problem does not arise in the case of Tla because the aberrant expression of TL antigen on leukemia cells is *not* accompanied by synthesis of virions.

The conversion $TL^- \rightarrow TL^+$ is an absolute criterion of oncogenic transformation in TL^- strains of mice. The conversion $G_{IX}^- \rightarrow G_{IX}^+$ in G_{IX}^- strains of mice however is not an absolute indicator of oncogenic transformation but more generally signifies productive infection with MuLV. This difference may perhaps be considered in terms of lysogeny: Thus the switch from MuLV⁻ to MuLV⁺, and the occurrence of oncogenic transformation, can be viewed as independent manifestations of the same integrated viral genome, both of them associated with $G_{IX}^- \to G_{IX}^+$ conversion; the Tla genome would accordingly correspond with defective lysogeny, so that only the former manifestation is not possible, — hence the lack of virions and the exclusive association of $TL^- \to TL^+$ conversion with oncogenic transformation.

Table 4

	circumstances associated with $\to +$ conversion of pheno-type
Lysogeny : G_{IX} system	$\left\{\begin{array}{l}\text{production of virions} \\ \text{oncogenic transformation}\end{array}\right.$
Defective lysogeny : TL system	oncogenic transformation

4. Comment

A definitive answer to the question whether either of the chromosomal loci regulating the expression of G_{IX} antigen is the site of MuLV integration must ultimately require a more direct approach, such as a demonstration that RNA in the MuLV genome can hybridize specifically with a defined region of the mouse genome, *e.g.* linkage group IX, or that it can direct the synthesis of G_{IX} antigen *in vitro*. In the meantime there are further points that can be established by existing immunogenetic methods in relation to the question whether G_{IX} is specified by an integrated MuLV gene. Thus, there are other MuLV-associated antigens whose inheritance and genetic linkage have not yet been adequately established. We have evidence that GCSA and G_{IX} are closely associated in segregation tests. Probably both of these however are non-virion components, so it will be of greater importance to the question of viral integration to find out whether the gene coding for gs antigen, which *is* a structural component of the virion, will show Mendelian segregation (as in the chicken [18]) and if so, whether gs antigen will segregate in company with G_{IX} and GCSA antigens. When we know more definitely what the segregation patterns of these antigens are we may be in a position to make stronger inferences about possible integration sites of MuLV genes.

E.A. Boyse

This will doubtless elucidate the inheritance of MuLV but there is no reason to think that it will help towards an understanding of how oncogenic transformation is mediated. It is remarkable that the two loci Tla and G_{IX} which have the exceptional relation to leukemogenesis that we have described should both be located in linkage group IX. As this may have more significance than fortuitous linkage, we have been especially interested in what the relation of G_{IX} to oncogenesis may be. It is certainly difficult to formulate worthwhile questions that are both relevant to this more general problem and can be tested experimentally. One which offers some prospect of solution is the question whether the maintenance of the oncogenic phenotype, in cells in which $TL^- \rightarrow TL^+$ or $G_{IX}^- \rightarrow G_{IX}^+$ conversion has taken place, is dependent on the function of the locus concerned in the aberrant expression of the respective antigens. It is possible to test this in the case of TL by using leukemias induced in the progeny of crosses which differ at the H-2 and Tla loci. Passage of such leukemias in either parental mouse strains selects out deletion variants which have lost one H-2 haplotype and so can escape the homograft reaction [review 19]. We have established that this may be accompanied by concomitant deletion of the Tla locus [20], and have already analyzed two reciprocal variants from one heterozygous TL^+ leukemia [20,21]. Thus the use of deletion variants is a feasible approach to establishing whether there is an essential connection between either or both Tla loci in the malignant lymphocyte and the maintenance of the oncogenic phenotype. The same approach should be valid for the G_{IX} locus since this also is linked with H-2, although it has yet to be established whether the deletion extends so far from H-2. If it does, it will be possible to select for variants in which one or the other G_{IX} locus has been excised, and so perhaps arrive at some firm statements about the relation of the G_{IX} locus to malignancy.

References

[1] G.D. Snell and J.H. Stimpfling, *In:* E.L. Green, The Jackson Laboratory, Biology of the Laboratory Mouse (McGraw Hill, Inc., 1966) p. 457.
[2] E.A. Boyse, L.J. Old and E. Stockert, *In:* P. Grabar and P. Miescher, Immunopathology, IVth Int. Symposium (Schwabe & Co., Basel, 1965) p. 23.
[3] E.A. Boyse and L.J. Old, Ann. Rev. Genetics 3 (1969) 269.
[4] E. Stockert, L.J. Old and E.A. Boyse, J. Exptl. Med. 133 (1971) 1334.
[5] F. Lilly, E.A. Boyse and L.J. Old, The Lancet 2 (1964) 1207.
[6] F. Lilly, *In:* R.M. Dutcher, Comparative leukemia research 1969 (S. Karger, New York, 1969) p. 213.
[7] E.A. Boyse, L.J. Old and E. Stockert, Proc. Natl. Acad. Sci. U.S. 60 (1968) 886.
[8] D.A.L. Davies, B.J. Alkins, E.A. Boyse, L.J. Old and E. Stockert, Immunology 16 (1969) 669.

[9] E.A. Boyse, E. Stockert and L.J. Old, J. Exptl. Med. 128 (1968) 85.
[10] W.M. Watkins, Science 152 (1966) 172.
[11] E.A. Boyse and L.J. Old, Transplantation 11 (1971) 561.
[12] D.W. Bailey, Transplantation 4 (1966) 482.
[13] G. Geering, L.J. Old and E.A. Boyse, J. Exptl. Med. 124 (1966) 753.
[14] L.J. Old, E.A. Boyse and E. Stockert, Cancer Res. 25 (1965) 813.
[15] T. Aoki, E.A. Boyse, L.J. Old, E. de Harven, U. Hämmerling and H.A. Wood, Proc. Natl. Acad. Sci. U.S. 65 (1970) 569.
[16] R.C. Nowinski, L.J. Old, E.A. Boyse, E. de Harven and G. Geering, Virology 34 (1968) 617.
[17] R.J. Huebner and G.J. Todaro, Proc. Natl. Acad. Sci. U.S. 64 (1969) 1087.
[18] L.N. Payne and R.C. Chubb, J. Gen. Virol. 3 (1968) 379.
[19] B. Bjaring and G. Klein, J. Natl. Cancer Inst. 41 (1968) 1411.
[20] E.A. Boyse, E. Stockert, C.A. Iritani and L.J. Old, Proc. Natl. Acad. Sci. U.S. 65 (1970) 933.
[21] E.A. Boyse, L.J. Old and E. Stockert, *In:* E. Mihich, Regulation of cell metabolism: organizational and pharmacological aspects on the molecular level (Academic Press, New York 1971) p. 145.

EXPRESSION OF MuLV-gs ANTIGEN IN MICE OF SEGREGATING POPULATIONS; EVIDENCE FOR MENDELIAN INHERITANCE[1]

Jo HILGERS,[2] Marina BEYA, Gayla GEERING, Edward A. BOYSE
and Lloyd J. OLD
Division of Immunology,
Sloan-Kettering Institute for Cancer Research, New York, N.Y. 10021, U.S.A.

1. Introduction

Payne and Chubb [1] found that a single dominant host gene is responsible for the presence of the group-specific (gs) antigen of the avian leukosis virus (AvLV) in normal chicken embryo cells. Bentvelzen [2] reported that a single gene controls the gamete-born transmission of a mammary tumor virus (MTV) in GR mice; his data indicate that a single cellular genetic locus governs the production of complete MTV.

Gamete-born transmission, as now seemingly demonstrated for MTV in GR mice, was first suggested for murine leukemia virus (MuLV) in AKR mice by Gross [3] [see also Law, ref. 4]. We have looked for evidence that the expression of gs antigen of MuLV may be under control by cellular genes.

2. Materials and methods

2.1. Animals and test cells

The mouse strains used are maintained at the Sloan-Kettering Institute. AKR and C58 have a high incidence of leukemia; all other strains used have a relatively low incidence.

The standard $MuLV^+$ (E♂G2) and $MuLV^-$ (EL4) mouse leukemias are transplanted in C57BL/6 mice. E♂G2 was induced in a C57BL/6 mouse by passage A Gross virus and is our G^+ reference cell (G = Gross cell surface

[1] This work was supported in part by NCI grant CA 08748 and a grant from the John A. Hartford Foundation, Inc.
[2] Present address: Department of Biology, The Netherlands Cancer Institute, Sarphatistraat 108, Amsterdam, The Netherlands.

antigen). EL4 is an ascites leukemia originally induced in a C57BL mouse by DMBA and is our standard G⁻ reference cell [5].

All mice were tested at ages from 2 to 8 months.

2.2. Rat anti MuLV serum

The antiserum was obtained from (W/Fu x BN)F$_1$ rats bearing a syngeneic leukemia W/FU(C58NT)D that was originally induced by murine Gross leukemia virus [6]. At a dilution of 1/16 or greater, this antiserum was found to be specific for MuLV-gs in the immunofluorescence test, and the fluorescence reaction could be blocked with a guinea pig anti-MuLV-gs serum (kindly provided by Dr. Gilden, NIH, Bethesda).

2.3. Indirect immunofluorescence (IF) and immunofluorescence absorption (IFA) tests

The IF test on fixed cells (10 minutes in acetone at room temperature) with the use of a counterstain (Evan's blue dye, 0.06% in distilled water) is described elsewhere [7].

For IFA tests antiserum was diluted two double dilutions below the endpoint of fluorescence (endpoint very distinct because of the applied counterstain) and incubated overnight at 4°C with an equal volume of serially diluted sonicated (6-10 seconds) spleen homogenate (17% weight extract in saline).

3. Results

Table 1 shows the distribution of MuLV-gs in several inbred mouse strains. Three categories of mouse strains can be identified on the basis of MuLV-gs expression in spleens:

(1) Mice with high levels of MuLV-gs. This corresponds with the overt production of MuLV in these mice. Examples are the high-leukemia-incidence strains AKR and C58. The usual titer of MuLV-gs antigen in IFA tests ranges from 1/4 to 1/8.

(2) Mice with intermediate levels of MuLV-gs. This is found in some low-leukemia-incidence strains (*e.g.* DBA/2 and C3H) that show viral activation with aging. The titer of MuLV-gs antigen ranges from 1/1 to 1/2 in positive mice.

(3) Mice with no MuLV-gs detectable by IFA in the spleens (*e.g.* C57BL, BALB/c, GR).

Table 2 shows tests of several hybrids between high-leukemia-incidence

Table 1

Quantitative IFA tests for MuLV-gs in extracts of spleens and leukemias from several inbred mouse strains.

Strain	Tissue used for absorption	Number pos./ number tested	Titer
C57BL/6	Leukemia (E♂G2)	1/1	1/32
C57BL/6	Leukemia (EL4)	0/1	
AKR	Spleen	22/22	1/4-1/16
AKR/H-2^b*	Spleen	5/5	1/4-1/8
C58	Spleen	14/14	1/2-1/8
NZB	Spleen	16/22	1/1-1/8
C57BL/6	Spleen	0/12	
C57BL/6/H-2^k*	Spleen	0/4	
BALB/c	Spleen	0/11	
GR	Spleen	0/7	
C3H/An	Spleen	1/5	1/1
DBA/2	Spleen	10/14	1/1-1/2
A	Spleen	0/6	
A/θ-AKR*	Spleen	0/5	

*Congenic strains.

Table 2

Quantitative IFA tests for MuLV-gs in spleen extracts from F_1 progeny of crosses between AKR or C58 (high leukemia incidence) and other mouse strains.

Hybrid ♀ × ♂	Tissue used for absorption	Number pos./ number tested	Titer
(C57BL/6 × AKR)F_1	Spleen	6/6	1/1-1/2
(BALB/c × AKR)F_1	Spleen	4/4	1/1-1/4
(T6 × AKR)F_1	Spleen	5/5	1/1-1/2
(C57BL/6 × C58)F_1	Spleen	11/14	1/1-1/2
(AKR × BALB/c)F_1	Spleen	3/6	1/1-1/4
(C58 × 129)F_1	Spleen	5/5	1/1-1/2
(C57BL/A × AKR)F_1	Spleen	2/8	1/1-1/2

strains (AKR, C58) and some low-incidence strains (C57BL, BALB/c, CBA/T6, 129). The titer of MuLV-gs ranges from 1/1 to 1/2 in positive mice; this is intermediate and comparable with the titers found in group 2 (above).

Fig. 1 shows the results of an experiment in which an AKR mouse, a C57BL mouse, and a (C57BL × AKR)F_1 mouse (of similar weight, and approximately 3 months of age) were injected intraperitioneally with equal volumes of the rat anti-MuLV serum. Each mouse was bled at intervals thereafter and the titer of anti-MuLV-gs measured by IF. Antibody disappeared rapidly in the AKR mouse, not as fast in the (C57BL × AKR)F_1 mouse, and very slowly in the C57BL mouse. This suggests that rat anti-MuLV-gs antibody may be absorbed *in vivo* by MuLV-gs antigen in the serum, and that the level of MuLV-gs in the serum of the F_1 hybrid is lower than in the AKR mouse. This would agree with the lesser amount of MuLV-gs in spleens of F_1 hybrids in comparison with AKR, as measured by IFA.

Table 3 shows the results of IFA tests in mice of 2 backcrosses and an F_2 generation derived from AKR or C58 (high leukemia incidence) and C57BL/6 (low leukemia incidence). Mice with titers of 1/4 or higher were scored as strong reactors, equivalent to AKR or C58. Mice with titers of 1/2 or lower were grouped together as weak-or-negative reactors. These data show a 1:1 ratio in the backcross and a 1:3 ratio in the F_2, suggesting that a single locus controls the expression of MuLV-gs.

There was a good correlation between IFA and CF (complement fixation) tests, which were carried out in parallel for almost all extracts. The same pool of antiserum was used in CF (after two preliminary absorptions of the undiluted serum with a homogenate of the MuLV$^-$ leukemia EL4). The IFA test was slightly more sensitive than the CF test.

4. Discussion

The segregation data in the crosses between leukemia-prone and leukemia-resistant mouse strains accord with the hypothesis that a single locus in the cellular genome controls expression of MuLV-gs (and presumably virus production). More extensive genetic studies are necessary to confirm this.

Since MuLV and MuLV-related antigens (including MuLV-gs) may appear spontaneously and can be induced in mice that normally do not express them [see 8,9] it seems that most if not all mice possess the MuLV genome. It follows that the locus identified as responsible for the invariable expression of MuLV-gs in AKR and C58 mice, and its non-expression in other mice, may have regulatory function and have alleles which govern expression *vs*. non-expression of the structural gs gene (which itself may be situated at the same locus or elsewhere).

The fact that expression of the group-specific antigen of AvLV can similarly

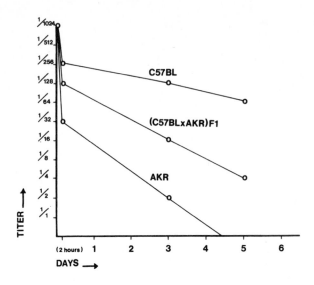

Fig. 1. The disappearance rate of rat anti-MuLV-gs in the serum of mice from a high and a low leukemia strain and their F_1 hybrid.

Table 3
Quantitative IFA tests for MuLV-gs in spleens of mice of segregating populations from crosses of AKR or C58 with C57BL/6.

Segregating populations ♀ × ♂	Total tested	Strong reactors*	Weak and negative reactors**	Significance in regard to 1:1 or 1:3 ratio
(C57BL/6 × AKR)F_1 × AKR	114	54 = 47%	60 = 53%	$p > 0.6$
(C57BL/6 × C58)F_1 × C58	37	17 = 46%	20 = 54%	$p > 0.6$
(C57BL/6 × C58)F_2	35	8 = 23%	27 = 77%	$p > 0.7$

*Titers from 1/4-1/16.
**Titers from negative to 1/1-1/2.

be induced in normal gs-negative chicken embryos [see Weiss, this volume] suggests that in case of the avian tumor viruses also the expression of gs antigen is governed by a regulatory locus distinct from the structural gs gene.

For arguments relating to the alternative possibility, *i.e.* that the segregating gene identified may itself be the gs structural gene, see ref. [10].

References

[1] L.N. Payne and R.C. Chubb, J. Gen. Virol. 3 (1968) 379.
[2] P. Bentvelzen, Genetical control of the vertical transmission of the Mühlbock mammary tumor virus in the GR mouse strain (Amsterdam, Hollandia, 1968).
[3] L. Gross, Oncogenic viruses (London, Pergamon Press, 1961).
[4] L.W. Law, Nat. Cancer Inst. Monograph 22 (1966) 267.
[5] L.J. Old, E.A. Boyse and E. Stockert, Cancer Res. 25 (1965) 813.
[6] G. Geering, L.J. Old and E.A. Boyse, J. Exptl. Med. 124 (1966) 753.
[7] J. Hilgers, W.C. Williams, B. Myers and L. Dmochowski, Virology 45 (1971) 470.
[8] L.J. Old, E.A. Boyse, G. Geering and H.F. Oettgen, Cancer Res. 28 (1968) 1288.
[9] R.J. Huebner and G.J. Todaro, Proc. Natl. Acad. Sci. U.S. 64 (1969) 1087.
[10] E. Stockert, L.J. Old and E.A. Boyse, J. Exptl. Med. 133 (1971) 1334.

IMMUNOCHEMICAL STUDIES OF THE MAJOR GROUP-SPECIFIC ANTIGEN OF MAMMALIAN C-TYPE VIRUSES

Raymond V. GILDEN
Flow Laboratories, Inc., Rockville, Md., U.S.A.

Studies of C-type viruses from four mammalian species have revealed striking similarities in virion polypeptide patterns obtained in alkaline SDS acrylamide gels [1, 2]. Generally three distinct low molecular weight zones which apparently consist only of protein and two higher molecular weight glyco-protein zones are obtained (fig. 1A). This pattern is very similar to that seen for avian viruses [3], although one additional low molecular weight polypeptide has been found [4, 5], and also the virus found in the VSW viper cell line [6].

Using the isoelectric focusing technique [7] with Tween-ether disrupted virus, we have isolated the major internal virion protein in high yield and in a highly purified state. A distinctive isoelelectric point was found for each species virus [1, 2, 6, 8] and on acrylamide gel electrophoresis, this protein corresponded to the third fastest migrating of the low molecular weight polypeptides [1, 2]; (fig. 1B).

Antiserum was prepared against the isoelectric focus (IEF) purified protein (generally in guinea pigs) for each species and the resulting sera were tested against various virus preparations including fractions from the isoelectric focusing separations and those eluted from the acrylamide gels. Also included in the various tests were sera from rats bearing, or immunized with, murine sarcoma virus induced tumors and dogs bearing feline sarcoma virus induced tumors [9]. The guinea pig antisera had the following general properties: (a) they were species specific and monospecific in gel diffusion (single line) and complement-fixation tests, although certain anti-mouse sera showed cross-reactions with concentrated cat virus; (b) they were group-specific in that whenever multiple isolates of a species were available for test they reacted equally with each isolate, and they could be used to titrate virus in CF induction tests (i.e., COMUL, COCAL, or COHAL) without necessitating absorption with normal cells; (c) whenever these sera reacted with cell lines in vitro, such cells always contained virus particles; (d) reactions with IEF or

193

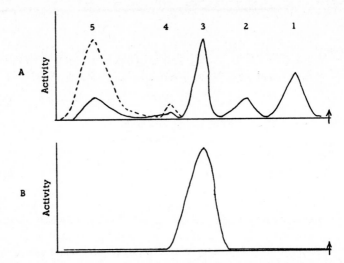

Fig. 1. Acrylamide gel electrophoresis of mammalian C-type viruses after disruption by SDS, urea and mercaptoethanol. 7.5% gels at pH 9.0. Arrow indicates marker dye front. (A) Total virion: Amino acid radioactivity (solid line); glucosamine activity (dotted line). Typical molecular weights of these components were (1) 13,000, (2) 18,000, (3) 30,000 (4) 40,000, and (5) 80,000. Slight differences in exact values were seen with each species virus. (B) Isoelectric focus purified antigen.

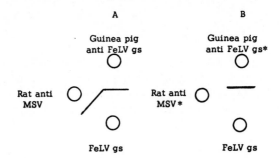

*Absorbed with MuLV gs

Fig. 2. Demonstration of species-specific and interspecific determinants on major polypeptide of feline leukemia virus. Drawn from actual figure [ref. 2]. This figure (A) shows that cross-reactive and species-specific antisera give a single line of identity with purified feline virus antigen. The two determinants are shown by the absorption of sera with MuLV-gs antigen. Here (B) the interspecies antibody is removed while the species-specific antibody is unaffected.

acrylamide gel fractions were superimposable with those of sera from tumored animals. On the basis of these features we could reasonably conclude that we had identified the major group-specific antigenic determinants, originally described as gs-1 [10] for the murine leukemia viruses.

Further studies using MSV rat sera which were cross-reactive with the several mammalian viruses [9] showed that the cross-reactive determinants, apparently identical to gs-3 [11, 12] and interspec [13] resided as well on the same polypeptide which carried the species specific determinant (fig. 2). Among the lines of evidence which support this view was the finding that complete precipitation of the feline virus antigen was possible with both specific anti-feline serum and cross-reactive MSV rat serum. As of this writing, the immunologic relationships between the other virion polypeptides and the major polypeptide, both on an intra- and inter-species basis remain to be studied in detail. Since the four low molecular weight polypeptides of the avian viruses are each antigenically distinct [14], it would seem reasonable to assume that more than one species specific and interspecific antigenic determinant will be clearly demonstrated for the mammalian viruses.

The major antigens of the viruses from three vertebrate classes show no inter-class cross-reactions [15, 16], thus, it seems clear that the mammalian viruses are more closely related to each other than to the non-mammalian viruses. This suggests that the C-type viruses have a long evolutionary history, and have not arisen from a single species in the recent past. We speculate [17, 18], based on the evidence from studies of the natural biology of C-type viruses [19], that a common ancestral virus for the present day viruses must have existed in the common ancestor of reptiles, birds and mammals. This may be a conservative estimate since the generality of cancer would predict the origin of an "oncogene" [20] early in the development of metazoans. The hypothesis of co-evolution of virus and host species appears testable by comparison of amino acid sequences of the major virion polypeptide of the various viruses. A phylogenetic tree based on such data should parallel the known tree derived from paleontological data.

References

[1] S. Oroszlan, C. Foreman, G. Kelloff and R.V. Gilden, Virology 43 (1971) 665.

[2] S. Oroszlan, R.J. Huebner and R.V. Gilden, Proc. Natl. Acad. Sci. U.S., in press.

[3] P.H. Duesberg, H.L. Robinson, W.S. Robinson, R.J. Huebner and H.C. Turner, Virology 36 (1968) 73.

[4] D.P. Bolognesi and H. Bauer, Virology 42 (1970) 1097.

[5] P.P. Hung, H.L. Robinson and W.S. Robinson, Virology 43 (1971) 251.

[6] S. Oroszlan and R.V. Gilden, unpublished results.

[7] O. Vesterberg and H. Swensson, Acta Chem. Scand. 20 (1966) 820.

[8] S. Oroszlan, C. Fisher, T.B. Stanley and R.V. Gilden, J. Gen. Virol. 8 (1970) 1.

[9] R.V. Gilden, S. Oroszlan and R.J. Huebner, Nature, in press.

[10] A. Gregoriades and L.J. Old, Virology 37 (1969) 189.

[11] G. Geering, W.D. Hardy, Jr., L.J. Old and E. DeHarven, Virology 36 (1968) 678.

[12] G. Geering, T. Aoki and L.J. Old, Nature 226 (1970) 265.

[13] W. Schafer, V. Lange, L. Pister, E. Seifert, F. De Noronha and F.W. Schmidt, Z. Naturforsch. 25 (1970) 1024.

[14] H. Bauer and D.P. Bolognesi, Virology 42 (1970) 1113.

[15] R.V. Gilden, Y.K. Lee, S. Oroszlan, J.L. Walker and R.J. Huebner, Virology 41 (1970) 187.

[16] R.V. Gilden and S. Oroszlan, unpublished results.

[17] R.J. Huebner and R.V. Gilden, this symposium.

[18] R.V. Gilden and R.J. Huebner, in preparation.

[19] R.J. Huebner, G. Kelloff, P.S. Sarma, W.T. Lane, H.C. Turner, R.V. Gilden, S. Oroszlan, H. Meier and D.D. Meyers, Proc. Natl. Acad. Sci. U.S. 67 (1970) 336.

[20] R.J. Huebner and G.J. Todaro, Proc. Natl. Acad. Sci. U.S. 64 (1969) 1087.

INHERITED RNA VIRAL GENOMES (VIROGENES AND ONCOGENES) IN THE ETIOLOGY OF CANCER

Robert J. HUEBNER and Raymond V. GILDEN
Viral Carcinogenesis Branch, National Cancer Institute, National Institutes of Health, Bethesda, Md., 20014, U.S.A.
Flow Laboratories, Inc., Rockville, Md., 20852, U.S.A.

Experts in differing cancer research disciplines have clearly delineated numerous different "causes" of cancer, as follows:

(1) Immunogeneticists have shown that identifiable host cell genes (both normal and mutational) are decisive determinants of spontaneous and induced cancers.

(2) Immunologists have determined that a variety of defective immunological mechanisms greatly influence the incidence of certain types of cancer.

(3) Carcinogenesis investigators have regularly induced many different cancers in experimental animals with numerous chemicals and various types of radiation; in addition many such carcinogens have been identified as causes of natural cancer in man.

(4) Endocrinologists have not only produced experimental cancers with hormones and identified hormones as determinants of certain natural cancers, but they have also utilized hormones for suppression of cancer.

(5) Epidemiologists and biostatisticians have shown most natural cancers in man and animals to be remarkably stochastic in occurrence; thus the proposition that infectious viruses or other infectious agents serve as significant factors in the generality of natural cancers has become to be regarded as less than credible.[1]

(6) Virologists, on the other hand, have not only produced cancer in many species of animals with tumor viruses, but have also delineated the C-type RNA tumor viruses as natural causes of leukemia and sarcoma in a number of species in 3 classes of vertebrates. B-type RNA viruses have been identified as causes of mammary tumor in mice and have been incriminated also in mammary tumors of rats and monkeys (table 1).

---

[1] Exceptions are lung cancers in smokers and certain lymphoproliferative "cancers" in which herpes type viruses have been incriminated.

R.J. Huebner and R.V. Gilden

Table 1
RNA tumor viruses.

C-type		
Chickens	Leukemia virus (ALV)	4 types, numerous strains
	Sarcoma virus (RSV)	4 types, 10 or more strains
	Endotheliosis and carcinoma viruses	
Mice	Leukemia virus (MuLV)	4 types, numerous strains
	Sarcoma virus (MSV)	3 types, numerous pseudotypes
Cats	Lymphoma virus (FeLV)	2-3 types, several strains
	Sarcoma virus (FSV)	1 type, several strains
Hamsters	Leukemia virus (HaLV)	1 type, several strains isolated from MSV(HaLV)
Rats	Leukemia virus (RaLV)	2 strains, 1 isolated from M-MSV(RaLV); another from cultures of rat thymus
Snakes	Russell's viper sarcoma virus; replicates in established tumor cell line	
Swine	Virus particles in pig kidney cultures	
Cattle	Virus particles isolated and grown in bovine tissue culture	
Primates	Several monkey and human tumor cell cultures reportedly replicate C-like particles	

B-type		
Mice	Mouse mammary tumor virus (MTV), Bittner milk agent, and nodule inducing virus	
Monkey	Rhesus mammary tumor cell culture replicating B-like particles	
Human	B-type particles observed in milk specimens from close relatives of mammary tumor patients	

Some cancer "authorities" interpret these differing but quite valid observations to mean that cancer represents many quite different diseases, caused by a bewilderingly large number of totally different etiological entities. Perhaps the most debilitating point of view was that echoed in a recent editorial in *Science* [1] in which it was emphatically stated that cancer represents 100 or more different diseases having equivalent numbers of different causes, and that any "all-out" attempt to conquer so many different diseases is almost by definition unlikely to succeed. We believe the facts do not justify such a pessimistic view. Recent exciting new discoveries have led to greater understanding of the fundamental molecular factors in cellular behavior and new concepts which view cancer as part of the natural evolutionary biology of vertebrates, and the cancer cell as the result of derepression or mutation of inherited genes (oncogenes) [2-4].

Recently we and our associates proposed the viral oncogene theory of cancer which we believe provides unifying explanations of the various seemingly paradoxical observations made by investigators working more or less exclusively in differing disciplines (*vide supra*). This theory is based on a central working hypothesis which postulates that most if not all cancers of vertebrates are specified by oncogenes of RNA tumor virus genomes which are inherited as part of the natural gene pools of vertebrates [2, 5-8]. In addition we view the genetic and morphological neoplastic changes which result in cancer as most likely the result of a breakdown in host gene regulation of the operator genes of the RNA tumor virus; a breakdown that could be induced by natural aging (senescence), by genetic defects, by endogenous hormonal and immunological aberrations, or by exogenous environmental carcinogens [2, 5].

Therefore, while we may agree that the many different factors implicated in the etiology of cancer are certainly valid, we believe that these differences are more apparent than real, and hope to show in this presentation that many differing etiological factors can be accommodated within the viral oncogene theory [2,5], a theory recently reinforced by the demonstrations of C-type group-specific (gs) antigens in embryonic tissues of two classes and four species of vertebrates as well as in their tumors. The more recent discovery in RNA tumor viruses by Temin and Mizutani [9] and Baltimore [10] of reverse transcriptases (RNA dependent polymerases) which specify complementary DNA provide useful mechanisms by which the RNA tumor virus information could be integrated into host DNA. We feel that the unitary oncogene theory provides a "fit" for much of the new as well as of old data. It seems to us that the available data require such a theory (or something like it) to explain the numerous different apparent causes of many differing types of cancer. Bentvelzen and associates [11,12] have proposed a very similar hypothesis for the mammary tumor viruses of mice. Temin [13], Spiegelman [14], Payne [15], Axelrad [16], Weiss [17], as well as others in this conference will also discuss the intimate interactions of RNA tumor viruses and host genes.

Since the premises of the RNA viral oncogene theory of cancer are (1) genetic inheritance of both structural and regulator genes which serve as determinants of cancer expressions, and (2) tumor inductions by derepression of the endogenous tumor-inducing RNA viral oncogenes by both endogenous and exogenous factors,[2] our first chore is to consider the contemporary evidence which we believe supports these central premises.

Evidence for vertical and genetic transmission of the RNA tumor virus genomes[3]

Studies of the natural histories of C-type RNA tumor virus genomes were greatly facilitated by discovery of group-specific (gs) and other virion and non-virion antigens of the RNA viruses of the chicken, mouse, rat, hamster and cat (see tables 1 and 2) [23-36]. Complement-fixation (CF), fluorescent antibody (FA) and gel diffusion studies demonstrated gs antigens in tumorous and normal tissues as well as infected tissues, thus providing directly detectable specific markers for expression of the RNA viral genome, markers which could be used to determine the natural prevalences of this genome despite the fact that fully infectious virus could rarely be demonstrated in many or most natural species [5,37-39].

Using these and other serological procedures (table 2), Old and Abelev and their associates [31,33,36,39], several of our associates and we [5,37] demonstrated widespread high prevalences of gs antigen in many tumorous and normal tissues of mice. More recently we demonstrated gs antigen in embryonic tissues of mice 10 to 18 days *in utero* [6,7,37,39], in hamsters at 10 to 11 days [7,34,40], in chickens 4 to 20 days *in ovo* [6,7,41] and in embryonic cats [7,38] (tables 3, 4 and 5). These interesting observations took on additional significance when we demonstrated immunological tolerance to gs antigens in all of these animals (table 6); thus mice, hamsters, cats and chickens were

---

[2] In the Jacob and Monod theory [18] these factors would liberate "operator" oncogenes from repressive control of normal "regulator" genes.

[3] It is necessary to distinguish between vertical transmission of infectious virus and genetic transmission of a DNA copy of the RNA viral genome. The first instance represents cytoplasmic "inheritance", the infectious agent being transmitted by an immunologically tolerant female who herself is the progeny of a tolerant infected female. Rubin, in an elegant study, described the stability of this pattern of vertical infection in 10% of the females in a large flock of chickens [19]. Gross [20] observed a similar female-determined vertical transmission pattern in AKR and C58 mice. In both mice and chickens the transmission of infectious virus is viewed as superinfection of cells carrying the normally inherited genome. Interestingly enough those chickens and mice shown to have universal infectious C-type RNA virus experience extremely high rates of leukemia early in life (see table 7). Similar vertical transmissions of conventional and non-oncogenic viruses such as LCM and cytomegaloviruses have also been established in mice; again, the infected female tolerant for the infectious virus is the determinant of vertical transmission [21,22].

Table 2
Antigen expressions in RNA tumor virus infected and transformed cells.

Virion expression

Envelope
Type-specific, susceptible to ether and chloroform
Detected by CF, FA and gel diffusion

Group-specific (gs)
Mammalian viruses
gs-1 — intraspecies specific; shared in common by all isolates within species

gs-3 — interspecies specific; shared by all known mammalian viruses

gs antigens are ether and alcohol stable, and small (30,000 mw). In mouse virus, both antigens on same molecule. Detected by CF, FA, gel diffusion, and autoradiographic tests

---

Non-virion expression

Cell associated antigens (GSA) (GSA of Aoki *et al.*) [35, 36]
Soluble antigens detected by cytotoxic tests on cell membranes and in plasma of virus infected mice. Specified by virus genome and may be similar to RNA virus-specified transplantation antigens. Not found on virus particle

H-2 histocompatibility antigens
Natural antigens located at different sites on infected cell membrane; not found on virus particle

Alloantigens and zenoantigens
Membrane isoantigens found attached to RNA virion particle surface [Aoki, unpublished data]

---

unable to respond with antibodies to their homotypic species-specific gs antigens, although they regularly developed antibodies to viral envelope and other cell surface antigens [6,7]. In addition, two of our associates, Drs. M.L. Vernon and M. Gardner and their associates [42,43] reported the presence of C-type particles observed by electron microscopy in those embryonic mouse tissues which were positive for gs antigen (thymus, spleen, hematopoietic and liver and intestinal tissues), and their absence in non-replicating CF-negative tissues such as skeletal and cardiac muscle. It should be pointed out, however, that embryonic tissues of most mice, hamsters, cats and of some chickens (shown in tables 3, 4 and 5) failed to yield infectious C-type viruses despite very extensive tests [7,40,41,44,45], infectious virus being found only in those strains of mice and chickens in which breeding practices led to segregation of

Table 3
Complement fixing antigens[a] in mouse embryo tissues[b] reactive with rat sera having high-titered antibodies to the murine gs antigen.

Strain	Specimen	Age range (days)	No. /no. pos./ tested	Range in titers	Virus isolated	Virus parti-cles seen[e]
BALB/c	Whole embryo	10-11	24/24	1:20 to 1:80[c]	No	+
	Whole embryo	13	0/23			+
	Individual[d]	18	51/62			+
	Muscle	18	0/9			0
C₃H/Bi	Whole embryo	13	13/18	1:20 to 1:160	No	+
	Individual	18	28/41			+
	Muscle		0/7			0
C57BL/Cum	Whole embryo	10-11	16/20	1:20 to 1 : 80	No	+
	Individual	17-18	3/12			+
	Muscle	17-18	0/10			0
NIH Swiss	Whole embryo	10-14	132/137	1:40 to 1:160	No	+
	Individual		28/42			+
	Muscle		0/20			0

a Representative CF positive antigen confirmed in gel diffusion as having identity with purified viral gs antigens by Dr. R. Gilden.
b From mouse strains having low natural incidences of lymphoma and cancer, and little or no infectious virus expressions.
c Final dilutions v/w of tissue extracts.
d Spleen, thymus, liver.
e In CF antigen positive tissues [42].

permissive host genes *(vide infra)*. C-type viruses have also been seen by electron microscopy in antigen-positive tissues of chicken [46] and cat [47] embryos.

Host gene regulation of virus and antigen expressions

Postnatal studies of normal spleens, thymuses, intestines and reproductive tissues of spontaneous and chemically induced mouse tumors have uncovered variable prevalences of gs antigen and infectious C-type viruses. Although in

Table 4
Hamster C-type virus gs antigen expression in embryos of hamsters (Graffi strain).

| | Guinea pig anti-hamster gs sera | |
	2[a]	4[a]
Maternal tissues		
Spleen	0/4[b]	–
Liver	0/4	–
Thymus	0/4	–
Ovaries	0/4	–
Uterus	0/4	–
Whole embryos		
(8-9 days old)	36/40	11/40

[a] Reciprocal of antigen dilution.
[b] No. positive/no. tested of 10% tissue extracts at indicated dilution vs. 4 units of antisera.

Table 5
Complement fixation antigens[a] detected by antisera[b] to purified GSA antigen in chick embryo tissues.

Tissue specimen	Age range (days)	No. /no. pos./ tested[c]
Whole embryo	4-10	11/18
Liver	10-20	13/18
Spleen	10-20	6/8
Intestine	11-15	4/6
	12-19	2/5
Yolk sac	6-10	5/5
Chorioallantoic membrane	8-11	3/6
Amniotic membrane	6-11	6/8

[a] Range of titers 1:20 to 1:160; final tissue dilution v/w.
[b] Rabbit antisera produced by Allen [112]. Nearly identical results were obtained with the same specimens when tested with antisera made in hamsters carrying sarcomas induced by SR-MSV (Schmidt-Ruppin variant).
[c] Five specimens of each tissue pooled.

Table 6
Immunological tolerance to gs antigen in various virus-infected, tumored, or "immunized" animals.

Sera	No. / no. pos./ tested[e]
From *mice* carrying gs positive MSV tumors[a]	0/120
From *mice* carrying gs positive pseudotype MSV tumors[b]	0/175
From C57BL *mice* infected with gs positive RADLV	0/10
From *mice*(10) carrying gs positive MC-induced tumors	0/100 or >
From immune *chickens*[c] [113]	0/13
[c] [114]	8/72
From virus-infected *cats*[d]	0/47
From immunized or virus-infected *hamsters*	0/42

[a] NIH Swiss, BALB/c, C57BL, feral mice.
[b] Five different pseudotypes of MSV.
[c] Chicken sera positive for envelope antibody and/or neutralizing antibody; gs antibody determinations by FA and gel diffusion.
[d] All cats with gs positive tumors; gs antibody tests were done in complement fixation.
[e] Except where indicated differently, the specimens were tested in CF.

certain strains of mice the prevalence of antigen and virus increased with increasing age [5,37] and/or were switched on in induced tumors [5,8,48-50], it was quite apparent, particularly in inbred mice, that the major factors controlling virion and oncogenic expressions were determined by host strain genotypes. A number of strains having well identified host genes which influence or specifically regulate the independent virogene and oncogene expressions of the RNA viral genome have been identified and some are shown in table 7. Tissues of mice carrying the k, s and q alleles were generally positive for gs antigen throughout life, whereas the b and d alleles of the H-2 locus were associated with resistance to expression of gs antigens, at least in early life, and were also decisive in helping to suppress the natural oncogenic (oncogene) expressions as well. We should point out (table 7), however, that there are notable exceptions to this rule and that expressions of RNA genome specified antigens and tumors are controlled by other genes as well [51].

Recently discovered allelic genes, dominant for resistance to infectious C-type virus, were demonstrated on major gene loci by Lilly *et al.* [52,53], Axelrad [16] and Pincus *et al.* [54,55]; on the other hand, dominant genes which specify gs antigen expressions in chicken and mouse tissues have been described by Payne and associates [15,56] and by Taylor *et al.* [57]. A number of mutant

Table 7
Some known host gene controls of virogene and oncogene expressions of RNA tumor virus in inbred mouse strains.

Host genes	Strain	Infectious virus	gs antigen	Early lymphoma	Late cancer
H-2^k	AKR/J	+++	+++	95%	Dead at 12 mth
	C58/J	+++	+++	90%	
H-2^k	C$_3$H/Fg	++	++	90%	Dead at 12-15 mth
	C$_3$H/Bi	–	++	< 1%	Low
	C57BR/J	–	+	< 1%	35%
H-2^s	SJL/J	+	+	Reticulosarcoma	78%
H-2^d	BALB/c	Low, early life; high, late life		< 0.1%	20%
H-2^b	C57BL/J	±	+	< 0.1%	6%
	C57L/J	–	–	< 0.1%	7%
	129/J	–	–	< 0.1%	Low
hr/hr	HRS congenic	++	++	45%	70%
hr +	lines	++	++	1%	20%
hr ++		++	++	< 1%	Not tested

genes, examples of which have been described by Heston and associates [58,59] and Meier and associates [60] are also clearly decisive host cell factors specifying different cancers.

Since most leukemia and other cancers in mice, hamsters and cats (as in man) occur in stochastic patterns [5,37], and since definitive efforts to detect horizontal spread of C-type viruses were mostly negative, we concluded that the high prevalences of gs antigen in virus-free embryos, lifelong immunological tolerance to gs antigen, and the visible presence of frequently non-infectious C-type particles could only be satisfactorily explained by postulating genetic transmission of RNA virus genomes in resistant animals exhibiting varying degrees of gene regulated suppression of the virogenes and oncogenes of these genomes.

Is the RNA virus genome integrated within the cell DNA?

There is general agreement that at least a portion of the C-type viral RNA base sequences can be readily detected in cellular DNA. This has been demonstrated by two hybridization techniques: (a) viral RNA to cellular DNA [61-65] and (b) DNA product of reverse transcriptase to cellular DNA [66]. Two critical features of the results published to date are lack of species specificity of the hybridization reactions within vertebrates and that, with minimal exception [65], both normal and transformed cells contain roughly equivalent genome (or portions thereof) copies. This of course satisfies one condition of the oncogene, namely that it be present in all vertebrate cells. Some variability in results is certainly expected in interspecies tests since both endogenous oncogenes and viral genomes should show some degree of divergence due to normal mutational events. Recently, using the reverse transcriptase product DNA, it has been possible to show virus-specific RNA in both virus producing and non-producing transformed cells while normal cells did not show such RNA [67]. Thus, while normal cells may possess the genome, it is only transcribed in the transformed cells. This again is consistent with the concept of derepression, "switch on", of the oncogene as the fundamental lesion in oncogenesis.

    While the results of such studies are not presented as proof of the oncogene hypothesis, it is interesting to note the consistency of the theory derived solely on biological grounds, with the molecular "facts". Recently Hatanaka *et al.* [68] demonstrated DNA synthesis in the cytoplasm of newly infected cells by sensitive autoradiographic techniques. The specificity and fate of this DNA remains to be determined but the finding does emphasize the lack of definitive knowledge of the mechanism of *in vivo* replication and transformation by C-type viruses.

    As mentioned above, the discovery of the RNA dependent DNA polymerase provided a logical mechanism (reverse transcription) whereby the RNA genome could have been incorporated in the cells of the progenitors of the several different classes of vertebrates (reptilian, avian and mammalian) and nine different orders of mammals (table 1) which have been shown to have RNA tumor viruses; an event which would have had to occur more than 300 million years ago [69]. Our reasoning for this proposition goes as follows: (1) the major gs polypeptides in the viper and chicken RNA tumor viruses, while chemically almost identical to those found in mammalian viruses, are immunologically completely distinct from the latter as well as from each other; and (2) the interspecies antigenic determinants of all the four well established mammalian viruses are cross reactive. The mammalian species, therefore, share specific viral genes as well as certain equally specific regulating host specific genes (see above), thus suggesting in mammals co-evolution of both the RNA virus and host genomes. The differing major gs antigen demonstrated in chickens and vipers suggests that the RNA genome must have been already present prior to the evolution of the more primitive classes of vertebrates.

Activation of virogene expressions of the murine C-type viruses concomitantly with spontaneous tumorigenesis, and tumorigenesis induced by radiation and carcinogenic chemicals

The reports by Gross in 1958 [70] and Lieberman and Kaplan in 1959 [71] of the activation of leukemia-inducing C-type RNA viruses in low leukemic strains of mice (C_3H/BI, C57BR and C57BL) provided the initial concepts which led our associates and us in the late 1960's to consider the possibility of genetic transmission of the RNA tumor virus genome.

Our tests of spontaneous leukemias and solid tumors in mice and other species clearly indicated that gs antigen expressions were more frequently demonstrated than infectious virus [5,6,72]. Subsequent systematic investigations by Whitmire [8], Meier [49] and Gardner [43] and their associates of subcutaneous sarcomas induced by 3-methylcholanthrene (3MC) and other chemical carcinogens revealed expressions of gs antigens at various detectable levels which appeared to a considerable extent to be predetermined by host gene regulatory systems known to specify resistance or susceptibility to expression of the RNA tumor viruses. Table 8 illustrates variable incidences of complement-fixing gs antigens in extracts of tumors induced by 3MC in 16 genotypically different strains of inbred and outbred mice, using intraspecies gs specific guinea pig and MSV-26 rat antisera. As can be seen the incidence of antigen-positive tumors varied from 0% in the resistant C57L strain to 100% in the susceptible AKR and C58 strains. The results revealed differences which appeared to reflect in part H-2 genotype differences in the inbred strains.

Since extracts of normal muscle and subcutaneous tissues taken from areas adjacent to the chemically induced tumors and from other sites as well were uniformly negative for both gs and other CF antigens, and since tissues such as spleen and thymus of tumored animals showed no evidences of increased incidences or titers of gs antigen, we were inclined towards the view that the new antigens found in the tumors were specified by RNA virus genomes endogenous to the tumor cells.

Alternative hypotheses suggesting that the antigens represented infectious virus picked up from hematopoietic tissues by tumor cells after their transformation, or that the CF-positive cells were not tumor cells but cells of the hematopoietic system, seemed unlikely because the antigen content of the tumors more often than not were more strongly positive than the hematopoietic tissues in the same host, and infectious virus was rarely detected in the genotypically "resistant" strains. Also, the gs antigens were observed in titers at level much higher than could be attributed to the minute amount of infectious virus detected in those instances where virus was isolated from the

Table 8

Incidences of tumors and gs antigen in the tumors of mice induced with 150 μg methylcholanthrene given subcutaneously at four weeks of age.

Mouse strain		H-2 alleles	Tumor incidence		gs antigen in tumors[a]							
			Tumors/total	%	(using guinea pig serum)				(using serum pool MSV 26)			
					1:2		1:4		1:2		1:4	
					No. pos./no. tested	%	No. pos./no. tested	%	No. pos./no. tested	%	No. pos./no. tested	%
Inbred	C57BL/6Cum	b	26/27	96	2/14	14	2/14	14	3/15	20	1/15	7
	C3H/fMai	k	27/30	90	15/17	88	13/17	76	15/17	88	11/17	65
	BALB/cCr	d	35/49	71	5/13	38	2/13	15	4/13	31	2/13	15
	C57BR/cdJ	k	18/27	67	0/16	0	0/16	0	2/11	18	1/11	9
	C3H/He	k	33/53	62	9/16	56	8/16	50	10/16	63	7/16	44
	SWR/J	q	11/22	50	5/9	56	1/9	11	6/9	67	3/9	33
	C58/J	k	11/22	50					10/10	100	10/10	100
	C57L/J	b	13/28	46	1/12	8	0/12	0	0/10	0	0/10	0
	SJL/J	s	13/35	37	7/9	78	6/9	67	11/15	73	6/15	40
	AKR/J	k	5/24	21	5/5	100	5/5	100	5/5	100	5/5	100
	DBA/2J	q	5/35	14	5/5	100	4/5	80	5/5	100	4/5	80
	DBA/1J	d	2/26	8	2/2	100	1/2	50	2/2	100	1/2	50
Random bred	NIH Swiss		26/35	74	11/15	73	0/15	0	8/15	53	0/15	0
	Ha/ICR		46/63	73	5/11	45	2/11	18	11/15	73	5/15	33
	CFW		21/29	72	3/7	43	0/7	0	9/13	69	3/13	23
	CF-1		37/66	56	5/5	100	4/5	80	15/15	100	13/15	87

a Equal to or greater than 3+ fixation of complement at designated dilution of 10% tumor extracts were considered positive for gs antigen. Guinea pig and MSV 26 antisera react primarily with gs-1 antigen, having little or no reaction with interspecies antigen.

virus resistant strains. Tests of those wild type viruses isolated from the subcutaneous sarcomas for sarcoma-inducing potential in newborn isogenic mice were uniformly negative, a finding which was not unexpected since, with one exception, all previous such studies for sarcoma-inducing virus in carcinogen-induced tumors were also negative [73-75]. C-type RNA viruses isolated from spontaneous sarcomas of mice also failed to produce sarcomas when transmitted to homotypic newborns [5,8,72]. Despite the ubiquitous prevalence of C-type RNA tumor viruses, wild type sarcoma-inducing viruses have been extremely rare; only one (MSV-FBJ) has ever been isolated directly from the mouse, two have been isolated from the cat, several from chickens, and none have been recovered thus far from sarcomas of hamsters and rats, thus suggesting that the well established sarcoma viruses (table 1) could not be responsible for any significant numbers of either spontaneous or chemically induced sarcomas in these species. In addition, no outbreaks of sarcomas have ever been reported, and exhaustive attempts to recover sarcoma- or focus-inducing viruses from sarcomas of many other species including those of man have been completely fruitless.

We suggest therefore that the endogenous RNA genome, which we have postulated to be universally present in vertebrate cells, provides the oncogene(s) responsible for sarcomagenesis as well as for the virogenes responsible for the structural antigens (gs and the envelope G^+) of the RNA tumor viruses detected in such tumors. In our view it seems likely that the histologic character of the target cell represents the chief determinant of the histologic type of tumor finally induced; for example, if the genome is derepressed in a fibroblast, the tumor most likely would turn out to be a fibrosarcoma; other tumors would be expected to turn out to be carcinomas or lymphomas in the event that epithelial or lymphoid cells were the targets. Although this explanation needs a great deal of substantiation, it provides a rational working hypothesis capable of explaining the available observations and data *(vide supra)*.

Activation and isolation of endogenous hamster and rat C-type RNA viruses as "helpers" for the MSV(0) genome

The recent activation and isolation of hamster and rat viruses provide useful examples of the application of the newer concepts and methods that are likely to prove useful in evaluating the validity of a unitary theory. Although RNA tumor-like viruses had been visualized in infectious virus-free hamster and rat tumors carried by transplantation in their respective hosts [76-79], until very recently all attempts to isolate infectious hamster and rat specific viruses failed.

In 1970 Kelloff *et al.* [80,81] reported the rescue of the MSV(O) sarcoma genome by hamster C-type virus (HaLV) in MSV hamster tumors transplanted in newborn hamsters. Identical hamster helper viruses were recovered by endpoint dilutions from three MSV(O) tumor lines induced by three different MSVs. Analysis of the viral properties revealed envelope and gs-1 (intraspecies) antigen properties distinct from those of the mouse, cat and chicken; however, interspecies gs antigens [82] were found which were cross reactive with the gs antigenic counterparts of the other mammalian viruses. Recently Nowinski *et al.* [34] confirmed these findings on the hamster specificity of C-type viruses isolated from hamsters by genome rescue procedures.

Similar results have also been obtained with sarcomagenic virus preparations derived from a M-MSV induced tumor in a Brown-Norway rat. This virus possesses a gs antigen reactivity distinct from that of the other known species specific C-type viruses, but at the same time contains the interspecies gs determinant [29]. This adds to the previous demonstration of a distinct envelope type for this virus [83]. Recently Aaronson [84] and Sarma *et al.* [85] have isolated rat specific helper viruses from these sarcoma virus stocks, thus we presume *in vivo* rescue of the MSV genome by the indigenous rat C-type virus, thus the sarcoma virus is designated MSV(RaLV). The C-type virus described by Teitz *et al.* [86] in cultures of rat thymus cells shares the species specific antigenic reactivity with MSV(RaLV) [87].

Thus rescue procedures and helper factors uncovering previously covert hamster and rat as well as mouse and chicken C-type virus expressions [17,84,88-92] provide promising new procedures that may prove useful when applied in similar efforts to activate infectious C-type viruses in human cells [93,94].

In vitro activation of C-type virogenes and oncogenes: I. In long and short term cultures of embryonic mouse fibroblasts

Spontaneous and chemical transformations of C_3H mouse cells grown in culture were observed as early as 1943 by Earle [95]. In 1967 Hall *et al.* [96] demonstrated gs antigen and infectious C-type virus in the majority of cell lines derived from Earle's C_3H cell lines. In 1969 Aaronson, Hartley and Todaro [97] reported spontaneous derepression of gs antigen and infectious C-type virus in 3T6 and 3T12 BALB/c and Swiss mouse cells grown *in vitro* for 50 to 100 subcultures. Spontaneous transformation and transplantability in mice developed concurrently with the "switch on" of the virogenic properties.

Recently Hartley *et al.* [98] observed derepression of C-type gs antigen and infectious virus in two lines of embryonic wild (feral) mouse cells in early subculture. In one cell line the viral expression appeared spontaneously; in the other, viral expression was activatable only after treatment with 3MC; untreated sister cultures remained negative for virus. These represent the first successful isolations to be made from wild mice despite numerous exhaustive attempts. Like all other wild type isolates from laboratory mice, the wild mouse isolates have immunologic properties of the Gross serotype and the presence of virus was predicted by the demonstration of gs antigens in the cells prior to testing for virus. Specific gs antigens have recently been demonstrated in most spontaneous tumors occurring in wild mice in extreme old age (25-32 months) and in some tumors induced earlier in life by 3MC [43].

In vitro activation of C-type virogenes and oncogenes: II. In hamster tumors produced by hamster cells transformed in vitro by carcinogenic chemicals

Recently Freeman and his associates [99] found that hamster cells transformed by 3MC and several fractions of cigarette smoke residues yielded hamster specific C-type virus (HaLV) and gs antigen after transplantation of the cells into newborn hamsters and subsequent re-culture of the tumor cells *in vitro*. Although the mechanisms of virus induction are unknown, the inductions were predictable, since the transformed cell lines yielded infectious virus in 5 of 6 attempts (see table 9). In the same report they described the isolation of HaLV from cell lines established in culture from sarcomas induced in hamsters by injection of DMBA (dimethylbenz(a)anthracene); again the presence of infectious virus was indicated by the appearance of HaLV specific gs antigens in the tumor tissue and the cultured cells.

In vitro activation of oncogenes in cells infected with nontransforming C-type virus and treated with carcinogenic chemicals

One of the objections to the postulate that endogenous C-type genomes and their oncogenes were responsible for sarcomatous changes induced in cells by chemicals was the fact that when infectious C-type viruses were isolated from spontaneous and induced sarcomas or transformed cells, such viruses uniformly lacked the ability to reproduce such neoplastic events on transmission despite their ready infectiousness. This disconcerting observation was not, of course, new, since only a handful of sarcoma viruses have ever been directly isolated from spontaneous sarcomas and none from induced sarcomas *(vide supra)*. It appears that the focus-producing sarcoma viruses of mice (M-MSV, H-MSV and Ki-MSV) utilized extensively for experimental model studies are mutants of the established nontransforming leukemia viruses (Moloney, Harvey, Kirsten) (table 1).

The generally defective nature of the sarcoma genome and its need for helper C-type virus provides a possible explanation for its paradoxical behavior. We have referred to the noninfectious but rescuable MSV(O) as a movable oncogene, i.e., oncogenes rescuable from the HT-1 sarcoma cell line [44,90,100], an MSV(O) which lacks all evidence of phenotypic virion expression. The HT-1 MSV genome, for instance, was incorporated in helper virus coats of numerous mouse, hamster and cat RNA tumor viruses [90,101,102]. The "movable" sarcoma oncogene (with the use of infectious helpers) was then readily introduced into hamster, rat, cat, dog, monkey and human cells, events leading to sarcomatous transformation of the recipient cells. The genome can be rescued again with the same helpers, following which the process can be repeated. Since most of the extant murine sarcoma viruses (and no doubt some of the avian) are mutant derivatives from and also mixtures with nontransforming virus, it occurred to us that the nontransforming C-type viral genomes must contain generally repressed but activatable oncogenes for transforming mesenchymal cells into sarcoma cells.[4]

Activation in vitro of RNA tumor virus by carcinogenic chemicals

In a recent series of experiments, Freeman, Rhim and their associates [8,103-107] attempted to find out if the sarcoma oncogene of nontransforming C-type viruses could be derepressed in hamster, rat and mouse cells infected in culture with a variety of these viruses; we presumed that such cells would be "primed" with numerous viral oncogenes having the potential for transforming the cells and thus might well be subject to accelerated and more efficient transformation, when treated with carcinogenic agents. Our anticipations were amply supported as can be seen in tables 9, 10 and 11.

---

[4] This, of course, was previously suggested by the association of C-type viruses or viral antigens with spontaneous and chemically induced sarcomas as well as with spontaneous transformation of mouse cells *in vitro* as was described above, and exemplified by the concomitant switch on of the C-type genome with spontaneous and chemical transformations of mouse and hamster cells.

General discussion

Considerable direct evidence was presented during this conference which provided support for the oncogene theory which postulates inherited transmission of the C-type RNA genome or its presence in a provirus or protovirus state, and its apparently critical importance in the etiology of spontaneous and induced cancer [2,13,15-17]. Contemporary information on host gene regulation of the expressions of both these genomes renders something like the Jacob and Monod gene regulation theory increasingly likely as the mechanism by which the host cells control the oncogenes and virogenes (operons) of the RNA tumor virus genomes.

Recent reports of B-type virus in human milk [14,108] and of C-type virus particles in human tumor cell cultures [109] if confirmed should accelerate progress towards a more complete understanding of the genetic alterations which take place in normal human cells at the time neoplastic transformation is initiated, and also of the mechanisms which must be involved in maintaining the heritable neoplastic state in daughter cancer cells and occasional reversions from this state. The significance of widespread prevalence of unassembled internal antigenic proteins of the C-type RNA virus in embryonic tissues as well as in tumor tissues should also soon be clarified. The vastly important reverse transcriptase of Temin and Baltimore, which has also been shown to be antigenic [110, 111], should also be elucidated in relation to cancer induction in all of the species discussed. My associates have suggested *(vide supra)* that one of its chief functions was perhaps to integrate the RNA tumor viruses into the DNA of germ cells prior to the evolution of vertebrates.

We realize that the central question concerning the integration of the RNA viral genetic information in the host genome requires definitive proof in molecular and classical genetic terms. We believe this determination should be possible within a relatively short period at least in the avian and murine systems. In the meantime, however, the oncogene theory as we have proposed [2], Temin's protovirus theory [13], and Bentvelzen's genetic inheritance theory for the B-type RNA mammary virus [11] provide working hypotheses which in various degrees are consistent with the natural histories of both natural cancer and of the natural distributions of the RNA tumor viruses.

Table 9

Transformation of hamster cells by carcinogenic chemicals.

Chemical or virus	Virus status	Trans- formation	Transplant	Activation of HaLV[a]
BZP (1.0 µg/ml) (4 experiments)	No virus	+	+ (cloned cells)	NT[b]
MC (0.1 µg/ml) (12 experiments)	No virus	+	+	+[c]
3 Cigarette smoke fractions (1.0 µg/ml)	No virus	+	+	+[c]
City smog (crude extract)	HaLV[+]	++	−	NT
	HaLV[−]	+	NC[d]	NT

[a] HaLV = hamster RNA virus.
[b] NT = not tested.
[c] Five of six tumors yielded HaLV in subcultured cells.
[d] NC = not complete.

Table 10

Rat cell transformation by the combined action of carcinogenic chemicals and RNA viruses.[a]

Chemical or virus	Virus status	Transformation	Transplant
DENA (0.1 mM)	RLV[+]	+	−
	RLV[−]	−	−
3MC (0.01 to 1.00 µg/ml) (2 separate cell lines)	RLV[+]	+	+
	RLV[−]	−	−
DMBA (0.01 to 1.00 µg/ml)	RLV[+]	+	+
	RLV[−]	−	−
BZP (10.0 µg/ml)	RLV[+]	+	·+
	RLV[−]	−	−

[a] Data from Freeman, Price, Rhim and associates.

Table 11

Mouse cell transformation by the combined action of carcinogenic chemicals and RNA viruses.[a]

Chemical or virus	Virus status	Transformation	Transplant
3MC (0.10 to 1.00 μg/ml)	AKR/LV$^+$	+	+
	AKR/LV$^-$	−	−
BZP (1.0 to 5.0 μg/ml)	AKR/LV$^+$	+	NC[b]
	AKR/LV$^-$	−	NC

[a] Data from Rhim and associates.
[b] NC = not complete.

Table 12

Incidence of spontaneous cancers in wild mice.

Time observed (months)	Total observed for time period	Tumors	Rate of tumors/100
1-3	192	0	0.0
4-6	150	0	0.0
7-9	147	0	0.0
10-12	129	1	0.8
13-15	100	0	0.0
16-18	88	1	1.1
19-21	65	1	1.5
22-24	39	3	7.7
25-27	27	4	14.8
28-30	24	1	4.2

References

[1] P.H. Abelson, Editorial, Science 172 (1971) 989.
[2] R.J. Huebner and G.J. Todaro, Proc. Natl. Acad. Sci. U.S. 64 (1969) 1087.
[3] F.M. Burnet, Lancet i (1968) 1383.
[4] C.D. Darlington, Genetics and Man (McMillan Co., New York, 1964) p. 149.
[5] R.J. Huebner, G.J. Todaro, P. Sarma, J.W. Hartley, A.E. Freeman, R.L. Peters, C.E. Whitmire, H. Meier and R.V. Gilden, *In:* Defectiveness, rescue and stimulation of oncogenic viruses (No. 183), Second International Symposium on Tumor Viruses (Editions du Centre National de La Recherche Scientifique, Paris, 1970) p. 33.

216   *R.J. Huebner and R.V. Gilden*

[6] R.J. Huebner and H.J. Igel, *In:* M. Pollard (ed.), Perspectives in virology VII (Academic Press, New York, 1971), p. 55.
[7] R.J. Huebner, G.J. Kelloff, P.S. Sarma, W.T. Lane, H.C. Turner, R.V. Gilden, S. Oroszlan, H. Meier, D.D. Myers and R.L. Peters, Proc. Natl. Acad. Sci. U.S. 67 (1970) 366.
[8] R.J. Huebner, A.E. Freeman, C.E. Whitmire, P.J. Price, J.S. Rhim, G.J. Kelloff, R.V. Gilden and H. Meier, *In:* Proc. of the 24th Annual Symposium on Fundamental Cancer Research, Environment and Cancer (1971), in press.
[9] H. Temin and S. Mizutani, Nature 226 (1970) 1211.
[10] D. Baltimore, Nature 226 (1970) 1209.
[11] P. Bentvelzen and J.H. Daams, J. Natl. Cancer Inst. 43 (1969) 1025.
[12] P.A.J. Bentvelzen, this Symposium.
[13] H.M. Temin, J. Natl. Cancer Inst. 46 (guest editorial, 1971), p. III.
[14] S. Spiegelman, this Symposium.
[15] L.N. Payne, this Symposium.
[16] A.A. Axelrad, this Symposium.
[17] R.A. Weiss, this Symposium.
[18] F. Jacob and J. Monod, J. Mol. Biol. 3 (1961) 318.
[19] H. Rubin, A. Cornelius and L. Fanshier, Proc. Natl. Acad. Sci. U.S. 47 (1961) 1058.
[20] L. Gross, Proc. Soc. Exptl. Biol. Med. 107 (1961) 90.
[21] V.H. Haas, Public Health Rep. 56 (1941) 285.
[22] M.G. Smith, Progr. Med. Virol. 2 (1959) 171.
[23] R.J. Huebner, D. Armstrong, M. Okuyan, P.S. Sarma and H.C. Turner, Proc. Natl. Acad. Sci. U.S. 51 (1964) 742.
[24] H. Bauer and W. Schäfer, Z. Naturforsch. 20b (1965) 815.
[25] P.S. Sarma, H.C. Turner and R.J. Huebner, Virology 23 (1964) 313.
[26] G. Geering, L.J. Old and E.A. Boyse, J. Exptl. Med. 124 (1966) 753.
[27] G. Geering, W.D. Hardy, L.J. Old and E. De Harven, Virology 36 (1968) 678.
[28] G. Kelloff, R.J. Huebner, S. Oroszlan, R. Toni and R.V. Gilden, J. Gen. Virol. 9 (1970) 27.
[29] R.V. Gilden, S. Oroszlan and R.J. Huebner, Virology 43 (1971) 722.
[30] W. Schäfer, Presented at the Colloquium on Selected Feline Viruses (Cornell University, Ithaca, N.Y. 1970).
[31] W. Hardy, G. Geering, L.J. Old, E. De Harven, R. Brodey and S. Mc Donough, Science 166 (1969) 1019.
[32] L.J. Old and E.A. Boyse, Fed. Proc. 24 (1965) 1009.
[33] L.J. Old, E.A. Boyse, G. Geering and H.F. Oettgen, Cancer Res. 28 (1968) 1288.
[34] R.C. Nowinski, L.J. Old, P.V. O'Donnell and F.K. Sanders, Nature New Biol. 230 (1971) 282.
[35] T. Aoki, E.A. Boyse and L.J. Old, J. Natl. Cancer Inst. 41 (1968) 89.
[36] T. Aoki, E.A. Boyse and L.J. Old, J. Natl. Cancer Inst. 41 (1968) 97.
[37] R.J. Huebner, *In:* R.M. Dutcher (ed.), Comparative leukemia research 1969, Bibl. Haemat. (Karger, Basel/München/New York, 1970) p. 22.
[38] R.J. Huebner, P.S. Sarma, G.J. Kelloff, R.V. Gilden, H. Meier, D.D. Myers and R.L. Peters, *In:* H. Friedman (ed.), Immunological tolerance to microbial antigens, Ann. N.Y. Acad. Sci. 181 (1971) 279.
[39] G.I. Abelev and D.A. Elgort, Int. J. Cancer 6 (1970) 145.
[40] G. Kelloff, R.J. Huebner and R.V. Gilden, J. Gen. Virol. 13 (1971) 289.

[41] P.S. Sarma, D.W. Allen and R.J. Huebner, unpublished data.

[42] M.L. Vernon, unpublished data.

[43] M.B. Gardner, J.E. Officer, R.W. Rongey, J.D. Estes, H.C. Turner and R.J. Huebner, Nature 232 (1971) 617.

[44] J.W. Hartley, W.P. Rowe, W.I. Capps and R.J. Huebner, J. Virol. 3 (1969) 126.

[45] J.E. Officer, M.B. Gardner, J.D. Estes, J.W. Hartley and R.J. Huebner, unpublished data.

[46] R.M. Dougherty, H.S. Di Stefano and F.K. Roth, Proc. Natl. Acad. Sci. U.S. 58 (1967) 808.

[47] M.B. Gardner, P. Arnstein, J.D. Estes and R.J. Huebner, unpublished observations.

[48] H.J. Igel, R.J. Huebner, H.C. Turner, P. Kotin and H.L. Falk, Science 166 (1969) 1624.

[49] H. Meier, D.D. Myers and R.J. Huebner, presented at the Vth International Symposium on Comparative Leukemia Research in Padova, Italy, September 1971.

[50] C.E. Whitmire, R.A. Salerno, L. Rabstein, R.J. Huebner and H.C. Turner, in preparation.

[51] H. Meier and R.J. Huebner, Proc. Natl. Acad. Sci. U.S. 68 (1971) 2664.

[52] F. Lilly, J. Natl. Cancer Inst. 45 (1970) 163.

[53] F. Lilly, this Symposium

[54] T. Pincus, J.W. Hartley and W.P. Rowe, J. Exp. Med. 133 (1971) 1219.

[55] T. Pincus, W.P. Rowe and F. Lilly, J. Exp. Med. 133 (1971) 1234.

[56] L.N. Payne and R.C. Chubb, J. Gen. Virol. 3 (1968) 379.

[57] B.A. Taylor, H. Meier and D.D. Myers, Proc. Natl. Acad. Sci. U.S. (1971) in press.

[58] G. Vlahakis, W.E. Heston and G.H. Smith, Science 170 (1970) 185.

[59] W.E. Heston, this Symposium.

[60] H. Meier, D.D. Myers and R.J. Huebner, Proc. Natl. Acad. Sci. U.S. 63 (1969) 759.

[61] M. Hatanaka, Nippen Rinsho 22 (1964) 1203. (In Japanese.)

[62] H.M. Temin, Proc. Natl. Acad. Sci. U.S. 52 (1964) 323

[63] L. Harel, J. Harel and J. Huppert, Biochem. Res. Comm. 28 (1967) 44.

[64] D.E. Wilson and H. Bauer, Virology 33 (1968) 745.

[65] M.A. Baluda and D.P. Nayak, Proc. Natl. Acad. Sci. U.S. 66 (1970) 329.

[66] L.D. Gelb, S.A. Aaronson and M.A. Martin, Science 172 (1971) 1353.

[67] M. Green, H. Rokutanda and M. Rokutanda, Nature New Biol. 230 (1971) 229.

[68] M. Hatanaka, T. Kakefuda, R.V. Gilden and E.A.O. Callan, Proc. Natl. Acad. Sci. U.S. (1971) in press.

[69] R.V. Gilden and R.J. Huebner, this Symposium.

[70] L. Gross, Acta Haematol. 19 (1958) 353.

[71] M. Lieberman and H.S. Kaplan, Science 130 (1959) 387.

[72] R.L. Peters, L.S. Rabstein, R.M. Madison, G.J. Spahn, W.T. Lane, H.C. Turner and R.J. Huebner, in preparation.

[73] B. Toth and P. Shubik, Cancer Res. 27 (1967) 43.

[74] C. Heidelberger, *In:* Canadian Cancer Conference 1966, 7 (Pergamon Press, New York, 1967) p. 326.

[75] R.T. Prehn, J. Natl.Cancer Inst. 32 (1964) 1.

[76] W.A. Stenback, G.L. van Hoosier, jr. and J.J. Trentin, Proc. Soc. Exptl. Biol. Med. 122 (1966) 1219.

[77] G. Geering, T. Aoki and L.J. Old, Nature 226 (1970) 265.

[78] H.C. Chopra, A.E. Bogden, I. Zelljadt, E.M. Jensen and D.J. Taylor, European J. Cancer 6 (1970) 287.

[79] R.S. Weinstein and W.C. Moloney, Proc. Soc. Exptl. Biol. Med. 118 (1965) 459.

[80] G. Kelloff, R.J. Huebner, Y.K. Lee, R. Toni and R.V. Gilden, Proc. Natl. Acad. Sci. 65 (1970) 310.

[81] G. Kelloff, R.J. Huebner, K.H. Chang, Y.K. Lee and R.V. Gilden, J. Gen. Virol. 9 (1970) 19.

[82] R.V. Gilden, S. Oroszlan and R.J. Huebner, Nature 231 (1971) 107.

[83] R.C. Ting, J. Virol. 2 (1968) 865.

[84] S. Aaronson, Virology 44 (1971) 29.

[85] P.S. Sarma, T. Log, R.J. Huebner and R.V. Gilden, Virology (1971) in press.

[86] Y. Teitz, E.H. Lennette, L.S. Oshiro and N.E. Cremer, J. Natl. Cancer Inst. 46 (1971) 11.

[87] R.V. Gilden and R.J. Huebner, unpublished data.

[88] H. Hanafusa, T. Hanafusa and H. Rubin, Virology 22 (1964) 591.

[89] P.K. Vogt, *In:* K.M. Smith and M.A. Lauffer (eds.), Advances in virus research (Academic Press, New York, 1965) p. 293.

[90] R.J. Huebner, Proc. Natl. Acad. Sci. U.S. 58 (1967) 835.

[91] H. Hanafusa, this Symposium.

[92] V. Klement, J.W. Hartley, W.P. Rowe and R.J. Huebner, J. Natl. Cancer Inst. 43 (1969) 925.

[93] S. Aaronson, Nature 230 (1971) 445.

[94] R.M. Mc Allister, J.E. Filbert, M.O. Nicolson, R.W. Rongey, M.B. Gardner, R.V. Gilden and R.J. Huebner, Nature New Biology 230 (1971) 279.

[95] W.R. Earle, J. Natl. Cancer Inst. 4 (1943) 165.

[96] W.T. Hall, W.F. Andresen, K.K. Sanford, V. Evans and J.W. Hartley, Science 156 (1967) 85.

[97] S.A. Aaronson, J.W. Hartley and G.J. Todaro, Proc. Natl. Acad. Sci. U.S. 64 (1969) 87.

[98] J.W. Hartley, A.E. Freeman, J.E. Officer and M.B. Gardner, unpublished data.

[99] A.E. Freeman, G.J. Kelloff, R.V. Gilden, W.T. Lane, A.P. Swain and R.J. Huebner, Proc. Natl. Acad. Sci. U.S. 68 (1971) 2386.

[100] S.S. Chang, R.V. Gilden and R.J. Huebner, J. Gen. Virol. 10 (1971) 107.

[101] P.J. Fischinger and T.E. O'Connor, Science 165 (1969) 714.

[102] P.S. Sarma, T. Log and R.J. Huebner, Proc. Natl. Acad. Sci. 65 (1970) 81.

[103] A.E. Freeman, P.J. Price, H.J. Igel, J.C. Young, J.M. Maryak and R.J. Huebner, J. Natl. Cancer Inst. 44 (1970) 65.

[104] P.J. Price, A.E. Freeman, W.T. Lane and R.J. Huebner, Nature New Biology 230 (1971) 144.

[105] A.E. Freeman, P.J. Price, R.J. Bryan, R.J. Gordon, R.V. Gilden, G.J. Kelloff and R.J. Huebner, Proc. Natl. Acad. Sci. U.S. 68 (1971) 445.

[106] J.S. Rhim, B. Creasy and R.J. Huebner, Proc. Natl. Acad. Sci. U.S. (1971) in press.

[107] J.S. Rhim, W. Vass, H.Y. Cho and R.J. Huebner, Int. J. Cancer 7 (1971) 65.

[108] D. Moore, J. Charney, B.Kramarsky, E.Y. Lasfargues, N.H. Sarkar, M.J. Brennan, J.H. Burrows, S.M. Sirsat, J.C. Paymaster and A.B. Vaidya, Nature 229 (1971) 611.

[109] E.S. Priori, L. Dmochowski, B. Myers and J.R. Wilbur, Nature New Biology 232 (1971) 61.

[110] S.A. Aaronson, W.P. Parks, E.M. Scolnick and G.J. Todaro, Proc. Natl. Acad. Sci. U.S. 68 (1971) 920.
[111] S. Oroszlan, M. Hatanaka, R.V. Gilden and R.J. Huebner, J. Virology 8 (1971) 816.
[112] D.W. Allen, P.S. Sarma, H.D. Niall and R. Sauer, Proc. Natl. Acad. Sci. U.S. 67 (1970) 837.
[113] G. Kelloff and P.K. Vogt, Virology 29 (1966) 366.
[114] D. Armstrong, M. Okuyan and R.J. Huebner, Science 144 (1964) 1584.

Part 5

GENETIC FACTORS IN LEUKEMIA

LOCI DETERMINING CELL SURFACE ALLOANTIGENS[1]

George D. SNELL and Marianna CHERRY
The Jackson Laboratory, Bar Harbor
Me. 04609, U.S.A.[2]

This review is based on two premises: (1) that the chemistry of the cell surface is genetically determined and, (2) that the cell surface plays a role in viral infection and oncogenesis. This is the rationale for discussing the murine loci which determine cell surface alloantigens at a symposium on RNA viruses and host genome in oncogenesis.

Cell surface alloantigens have been identified by 3 methods: histogenetic or transplantation methods (usually skin or tumor grafting), red cell agglutination (blood typing), and lymphoid cell cytolysis. There are other methods that might and in due course may be used, e.g., cell surface labeling with immunofluorescent antibody, but while these have been applied to the study of all surface alloantigens they have played little or no role in their initial identification.

The nomenclature for alloantigen-determining loci is very confused and in some instances does not conform to standard genetic usage [1]. We shall adopt here symbols which have recently been proposed [2], and to which some but not all investigators in this field have agreed. The symbols are based on the three methods of alloantigen demonstration. Histocompatibility genes, demonstrated by the rejection of transplants, are designated by an initial *H*, and erythrocyte alloantigen determining genes by an initial *Ea*. Alloantigens on lymphocytes are most characteristically indicated by an initial *Ly,* but additional symbols are used to deal with special cases. We shall indicate these in the appropriate places. In each case Arabic numbers are appended to identify

[1] The work included in this review which was done at The Jackson Laboratory was supported by National Institutes of Health Research Grant CA-01329 from the National Cancer Institute, and by a grant from the Virginia and D.K. Ludwig Foundation.
[2] The principles of laboratory animal care, as promulgated by the National Society for Medical Research, are observed in this Laboratory.

Table 1

Strain distribution of the known specificities of the non-H-2 alloantigen determining loci.

Strain	Ea-1*	Ea-2 (R-Z, H-14)	Ea-3 (λ)	Ea-4 (D)	Ea-5 (H-5)	Ea-6 (H-6)	Ea-7 (T)	Ly-1 (mu, Ly-A)	Ly-2 (Ly-B)	Ly-3 (Ly-C)	Pca-1	Thy-1 (θ)	Tla	H-2 allele
C57BL	$-^{h}$	2^{kq}	$-^{g}$	2^{io}	$-^{a}$	1^{a}	2^{s}	2^{be}	2^{b}	2^{c}	$-^{t}$	2^{n}	$-^{d}$	*b*
C57BL/Ks		2^{r}		2^{r}				2^{f}	2^{f}			2^{f}	2^{f}	*d*
SEC/1Re	$-^{p}$	2^{r}	1^{g}	1^{r}				2^{f}	2^{f}			2^{f}		*d*
C57L		2^{q}		1^{r}			2^{r}	2^{be}	2^{b}	2^{c}		2^{f}	$-^{d}$	*b*
DA/HuSn		2^{r}		1^{r}			2^{r}	2^{c}	2^{c}	2^{c}		2^{f}	$-^{f}$	*qp*
WB/Re		2^{q}		1^{ir}			2^{r}	2^{f}	2^{c}			2^{f}	$-^{f}$	*ja*
ST/bJ		2^{r}		1^{r}			2^{r}	2^{f}	2^{c}	2^{c}		2^{f}	$-^{d}$	*k*
C57BR/cd	2^{q}	2^{q}		1^{r}			2^{sr}	2^{b}	2^{b}	2^{c}				*k*
A	2^{kq}	$-^{g}$		1^{i}	1^{a}	1^{a}	2^{r}	2^{be}	2^{b}	2^{c}	$+^{t}$	2^{n}	$1,2,3^{d}$	*a*
HTI				1^{i}				2^{c}	2^{c}	2^{c}	$-^{t}$		$1,2,3^{d}$	*i*
NZB				1^{r}			2^{r}	2^{b}	2^{b}	2^{c}	$+^{t}$		$1,2,3^{d}$	*d*
SJL				1^{r}			2^{r}	2^{c}	2^{b}	2^{c}	$+^{t}$		$1,2,3^{d}$	*s*
SWR		2^{q}		1^{r}			2^{r}	2^{be}	2^{b}	2^{c}			$1,2,3^{d}$	*q*
BALB/c	2^{kq}	2^{kq}	$-^{g}$	1^{r}		$-^{j}$	2^{r}	2^{b}	2^{b}	2^{c}	$+^{t}$	2^{n}	2^{d}	*d*
HTG		2^{r}		1^{r}			1^{s}	2^{be}	2^{b}	2^{c}	$-^{t}$	2^{f}	$-^{d}$	*g*
129		2^{kq}		1^{i}	1^{a}	1^{a}	1^{r}	2^{be}	2^{c}	2^{c}		2^{n}	2^{d}	*b*
LP		2^{q}		1^{io}	$-^{a}$	1^{a}	1^{s}	2^{c}	2^{c}	2^{c}			2^{f}	*b*
C3H/He	$-^{p}$	2^{kq}	$-^{g}$	1^{r}			1^{s}	1^{be}	1^{c}	2^{c}	$+^{t}$	2^{n}	$-^{d}$	*k*
FL/2Re		2^{r}		1^{r}		1^{j}	2^{r}	1^{f}	2^{f}	2^{f}		2^{f}	$-^{f}$	*k*
CBA/J	$-^{h}$	2^{kq}		1^{i}		1^{j}	$1?^{r}$	1^{e}	1^{f}			2^{f}	$-^{d}$	*k*
C3H/St				1^{i}	1^{a}	$-^{a}$						2^{n}		*k*
DBA/1		2^{kq}		1^{i}	$-^{a}$	$-^{a}$	2^{r}	1^{be}	1^{b}			2^{m}	$-^{d}$	*q*
JK		2^{r}			$-^{a}$	$-^{a}$		1^{b}	1^{b}				$-^{d}$	*i*
DBA/2	$-^{p}$	2^{kq}		1^{o}			2^{r}	1^{be}	1^{b}	2^{c}	$-^{t}$		2^{d}	*d*
HRS		2^{r}		1^{r}			2^{r}	2^{f}	2^{f}			2^{f}	$-^{f}$	*k*

Strain													
SM/J	2^r				1^r	2^r	2^f	1^f	2^c	$+^t$	2^f	$\_f$	*v*
CE/J	2^r				1^r	2^r	2^c	1^c	2^c	$\_t$	2^f	$\_f$	*k*
I $\quad$ –p	2^r				1^r	2^r	2^b	1^b			2^f	$\_d$	*l*
YBR	2^k	1^a	1^a	1^a									*d*
C58	2^k	1^a	$\_a$	1^a	1^r	1^r	2^b	1^b	1^c	$\_t$	2^n	$1,2,3^d$	*k*
MA/J	2^q	1^a			1^r	2^r	1^f	1^f		$+^t$	1^f	$\_d$	*k*
AKR	2^{kq}			1^j	1^r	2^r	2^b	1^b	1^c	$+^t$	1^n	$\_d$	*k*
AKR.M					1^r	2^r	2^f	2^f			1^f	$1,2,3?^f$	*m*
PL	2^q				1^r	2^r	2^c	1^c	1^c	$+^t$	1^f	$1,2,3^d$	*u*
BDP	2^q				1^r	2^r	1^f	1^f			1^f	$1,2,3?^f$	*p*
BUB/Bn	2^r				1^r	1^r	2^f	2^f			1^f	$1,2,3?^f$	*q*
F/St	1^k	1^a	$\_a$	1^a	1^i							$1,2,3d$	*n*
RF/J	1^q	1^a	$\_a$		1^r	2^r	2^{be}	1^b	1^c	$+^t$	1^n	$\_d$	*k*
RFM	1^k										1^n		*f*
RIII	1^q				1^i	2^r	2^e						*r*

*All laboratory strains tested have null allele $Ea\text{-}1^o$.

Alleles $Ea\text{-}1^a$ and $Ea\text{-}1^b$ are found only in wild populations.

[a] Amos et al. [10].
[b] Boyse et al. [21].
[c] Boyse et al. [23].
[d] Boyse et al. [20].
[e] Cherry and Snell [22].
[f] Cherry and Snell (unpublished data).
[g] Egerov [11].
[h] Foster et al. [12].
[i] Klein and Martinkova [13].
[j] Palm (personal communication).

[k] Popp [14].
[l] Popp [15].
[m] Reif and Allen [24].
[n] Reif and Allen [28].
[o] Shreffler [16].
[p] Singer et al. [29].
[q] Snell et al. [17].
[r] Snell (unpublished data).
[s] Stompfling and Snell [18].
[t] Takahashi et al. [27].

224 G.D. Snell and M. Cherry

separate loci with similar effects (e.g., H-1, H-2, Ea-4, Ea-5, etc.). In accordance with standard genetic usage [1], alleles are indicated by superscript small letters (e.g., H-1ᵃ, H-1ᵇ). Specificities (synonymous with antigens in HL-A terminology) are designated by numbers, preceded, where necessary to avoid ambiguity, by the locus symbol (e.g., 2 or H-2.2, Ly-1.1, etc.) [3].

We shall summarize briefly the current state of knowledge concerning the three categories of loci. Additional information will be found in another recent review [2] and in table 1.

The number of known histocompatibility loci has stood from some time at 13 [4]. Of the loci currently designated by the symbol H, two, H-5 and H-6, were demonstrated by red cell typing. At least one of them, H-6, is probably without histocompatibility effect, at least on skin grafts (Lilly, personal communication). These belong in the Ea category. But the loss of these two is balanced by the addition of the X-linked and Y-linked loci [5,6]. These 13 known loci probably constitute only a fraction of the total H locus number [7,8]. Bailey has recently reported evidence for six more [9], and the number of new loci is still rising [Bailey, unpublished data]. Seven H loci are already located in the linkage map and Bailey is rapidly adding others.

The number of loci in the Ea category now stands at seven ([10-18], see [2] for a more detailed summary). The map position of two of them has been determined [12,19].

Five loci have been reported as a result of tests of the cytotoxic effect on lymphoid cells of alloantibody plus complement. The first locus to be described, Tla [20], is the subject of one of the papers presented at this Symposium. Ly-1 [21,22] (originally called Ly-A or μ), Ly-2 [21] (originally called Ly-B), and Ly-3 [23] (originally called Ly-C) are demonstrable on lymphocytes, especially thymic lymphocytes. Since Ly-2 and Ly-3 show complete linkage, they should actually be regarded as one locus. Thy-1 or θ [24] determines a strong thymic lymphocyte alloantigen. Anti-Thy-1 is turning out to be a useful agent for identifying [25] or selectively destroying [26] lymphocytes of thymic origin. Pca-1 [27] determines a plasma cell alloantigen.

There is of course some overlap between our three categories of loci. H-2 is the most notable example. Another example is Ea-2 which, as shown by Popp [15], can be demonstrated by cytotoxicity of thymocytes as well as by red cell agglutination. On the whole, however, the three categories seem to be surprisingly separate. We have summarized the evidence elsewhere [2].

The strain distribution of the known specificities of the non-H-2 alloantigen determining loci is shown in table 1. Except in the case of H-2, the table shows specificities, not alleles. The recommended convention is that specificity 1 correspond to allele a. For the three Tla alleles, the combination 1,2,3 is called *a*, — is called *b*, and *2* is called *c*. For *Tla* we give serotype of normal, not of leukemic, lymphocytes, which can be different. The proposed new designations for the various loci appear at the top of the table; just below them are the old designations which they replace. The last column in the table shows the *H-2* allele of each of the strains. *H-2* and *Tla* are placed adjacent to each other because they are linked and may therefore be expected to show some degree of association. Rather than arranging the strains alphabetically, we have arranged them so as to bring out similarities of serotype. In most cases these similarities reflect known relationships [30]. The sources of information are shown in the footnotes. A good deal of our own unpublished information is included.

We should add one word of caution in regard to the table. While the majority of the tests, both our own and those of other investigators, have been done with J (Jackson Laboratory) sublines, or sublines otherwise closely related, there may be some instances where widely separated sublines have been used. As shown by Amos *et al.* [10] in the case of the *Ea-5* and *Ea-6* serotypes of the He and St sublines of C3H, there can be major substrain differences. In most instances we have not indicated a subline in the table for the reason that this would not accurately reflect the diversity of sublines that have been used.

Information comparable to that given in table 1 on the strain distribution of blood group and lymphocyte group alleles has been given for histocompatibility alleles by Graff and Snell [31], and Graff *et al.* [32].

The total number of reported loci which determine cell surface alloantigens now stands at 32. And the number is rapidly rising. The rise is currently most rapid with respect to histocompatibility loci, but an extension of serotyping methods to cells other than erythrocytes and lymphocytes might touch off an information explosion in this area. Since each known locus must have a minimum of two alleles, this points to a substantial polymorphism of the cell surface. This minimum polymorphism can be compounded many times over by the existence of multiple alleles. Our information in this area merely scratches the surface. More than 20 *H-2* alleles have been identified in laboratory stocks, and studies of wild mice will rapidly increase this number [33]. While *H-2* may be unique in its complexity, all or nearly all the other *H* loci seem to have multiple alleles [32,34], and Bailey [7], on the basis of a mutation study, has emphasized the vastness of the murine histocompatibility gene system. The majority of the blood group and lymphocyte group loci seem at the moment to be simpler, but this may merely reflect our ignorance. Imperfect though our information is, we can say beyond question that the genetics, and hence also the chemistry, of the cell membrane is both extraordinarily complex and extraordinarily diverse. We know also that the diversity applies both to tissues and to individuals.

Our basic premise is that the function of the family of genes we are talking about is to provide the chemical building blocks for the cell membrane. If this premise is correct, than any further probing as to the functions of these genes turns into a question as to the functions of the cell membrane. This is a complex and speculative subject, but it seems to us that four functions can usefully be distinguished, namely, support, transport, cognition-reaction, and defense. We shall concern ourselves here only with the last two.

For the cells of multicellular organisms to perform their great diversity of functions, they must respond appropriately to each of the various intercellular environments to which they are exposed. The consequences of imperfect response are cell death, structural abnormality, or the overgrowth that we call cancer. There is a growing, though still very limited, body of evidence that the cell membrane plays a major role in governing this response. It is to this function of the membrane that we have applied the term cognition-reaction. By cognition-reaction we mean any response of the cell membrane to any aspect of the environment which in turn influences cell behavior. Most instances of cognition-reaction are probably governed by cell-to-cell contact, but interaction of the plasma membrane with the surrounding medium, *e.g.,* with specific hormones, also plays a role. We can cite here only two examples. Intravenously infused isogeneic thymocytes show a strong tendency to migrate out of the blood stream and into the lymph nodes and spleen. Berney and Gesner [35] have shown that thymocytes treated with neuraminidase, on the contrary, localize primarily in the liver. Presumably one or more sugars on the cell surface control or initiate this particular cognition-reaction of this particular category of cell. Contact inhibition provides the second example. Normal cells in tissue culture remain in single layers; cancer cells climb over one another and form multiple layers [36]. Mouse embryo cells maintained in tissue culture for 200 generations under conditions that minimize cell contact, do not loose the faculty of contact inhibition and do not become tumorogenic. Crowded cells do undergo these changes [37]. The cell surface is probably the controlling factor in these phenomena.

As a defensive structure, it is the function of the cell membrane to prevent the penetration of viruses, and to circumvent molecular mimicry of cell surface antigens by bacteria and other parasites. At least, these are the two functions that we know something about. Both of them are served by membrane polymorphism. If all houses have the same lock, the robber has no difficulty solving thè problem of entry. The evolution of diverse defenses requires a corresponding evolution of diverse attacks. We have reviewed this subject elsewhere [38] and at most can bring a few points up to date.

We have speculated that cell membrane alloantigens may play a role in viral penetration of the membrane; Crittenden *et al.* have shown that in at least one instance in poultry this is the case [39]. A dominant gene for susceptibility to early steps of cellular infection by subgroup B avian leukosis-sarcoma viruses is associated with the presence of an erythrocyte alloantigen. This gene appears to control both an alloantigen and a cell membrane receptor for an oncogenic virus.

The *H-2* locus seems to play a role in the later stages of susceptibility to viral oncogenesis [40]. This makes it unlikely that the *H-2* alloantigen is acting as a virus receptor. As we pointed out earlier [38], there are suggestive similarities between the relationship of *H-2* to viral tumor induction and the relation of McDevitt's closely associated *Ir-1* locus [41] to the immune response. The big question is whether this Ir effect is in fact an expression of *H-2* itself or whether it is due to a distinct locus just outside the *H-2* region or perhaps included within the D and K ends of *H-2*. Until this question is answered, any speculations start from very uncertain premises. It is perhaps significant that *H-4* and *H-7*, like *H-2*, affect viral leukemogenesis [42]. But this action is much weaker and probably occurs at an earlier stage. Whether or not *Ir* genes are an expression of *H* loci, they are quite likely to prove important in many infectious diseases. They seem to be turning up in a variety of contexts. If *Ir-1* is distinct from *H-2*, there is nevertheless quite possibly some significance in its association with *H-2*. We pointed out that the presence of the remarkable *T* locus in the IXth linkage group about 10 crossover units from *H-2* serves as a device for keeping this whole chromosome region heterozygous [38]. We suggested that there would be a selective advantage in the accumulation in this chromosome segment of other loci for which polymorphism is selectively beneficial. Quite possibly *Ir-1* belongs in this category.

Addendum

AKR/Cum, unlike other AKR sublines, is *Thy-2* (θ-C3H). (Schlesinger, M., and D. Hurvitz. 1969. Characterization of cytotoxic isoantisera produced in RIII mice. Transplantation 7:132-141.)

References

[1] The Committee on Standardized Genetic Nomenclature for Mice, J. Hered. 54 (1963) 159.
[2] G.D. Snell, *In:* Internat. Symp. on relationships between tumor antigens and histocompatibility systems, Paris, Transplantation Proc. 3 (1971) 1133.

[3] G.D. Snell, G. Hoecker, D.B. Amos and J.H. Stimpfling, Transplantation 2 (1964) 777.

[4] G.D. Snell, G. Cudkowicz and H.P. Bunker, Transplantation 5 (1967) 492.

[5] D.W. Bailey, Transplantation 1 (1963) 70.

[6] E.J. Eichwald, C.R. Silmser and I. Weissman, J. Natl. Cancer Inst. 20 (1958) 563.

[7] D.W. Bailey, First Internat. Cong. Transplantation Soc. p. 212 (1967)

[8] D.W. Bailey and L.E. Mobraaten, Transplantation 7 (1969) 394.

[9] D.W. Bailey, Transplantation 11 (1971) 325.

[10] D.B. Amos, M. Zumpft and P. Armstrong, Transplantation 1 (1963) 270.

[11] I.K. Egorov, Genetika, Mosk. 6 (1965) 80.

[12] M. Foster, M.L. Petras and D.L. Gasser, Proc. XII Internat. Cong. of Genetics, Vol. 1, p. 245.

[13] J. Klein and J. Martinkova, Folia Biol. 14 (1968) 237.

[14] D.M. Popp, Transplantation 5 (1967) 290.

[15] D. M. Popp, Transplantation 7 (1969) 233.

[16] D.C. Shreffler, Genetics 54 (1966) 362.

[17] G.D. Snell, G. Hoecker and J.H. Stimpfling, Transplantation 5 (1967) 481.

[18] J.H. Stimpfling and G.D. Snell, Transplantation 6 (1968) 468.

[19] F. Lilly, Transplantation 5 (1967) 83.

[20] E.A. Boyse, L.J. Old and E. Stockert, *In:* P. Grabar and P.A. Miescher (eds.), Immunopathology, IVth Internat. Symp. (New York) p. 23 (1965).

[21] E.A. Boyse, M. Miyazawa, T. Aoki and L.J. Old, Proc. Roy. Soc. Biol. 170 (1968) 175.

[22] M. Cherry and G.D. Snell, Transplantation 8 (1969) 319.

[23] E.A. Boyse, K. Itakura, E. Stockert, C.A. Iritani and M. Miura, Transplantation 11 (1971) 351.

[24] A.E. Reif and J.M.V. Allen, J. Exptl. Med. 120 (1964) 413.

[25] M.C. Raff and H.H. Wortis, Immunology 18 (1970) 931.

[26] M.C. Raff, Nature 226 (1970) 1257.

[27] T. Takahashi, L.J. Old and E.A. Boyse, J. Exptl. Med. 131 (1970) 1325.

[28] A.E. Reif and J.M. Allen, Nature 209 (1966) 521.

[29] M.F. Singer, M. Foster, M.L. Petras, P. Tomlin and R.W. Sloan, Genetics 50 (1964) 285.

[30] J. Staats, *In:* E.L. Green (ed.), The biology of the laboratory mouse, 2nd ed. (McGraw-Hill, New York, 1966) p. 1-9.

[31] R.J. Graff and G.D. Snell, Transplantation 8 (1969) 861.

[32] R.J. Graff, S.L. Polinsky and G.D. Snell, Transplantation 11 (1971) 56.

[33] J. Klein, Science 168 (1970) 1362.

[34] R.J. Graff, Transplant. Proc. 2 (1970) 15.

[35] S.N. Berney and B.M. Gesner, Immunology 18 (1970) 681.

[36] H. Rubin, *In:* M. Locke (ed.), Major problems in developmental biology (Academic Press, N.Y., 1966) p. 315-337.

[37] S.A. Aaronson and G.J. Todaro, Science 162 (1968) 1024.

[38] G.D. Snell, Folia Biol. 14 (1968) 335.

[39] L.E. Crittenden, W.E. Briles and H.A. Stone, Science 169 (1970) 1324.

[40] F. Lilly, *In:* S. Cohen, M. Cudkowicz and R.T. McCluskey (eds.), Cellular interactions in the immune response (S. Karger, New York, 1971).

[41] H.O. McDevitt and B. Benacerraf, Adv. Immun. 11 (1969) 31.

[42] A. Axelrad, *In:* J.F. Morgan (ed.), Proc. Eighth Canadian Cancer Research Conference, Honey Harbour, Ont. (Pergamon Press, 1969) p. 313.

ANTIGEN EXPRESSION ON SPLEEN CELLS
OF FRIEND VIRUS-INFECTED MICE[1]

Frank LILLY

Department of Genetics, Albert Einstein College of Medicine,
Bronx, N.Y. 10461, U.S.A.

In mice, H-2 genotype is a major determinant of the outcome of infection with any of several oncogenic murine RNA viruses [1-5]. In the search for insights into the mechanism of this effect of H-2, it seems reasonable to consider as strong candidates for investigation those aspects of leukemogenesis related to membrane phenomena, since the H-2 alloantigens themselves are membrane markers.

One such phenomenon is the appearance on the surfaces of infected cells of antigens presumably synthesized under the direction of the viral genome [6-7]. These substances have been referred to as tumor-specific transplantation antigens, although this nomenclature has begun to seem unsatisfactory: strictly speaking the appearance of these antigens seems to signify more that the cells bearing them are productively infected with the virus than that they have necessarily been transformed by the virus.

In the course of studies of the FMR antigen [8], detected abundantly on spleen cells of susceptible BALB/c mice inoculated with the F-B strain of Friend virus, we noted that such infected spleen cells tended to give reliable and reproducible results when used as targets for the assay of cytotoxic anti-FMR antisera only when the target cell donor had received the virus 7 to 14 days previously. The antigen was generally demonstrable on the cells by day 4, but the overall level of sensitivity of the cells to the cytotoxic effect of the antiserum was often not fully developed for 2-3 more days. However, it was puzzling that after day 14, the cells seemed to show a reduced sensitivity to

[1] The technical assistance of Messrs Richard L. Coley and Horace Graham is gratefully acknowledged. These studies were supported by a contract (65-612) within the Special Virus-Cancer Program of the National Cancer Institute, United States Public Health Service. I am a recipient of a Career Scientist Award of the Health Research Council of the City of New York, contract I-512.

229

lysis by the antiserum, as judged by the antibody-directed release from them of ^{51}Cr label.

This paper summarizes our investigation of this phenomenon of the appearance followed by the apparent H-2-associated loss of FMR antigen. activity from spleen cells as a function of time after inoculation with Friend virus.

Loss of cytotoxic sensitivity to anti-FMR and anti-H-2.31 antisera

We inoculated a group of 6 to 9 week old BALB/c mice intraperitoneally with a standard, strong dose of F-B virus (a BALB/c-adapted, NB-tropic strain of Friend virus); at intervals thereafter these mice were used three at a time as individual spleen cell donors for the titration of antisera by the ^{51}Cr-release method [9,10]. In this first experiment, we examined sensitivity to two antisera: anti-FMR (BALB/c anti-F-B virus) and anti-H-2.31 (an anti-BALB/c sarcoma Meth A, which monospecifically identifies specificity 31 of the K region of the H-2^d haplotype). Figure 1 illustrates the results, each line representing the mean values in three parallel titrations of the same antiserum on spleen cells of individual mice.

Sensitivity to anti-FMR serum was, of course, nil on day 0 (virus-free mice) and was still very low on day 4 after virus inoculation. During the second week after infection, sensitivity to anti-FMR was at maximum levels, but from day 18 the level of cytotoxic sensitivity declined significantly. This decline reflected both a decrease in the apparent titer of the antiserum (by a factor of >3) and a decrease in the maximum percentage of cells lysed by the antiserum.

The inclusion of anti-H-2.31 serum in this initial study of cytotoxic sensitivity was conceived as a control for the anti-FMR serum, since we had no reason to expect a significant variation in this sensitivity as a function of time after virus inoculation. The results, however, indicated that sensitivity to anti-H-2.31 increased slightly between day 0 and day 7 and thereafter decreased even more rapidly and to a greater extent than in the case of anti-FMR.

In general the rates of disappearance of cytotoxic sensitivity to these two antisera tend to be about the same; i.e., anti-FMR sensitivity often decreases somewhat faster than seen in this first experiment, whereas anti-H-2.31 sensitivity may decrease more slowly and less completely than seen here. However, there is *no* absolute correlation of the two rates of decline in individual mice.

It is relevant, also, to correlate this decline in cytotoxicity with the progress of the Friend virus disease syndrome in these mice. Splenomegaly, which is the

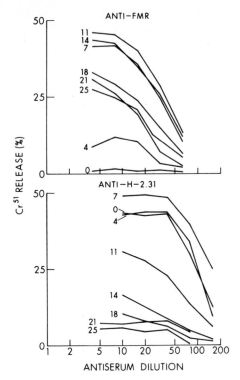

Fig. 1. Titration of anti-FMR and of anti-H-2.31 antisera by the ^{51}Cr-release method on spleen cells of BALB/c mice inoculated with the F-B strain of Friend virus. Each line represents the mean of the results from three spleen cell donors infected with virus the indicated number of days previously, and the same spleen cell preparations were used for both sets of titrations.

major gross symptom of the disease, proceeds as a regular, logarithmic increase in spleen weight during the interval from approximately day 3-4 through day 11-14 after large virus doses [8]. Thereafter spleen weight abruptly ceases to increase and may even decline somewhat. Usually the animals do not begin to look sick until around day 14, and the majority of them die between days 21 and 28, although a few may survive longer. It thus appears that a major qualitative change in the character of the disease begins to manifest itself around day 14, approximately the time when the loss of cell membrane antigens begins to be detectable.

This loss of sensitivity to cytotoxic antisera appears to be due to the loss from the membrane surface of the corresponding antigens, as demonstrated by the technique of quantitative absorption of the antisera with spleen cells. Figure 2 shows the results of one such experiment, again using as spleen cell

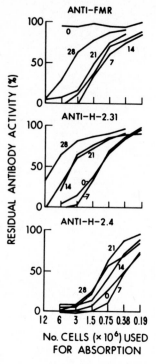

Fig. 2. Quantitative absorption of three antisera — anti-FMR, anti-H-2.31 and anti-H-2.4 — with spleen cells of BALB/c mice infected with F-B virus the indicated number of days previously. Counted numbers of cells from each of three donors were tested in parallel with each antiserum, and each line represents the mean of the three tests.

donors BALB/c mice inoculated with F-B virus at different intervals prior to the absorption studies. This experiment included a third antiserum, in addition to the same two used in the first experiment: anti-H-2.4 [(C57BL/6 x C3H/Bi) F_1 anti-A strain normal lymphoid tissues, which identifies alloantigen specificities 4 and 13 of the D region of the H-2^d haplotype]. As in the previous experiment, each line in the figure represents the mean value from three individual spleen cell preparations.

These results indicate that the number of antibody-accessible FMR antigen sites on spleen cells decreased significantly in the late stage of the Friend disease syndrome. The number of H-2.31 sites also decreased at an even faster rate on these same cells, but the number of H-2.4,13 sites on these cells decreased only slightly during this same period.

The isoantigens H-2.31 and H-2.4 map in closely linked subregions of the H-2 locus [11], but they are separable by rare recombination events. In previous studies of susceptibility to the Gross leukemia virus, the H-2 effect on leukemogenesis (Rgv-1) was found to be associated with the K region of H-2, where the determinant of H-2.31 maps, whereas the D region, the sublocus determining antigen H-2.4, appeared to be irrelevant to the phenomenon of leukemogenesis [12]. That this K region Rgv-1 locus is also the exact site of the H-2-associated influence on Friend virus susceptibility has not yet been directly demonstrated, but on the assumption that this is true, it may be of importance that the K region antigen 31 disappeared to a far greater extent than did the D region antigen 4.

Comparison of BALB/c and BALB.B mice

Earlier studies [3] of the effect of H-2 on the course of the Friend virus disease involved segregating generations of crosses of unrelated susceptible and resistant mouse strains. We have now partially completed, for the continuation of these studies, the breeding of a new congenic strain of mice, BALB/c-H-2^b (N7), hereafter called the BALB.B strain. It differs from the BALB/c strain H-2^d) almost exclusively with respect to its homozygosity for the region of linkage group IX bearing the H-2^b haplotype derived from C57BL/6, so that any differences observed in the pair of strains can be attributed with high probability to this difference in H-2 genotype.

BALB/c-grown F-B virus was titrated in matched animals of both strains by the spleen focus-formation assay [13], which is a measure of infectious centers induced by the given virus dose and which thus reflects largely the early events following virus inoculation. The titration curves obtained showed that BALB.B mice were less susceptible than BALB/c mice, but by a factor of less than 2 — a difference of minimal statistical significance.

When the same virus preparation was again titrated, this time by the criterion of splenomegaly in mice of the two congenic strains during a one-month observation period, a considerably more pronounced difference was seen. BALB.B mice appeared less susceptible to splenomegaly induction than BALB/c mice by a virus-dose factor of 10 or more. These findings seem to confirm our earlier conclusion that the H-2 effect on the Friend virus syndrome does not occur during the early events of cellular infection by the virus, but rather at some later stage in the evolution of the disease [3].

We then compared the time-course of cytotoxic sensitivity to anti-FMR and to selected anti-H-2 antisera in the two congenic strains of mice inoculated with a standard F-B virus dose. Spleen cells of BALB/c mice were again tested for sensitivity to anti-FMR, anti-H-2.31 and anti-H-2.4; spleen cells of BALB.B were tested for sensitivity to the same anti-FMR serum and to anti-H-2.33 [(B10.A × HTG) F_1 anti-C57BL leukemia E.L.4, which monospecifically identifies specificity 33 of the K region* of the H-2^b haplotype] and anti-H-2.2 [(BALB/c × HTI) F_1 anti-E.L.4, which monospecifically identifies specificity 2 of the D region of the H-2^b haplotype].

The data from these numerous cytotoxic assays were analyzed by computer (program devised in collaboration with Messrs Joseph Okun and Robert Curci) and are represented as mean cytotoxic titers in figure 3. Findings in BALB/c

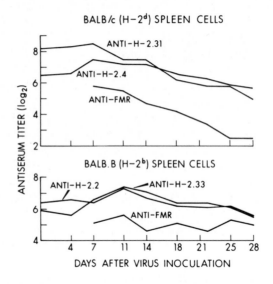

Fig. 3. Mean cytotoxic titers of antisera on spleen cells of F-B virus-infected BALB/c (H-2^d) and BALB.B (H-2^b) mice as a function of time after virus inoculation. The same anti-FMR serum was tested on both types of mice; the two anti-H-2 sera tested on each mouse strain detect a D region (anti-H-2.4 and anti-H-2.2) and a K region (anti-H-2.31 and anti-H-2.33) antigen of the H-2^d and H-2^b haplotypes, respectively.

---

*Whereas it appears reasonable to assume that the D region determinants of antigens H-2.2 and H-2.4 are in a true sense allelic to each other, there are reasons to suspect that the determinant of H-2.33 might not be strictly allelic with the K region determinant of antigen H-2.31. It is possible that *no* allelic equivalent of H-2.31 occurs in the H-2^b haplotype.

mice differed little from those of earlier experiments: sensitivity to anti-FMR and to anti-H-2.31 declined markedly and consistently from the second through the fourth week after virus inoculation; sensitivity to anti-H-2.4 declined only slightly in these same spleen cell preparations. By contrast, cytotoxic sensitivity to all three antisera tested on BALB.B spleen cells varied very little during the same time interval after virus inoculation.

Let us stress that the FMR antigen appeared on spleen cells of BALB/c and of BALB.B mice following virus infection at about the same rate, and that the level of antigen expression observed in both mice during the second week was very similar. The difference in the two kinds of mice, then, occurred thereafter and involved in H-2^d spleen cells the gradual loss of FMR antigen expression and simultaneously a similar loss of a K region H-2 antigen. H-2^b spleen cells showed no comparable loss of either the FMR antigen or the H-2 antigens tested.

Antigen expression on cells of a solid tumor line derived from a BALB/c mouse with Friend virus-induced leukemia

Buffett and Furth [14] and Friend and Haddad [15] showed that is was possible to establish lines of transplantable solid tumors by transferring fragments of spleen or liver from Friend virus-infected mice subcutaneously into normal, isogeneic recipients. However, this maneuver was generally successful only if the tissue donor was in a very *late* stage of the disease syndrome. In this case, not only did cells of the transplanted tissue proliferate *in situ* so that serial transfer was possible, but also a quantity of virus was transmitted along with the tumor tissue, so that a new primary infection developed simultaneously in the recipient. If, on the other hand, this tissue transfer was done using as donors mice in the *early* stages of the disease syndrome, the tissue fragments rarely proliferated and gave rise to solid tumors, although the virus contained in the inoculum induced the original disease again in the recipients.

The cells of such solid tumors might be considered as the ultimate progeny of those spleen cells in Friend virus-infected mice which we could examine only for about one month after infection, because the host rarely survived much longer than this. Proceeding on this working hypothesis, we established such a Friend virus-induced solid tumor line of BALB/c origin, and after 16 serial transfers we examined mechanically dispersed cells of the tumor for sensitivity to anti-FMR, anti-H-2.31 and anti-H-2.4. In the same experiment we compared the sensitivity to the same antisera of spleen cells from the same BALB/c mouse which provided the solid tumor cells and also spleen cells from a BALB/c mouse infected with cell-free F-B virus 8 days previously.

Cells of the solid tumor line were entirely resistant to cytolysis by anti-FMR serum (figure 4); spleen cells from the autochthonous host (which had a moderately enlarged spleen) were sensitive to anti-FMR serum, although at a considerably lower level than were spleen cells from the primary virus-infected mouse. With regard to their response to anti-H-2.31 and anti-H-2.4, solid tumor cells showed less cytotoxic sensitivity than autochthonous spleen cells, but the difference was small.

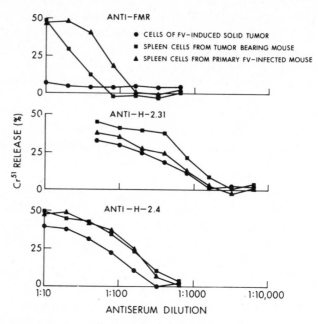

Fig. 4. Titration of three antisera on (1) cells of a transplanted solid tumor line derived from the spleen of BALB/c mouse with advanced Friend virus disease, (2) spleen cells from the same mouse used as donor of the solid tumor cells, and (3) a BALB/c mouse infected 8 days previously with cell-free F-B virus.

Discussion and summary

BALB/c ($H-2^d$) mice infected with F-B virus acquire whithin one week a new antigen specificity, FMR, demonstrable on their spleen cells by the use of antisera which lyse the antigen-bearing cells. Previous studies showed that, during the second week after infection, about 90 percent of the spleen cells sensitive to cytolysis by anti-H-2 sera were also sensitive to lysis by anti-FMR, indicating that the two antigens or sets of antigens coexist on the same cells [8].

However, it appears that the level of expression of FMR does not remain constant thereafter in the course of the disease, but rather that the antigen tends to disappear from the spleen cells during the third and fourth weeks after infection. Simultaneously, the K region antigen H-2.31 tends to disappear from these cells at about the same time and at the same rate or even faster. The level of expression of the D region antigen H-2.4 decreased only slightly during this same period of time. In the case of congenic BALB.B (H-2^b) mice, which are about equally susceptible to initial virus infection as BALB/c mice but significantly less susceptible to the disease syndrome induced by the virus, neither the FMR antigen nor any H-2 antigen tested decreased significantly on spleen cells.

The evidence that H-2 genotype apparently determines whether or not the FMR antigen remains at a high level or disappears leads to an obvious hypothesis concerning the mechanism of the H-2 influence on viral leuke- mogenesis. Perhaps, precisely because FMR levels remain high in H-2^b mice, these animals can more readily reject the cells by means of an immunological response to the antigen; by contrast, the same type and level of immune response in H-2^d mice might be less effective in overcoming the infected cells because these cells have become relatively resistant to the antibodies.

There is at present no obvious explanation for these changes in membrane antigen concentration. One would like to know if the antigen loss in the spleen occurred because the cells which possessed FMR gradually ceased to show it, or if a new cell population which perhaps never possessed the FMR antigen gradually replaced the antigen-bearing cell population. It is necessary to ask if the FMR antigen loss is due to its no longer being made by the cells, or if it is simply being masked in some manner, as perhaps by blocking, non-cytotoxic antibodies. The fact that our cytotoxic anti-FMR serum is routinely produced in BALB/c mice does not mean that they always produce such antibodies under different conditions of virus challenge. Finally, any such loss of antigen expression must evoke the phenomenon of antigenic modulation [16]; although some parallels could be drawn with the antibody-directed loss of TL antigens from leukemic cells, it is far from clear that the loss of FMR and of H-2.31 is an analogous process.

The apparent loss of a normal alloantigen, H-2.31, during the evolution of the Friend virus disease is a striking phenomenon. Since both FMR and H-2.31 are present concurrently at maximum levels on spleen cells about day 7 after infection, there is no reason to assume that they compete for the same site on the membrane, although a careful appraisal of their respective placement with respect to each other on the membrane surface [17] is in order. Nevertheless, it is difficult to believe that the simultaneous disappearance of the two antigens is

F. Lilly

entirely fortuitous, especially in view of the very close association of Rgv-1
with the K region of H-2. Thus the possibility exists that further studies of this
phenomenon will reveal the basic mechanism of the H-2 effect in viral
leukemogenesis.

References

[1] F. Lilly, E.A. Boyse and L.J. Old, Lancet ii (1964) 1207.
[2] J.R. Tennant and G.D. Snell, J. Natl. Cancer Inst. 41 (1968) 597.
[3] F. Lilly, J. Exptl. Med. 127 (1968) 465.
[4] S. Nandi, Proc. Natl. Acad. Sci. U.S. 58 (1967) 485.
[5] O. Mühlbock and A. Dux, Transpl. Proc. 3 (1971) 1247.
[6] L.J. Old and E.A. Boyse, Ann. Rev. Med. 15 (1964) 167.
[7] L.J. Old and E.A. Boyse, Federation Proc. 24 (1965) 1009.
[8] F. Lilly and S.G. Nathenson, Transpl. Proc. 1 (1969) 85.
[9] A.R. Sanderson, Brit. J. Exptl. Pathol. 45 (1964) 398.
[10] H. Wigzell, Transpl. 3 (1965) 423.
[11] D.C. Shreffler and J. Klein, Transpl. Proc. 2 (1970) 5.
[12] F. Lilly, Comparative Leukemia Research 1969 (S. Karger, Basel, 1970) p. 213.
[13] A.A. Axelrad and R.A. Steeves, Virology 24 (1964) 513.
[14] R.F. Buffett and J. Furth, Cancer Res. 19 (1959) 1063.
[15] C. Friend and J.R. Haddad, J. Natl. Cancer Inst. 25 (1960) 1279.
[16] E.A. Boyse, E. Stockert and L.J. Old, Proc. Natl. Acad. Sci. U.S. 58 (1967) 954.
[17] E.A. Boyse, L.J. Old and E. Stockert, Proc. Natl. Acad. Sci. U.S. 60 (1968) 886.

HOST CELL SUSCEPTIBILITY AND RESISTANCE
TO MURINE LEUKEMIA VIRUSES
AND THEIR GENETIC CONTROL*

A.A. AXELRAD, M. WARE and H.C. VAN DER GAAG

Division of Histology, Department of Anatomy,
University of Toronto, Canada

Introduction

In 1962, Odaka and Yamamoto [1] reported that a single major autosomal gene controls susceptibility to Friend leukemia virus (FV) in mice. The animals were scored as susceptible (RF strain) or resistant (C57BL/6 = B6 strain) on the basis of their spleen weights and number of nucleated cells in the peripheral blood 3 weeks after FV infection. Susceptibility appeared to be dominant over resistance at this locus. Odaka has since named the locus Fv [2]. The introduction of the spleen focus assay method [3] made it possible to score animals for their response to FV at 9 days after infection i.e. before they had developed disseminated disease. With this method, it was found by Odaka and ourselves [4-6] that the level of susceptibility of heterozygotes was intermediate between that of the susceptible and that of the resistant parent strain, and so it was concluded that the alleles for susceptibility and resistance at this locus were codominant. However, in other respects the data of both groups were in complete accord with the original hypothesis of Odaka and Yamamoto that FV-susceptibility and resistance are controlled primarily at a single autosomal gene locus.

To investigate this locus, it was evident that it would be useful to have the allele controlling FV-resistance and the allele controlling FV-susceptibility on the genetic background of each of the 2 parental strains. Therefore Odaka in Tokyo and we in Toronto each set about to produce 2 pairs of congenic strains which would differ at the locus that controlled the host response to FV. In what follows, my purpose will be to review what we have learned about the

*We acknowledge the excellent technical assistance of Mrs. Lottie Viezel and Miss Pat Doran. This work was supported by grants from the National Cancer Institute of Canada and from the Fraternal Order of Eagles through the Canadian Cancer Society.

239

genetic control of host cell responses to murine leukemia viruses *in vivo* and *in vitro* in the course of production and analysis of these congenic strains.

Production of FV-susceptible and FV-resistant congenic strains

Two series of backcrosses were carried out, one to the SIM strain, with repeated selection for FV-resistance, and the other to the B6 strain, with repeated selection for FV-susceptibility (fig. 1). At each generation, progeny tests were

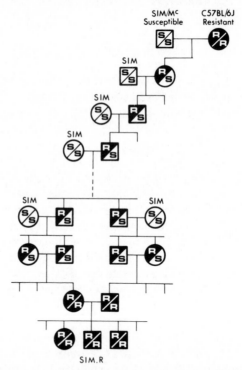

Fig. 1. Breeding and selection scheme used for introducing the FV-resistance allele R from the B6 (C57BL/6) strain into the genetic background of the FV-susceptible SIM strain, to produce the congenic strain SIM.R which differs from its SIM partner strain at an autosomal gene locus that controls the spleen focus response to Friend leukemia virus.

done and on the basis of these, presumptive genotypes were assigned to the parents. The breeding was then carried on with parents selected on the basis of these genotypes. The production of the SIM.R strain, carrying the allele for FV resistance from the B6 strain, and congenic with the susceptible SIM strain, will be discussed first. Since large doses of FV were used to test the progeny, those that were as susceptible as their SIM parents had confluent foci on their spleens. We made the decision at the beginning of the study to score as resistant any animal whose spleen did not have confluent foci. This turned out later to be a good decision. The progeny tests consistently gave 1:1 ratios for those that were apparently heterozygous and those that were apparently homozygous for FV-susceptibility [7]. After 8 such backcrosses, presumptive heterozygotes were intercrossed, and the genotypes of their progeny were determined by backcrossing them to SIM strain mice and testing the offspring with virus. Three classes were found: families in which all members were of intermediate susceptibility to FV, signifying that the parent was homozygous for resistance; those in which the members were all susceptible, signifying that the parent was homozygous for susceptibility; and those composed of both types i.e. in which the parent was heterozygous. The fact that in this intercross it was possible to recover mice homozygous for FV-resistance and mice homozygous for FV-susceptibility, both of which have since bred true constituted a reliable test for validity of the hypothesis that resistance to FV is under single gene control: the SIM.R and SIM strains could thus be regarded as congenic partners, with the allele for FV-resistance from the B6 strain having been incorporated into the genetic background of the SIM strain.

In order to have the allele from the SIM strain that controls FV-susceptibility on the genetic background of the B6 strain, we also repeated the breeding procedure in the reverse direction. In this instance we scored as susceptible any mouse whose spleen showed one focus or more, since the B6 parent strain was solidly resistant and never showed any foci, and since less than one focus could not be scored on an individual spleen.

The breeding scheme we used is shown in fig. 2. Initially, a mouse apparently homozygous for susceptibility was produced as one of the F_2 progeny of the cross between SIM and B6. This mouse was backcrossed to the B6 strain, and one of its apparently heterozygous progeny was again backcrossed to B6. This procedure was repeated until 7 backcrosses to the B6 strain, with selection for the heterozygote at each generation, had been produced. Then 2 presumptive heterozygotes were intercrossed. The progeny were tested by backcrosses to the B6 strain. Presumptive homozygotes for FV-susceptibility were selected and inbreeding was carried out with these. Tests on their progeny showed that these mice were breeding true for susceptibility for Friend virus; the B6.S and B6 strains could thus be regarded as congenic partners, with the allele for FV-susceptibility from the SIM strain having been incorporated into the genetic background of the B6 strain.

Table 1
Spleen focus responses of congenic strain mice to Friend leukemia virus (F-T).

Experiment	Dose of FV (FFU)*	No. of foci/spleen (mean ± S.E.)			
		SIM	SIM.R	B6	B6.S
C-33 B	6	5.4 ± 1.3			
	12	11.7 ± 2.5			
	120	Confluent	0		
	1200		1.6 ± 0.6	0	
	12000		6 to confluent	0	
C-54	1250				25.0 ± 19.7

*As assayed in SIM mice.

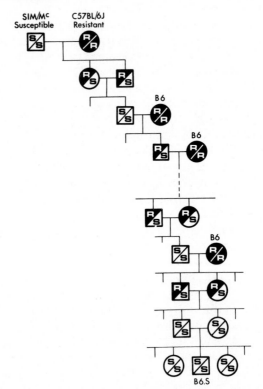

Fig. 2. Breeding and selection scheme used for introducing the FV-susceptibility allele S from the SIM strain into the genetic background of the solidly FV-resistant B6 strain, to produce the congenic strain B6.S, which differs from its B6 partner strain at an autosomal gene locus that controls the spleen focus response to Friend leukemia virus.

Responses of congenic strain mice to Friend virus

To determine the levels of susceptibility of the congenic partners to FV, known doses of the Toronto strain (F-T) of the virus were injected i.v. into the animals and their spleens were scored for foci 9 days later. The data obtained in 2 experiments are shown in table 1. They show that the SIM.R strain is resistant to the F-T strain of FV, and that the resistance is not absolute but relative, its susceptibility being about 750-fold lower than that of the SIM strain. The data also show that mice of the B6 strain developed no spleen foci even when given 12000 FFU of FV. In contrast, the B6.S congenic partner strain was clearly susceptible.

In the course of repeated backcrossing to the B6 strain with selection for susceptibility to spleen focus formation by FV, data from progeny tests made at each generation seemed to be at variance with the hypothesis that control of FV susceptibility resided at a single gene locus. Instead of the genotypic ratios in the (SIM x B6)F_1 x B6 backcrosses being 1:1, they were closer to 1:2. This led to the suspicion that more than one locus might be involved in the control of FV susceptibility [7]. Whether this was actually due to the operation of more than one gene could not, however, be determined at the time.

Genetic analysis of congenic strains

If one locus controlled the difference in susceptibility to FV between the SIM and B6 strains, then strain B6.S, homozygous for the susceptibility allele, should be as susceptible to FV as the SIM strain. That this is not the case is seen in table 1. The SIM strain seems, in fact, to be about 50 times as susceptible to FV as the B6.S strain. Similarly, if one locus controlled resistance to FV, then strain SIM.R, homozygous for the resistance allele, should be as resistant as the B6 strain. This is also not the case. B6 mice were apparently solidly resistant to the focus-forming action of the virus, while SIM.R mice gave low but definite focus-forming titers (table 1). It therefore seems that the simplest hypothesis to account for our data is that the difference between the SIM and B6 strains with respect to susceptibility to FV is controlled at more than one locus.

If 2 loci are considered responsible for the difference in FV susceptibility between the SIM and B6 strains, then the question follows: In the production of the SIM.R strain congenic with SIM and of the B6.S strain congenic with B6, was the gene locus isolated the same in both, or different?

To try to answer this question we examined the dominance relationships among the congenic strains and their partners. A series of crosses were carried out between the various strains and the FV susceptibility of the F_1 progeny was compared with that of either parent strain. (SIM.R x SIM)F_1 hybrids were found to behave like SIM.R (table 2); thus R was in this case dominant. (B6 x B6.S)F_1 hybrids behaved like B6.S (table 3); therefore S was in this case dominant. It can also be seen that the F_1 progeny of the cross B6 x SIM.R were no more resistant than were SIM.R mice (table 4). Thus the SIM strain must contribute a gene for susceptibility, and it must be dominant to whatever is contributed by B6.

Table 2

Relative sensitivities of congenic mice and their F_1 hybrids to Friend leukemia virus (F-T) *in vivo* (exp. C56).

Strain	Spleen focus-forming efficiency (FFU/ml)
SIM	$6.0 \pm 2.8 \times 10^4$
SIM.R	$1.1 \pm 0.2 \times 10^2$
(SIM.R × SIM)F_1	$4.1 \pm 1.1 \times 10^2$

Table 3

Relative sensitivities of congenic mice and their F_1 hybrids to Friend leukemia virus (F-T) *in vivo* (expts. C 48,54).

Strain	Spleen focus-forming efficiency (FFU/ml)
B6	0
B6.S	$2.0 \pm 1.0 \times 10^3$
(B6 × B6.S)F_1	$9.8 \pm 2.1 \times 10^2$

Table 4

Relative sensitivities of congenic mice and their F_1 hybrids to Friend leukemia virus (F-T) *in vivo* (exp. C50).

Strain	Spleen focus-forming efficiency (FFU/ml)
SIM.R	$2.3 \pm 0.9 \times 10^2$
(B6 × SIM.R)F_1	$2.1 \pm 0.6 \times 10^2$

The picture that emerges is that the difference between the SIM and B6 strains with respect to FV susceptibility appears to be best accounted for by the hypothesis that 2 loci are involved. At one locus, resistance is dominant and relative, and it is at this locus that SIM.R differs from SIM. At the other locus, susceptibility is dominant and it is at this locus that B6.S differs from B6. The resistance of B6 is absolute.

It is of interest that what previously appeared as single locus control of the response to FV in crosses, backcrosses and inter-crosses between SIM and B6 parental strains, with susceptibility and resistance behaving as codominant alleles, can now be explained on the basis of this concept. It can be shown that if 2 gene loci are responsible for a phenotypic character, and the negative allele (*e.g.* resistance) is dominant at one locus and recessive at the other, while the positive allele (*e.g.* susceptibility) behaves in reciprocal fashion, then the phenotypic ratios turn out to be indistinguishable from those that are seen if a single gene locus controls the character and the alleles at that locus are codominant.

In the production of our 2 congenic strain pairs, the fact that in both instances it was the dominant, rather than the recessive, allele at each locus that was transferred to the background of the other strain was a consequence of the breeding and selection scheme we used. At each backcross generation, to select a parent that carried the gene for resistance, the progeny test we used was a backcross to the susceptible SIM strain. If the allele for resistance were recessive, it would not have been detected. Similarly, at each backcross generation, to select a parent that carried the gene for susceptibility, the progeny test we used was a backcross to the resistant B6 strain. Dominance of the susceptibility allele thus ensured its transfer to the B6 background.

When Odaka tested his congenic strains derived from the FV-susceptible strain DDD and the FV-resistant strain B6 [2,8], the data he obtained did not agree with ours. His 2 pairs of congenic partners appeared to differ from each other with regard to FV-susceptibility at a single gene locus; susceptibility was dominant at this locus, and resistance was absolute.

To unravel this involved situation we must go back in time and follow another line of investigation.

Control of FV-induced spleen focus formation by two gene loci

In 1967, Lilly [9] reported the isolation of 2 strains of FV that differed in their host strain specificity although they gave the same disease and were antigenically indistinguishable. The first of these he called F-S virus; it gave high titers by the spleen focus assay method in Swiss ICR and DBA/2 but very low titers in BALB/c mice. The second strain of FV was derived from the F-S strain by passage through BALB/c mice, which were relatively resistant to the parental strain virus; he called this F-B virus. F-B virus behaved like F-S except that it could produce high spleen focus titers in BALB/c mice. Neither the F-S virus nor the F-B virus gave spleen foci in B6 mice.

Lilly tested the spleen focus response to the 2 virus strains in the progeny of crosses and backcrosses between the DBA/2 and the B6 strains [10]. The data he obtained clearly fitted a 2-gene model. Lilly named the loci Fv-1 and Fv-2. At first it seemed as if Fv-1 was concerned with control of the host response to F-S virus, and Fv-2 with control of the host response to F-B virus. At Fv-1, resistance to the F-S strain of FV was dominant; at Fv-2, susceptibility to the F-B strain of FV was dominant. However, The Fv-2 locus also seemed to have a strong influence on the response to F-S virus, but the Fv-1 locus had no influence on the response to F-B virus. Further clarification of this situation came from work in tissue culture.

Identification of loci isolated in congenic FV-susceptible and FV-resistant strains

In 1970, Hartley *et al.* [11] showed that it was possible to classify all murine leukemia viruses with respect to their host range on the basis of their relative infectivity titers in cells from NIH Swiss and BALB/c strain mice. Host cell responses to infection were compared by plaque assay on XC cells co-cultivated with secondary embryo cell cultures [12] prepared from the respective strains. Those virus strains that gave 2-3 log higher titers in NIH Swiss than in BALB/c cells were designated as "N-tropic", those that gave 1½ - 2 log higher titers in BALB/c than in NIH Swiss, as "B-tropic", and those that gave similar titers in both, as "NB-tropic".

We wished to determine whether either the SIM and SIM.R strains or the B6.S and B6 strains differed from one another in their responses *in vivo* and *in vitro* to infection with murine leukemia viruses of different tropism. The virus strains we used were Lilly's N-tropic F-S strain of FV, an N-tropic Bethesda strain of FV, Lilly's NB-tropic F-B strain of FV, and the B-tropic C57MC strain of murine leukemia virus, all kindly provided to us by Drs. Rowe and Hartley.

The pools of F-S and F-B strains of FV used for the studies *in vivo* were filtered supernatants of homogenates prepared from spleens of SIM mice infected with the respective virus strains. Those used for the studies *in vitro* were harvested from secondary or continuous embryo cell cultures of the appropriate mouse strains.

Relative sensitivities *in vivo* were assessed by the spleen focus assay method: Macroscopic foci on the fixed spleens of the animals were counted 9 days after *i.v.* injection of titrated doses of virus. The relative spleen focus-forming efficiencies of a given virus strain (expressed as FFU/ml) in the respective hosts were taken as a measure of the relative sensitivities of these hosts. Host cell responses to infection *in vitro* were compared by plaque assay on XC cells co-cultivated with secondary embryo cell cultures prepared from the respective congenic strains, and their relative plaque-forming efficiencies were expressed as PFU/ml.

The results are presented in tables 5 to 9 and in figs. 3 to 5. They show that both *in vivo* and *in vitro* the cells of SIM mice were highly sensitive to Lilly's N-tropic strain of FV, while those of SIM.R were around 3 logs less sensitive to the same virus strain. Similar results were obtained with Rowe and Hartley's N-tropic strain of FV *in vitro*. In contrast, Lilly's NB-tropic strain of FV gave about the same infectivity titers in SIM and SIM.R, both *in vitro* and *in vivo*. Furthermore, the data in table 7 show that cells from the SIM.R strain were highly sensitive to B-tropic C57MC virus but cells from the SIM congenic partner strain were resistant to this virus.

Cells from the B6.S strain had about the same high plaque-forming efficiencies as the cells from their B6 congenic partners when infected with the B-tropic C57MC virus, and both had the same low plaque-forming efficiencies with the N-tropic viruses *in vitro* (table 9). *In vivo*, however, there was an absolute difference between the B6.S and B6 strains that was not seen *in vitro*;

Table 5

Relative sensitivities of congenic partners to different strains of Friend leukemia virus *in vivo* (exp. C61).

Host	Spleen focus-forming efficiency (FFU/ml)	
	F-S strain	F-B strain
SIM	$1.0 \pm 0.3 \times 10^5$	$7.0 \pm 2.0 \times 10^4$
SIM.R	$3.1 \pm 0.8 \times 10^2$	$3.6 \pm 0.9 \times 10^4$

Table 6

Relative sensitivities of cells from SIM and SIM.R congenic mice to N- and NB-tropic strains of Friend leukemia virus *in vitro* (exp. P14).

Host	Plaque-forming efficiency (PFU/ml)	
	F-S strain (N-Tropic)	F-B strain (NB-tropic)
SIM	$7.2 \pm 1.8 \times 10^4$	$1.3 \pm 0.1 \times 10^6$
SIM.R	$8.0 \pm 2.0 \times 10^1$	$3.6 \pm 0.4 \times 10^5$

B6.S showed sensitivity to both the N-tropic and the NB-tropic strain of FV, while the B6 congenic partner was solidly resistant to both viruses *in vivo*.

While this work was in progress, Pincus *et al.* [13] were investigating the inheritance of host cell response to naturally occurring murine leukemia viruses. They began with mouse strains of N-type whose cells behaved like those of NIH Swiss, i.e. highly sensitive to N-tropic, but relatively resistant to B-tropic virus, and mouse strains of B-type, whose cells behaved like those of BALB/c, i.e. highly sensitive to B-tropic, but relatively resistant to N-tropic viruses *in vitro*. They then performed crosses, backcrosses and intercrosses between these strains and obtained an extensive body of data on the behaviour of mouse embryo cell cultures prepared from the progeny of these crosses. The data were best accounted for on the hypothesis that a single autosomal gene locus controls the host cell response to N- and B-tropic viruses. Heterozygotes produced by crossing mice of N-type with mice of B-type yielded cells that were resistant to both types of viruses. Pincus *et al.* [14] then found that the results *in vitro* were parallel to those *in vivo*. Lilly's F-S virus was shown to be N-tropic and his F-B virus, NB-tropic. The responses of cells from inbred and partially congenic mice were correlated with Fv-1 genotypes; those sensitive at Fv-1 showed the N-type of sensitivity and those resistant at Fv-1 showed the B-type of sensitivity. Thus although the Fv-1 locus has not yet been mapped, it is clear that it is this locus that controls the response to N- or B-tropic viruses. Resistance at the Fv-1 locus is dominant and relative. The 2 alleles so far recognized have recently been designated $Fv-1^n$ (sensitive to N-tropic but relatively resistant to B-tropic viruses) and $Fv-1^b$ (sensitive to B-tropic but relatively resistant to N-tropic viruses) [15]. Allelic differences at the Fv-1 locus had no effect on the response to NB-tropic viruses.

The Fv-2 locus was originally identified on the basis of the host response to F-B strain of FV in terms of spleen focus formation *in vivo* [10]. DBA/2 or Swiss mice which were sensitive to the spleen focus-forming activity of the F-B virus were designated as $Fv-2^s$, while those which developed no spleen foci in response to this virus *in vivo*, as $Fv-2^r$. *In vitro*, however, it was found that the F-B virus did not distinguish between B6 and NIH Swiss mouse embryo cells; XC plaque titers were similar in both types of cells [14].

The present findings are compatible with the hypothesis that the difference between the SIM and SIM.R congenic strains is at the Fv-1 locus; SIM may be considered to be $Fv-1^n$, and SIM.R, $Fv-1^b$. The locus controlling the difference between the B6.S and B6 strains evidently does not control the host range of these viruses in embryo cells *in vitro*; it is thus clearly not Fv-1 (both congenic partners are $Fv-1^b$). However, it is obviously another locus that is important for spleen focus formation *in vivo*. The relationship between that locus, which we call Fv-U, and the Fv-2 locus remains to be investigated.

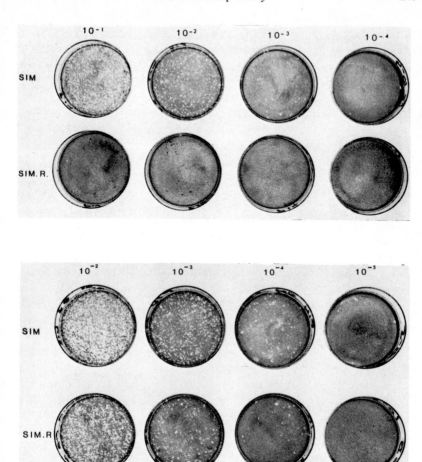

Figs. 3 and 4. Photographs of petri dishes showing titrations of Friend leukemia virus F-S and F-B strains in SIM and SIM.R embryo cell cultures by the XC plaque assay method.

Table 7

Relative sensitivities of cells from SIM and SIM.R congenic mice to B-tropic C57MC virus *in vitro* (exp. P34).

Host	Plaque-forming efficiency (PFU/ml)
SIM	< 20
SIM.R	$2.8 \pm 0.3 \times 10^4$

Table 8
Relative sensitivities of cells from B6 and B6.S congenic mice to different strains of murine leukemia virus *in vitro* (exp. P38).

Host	Plaque-forming efficiency (PFU/ml)		
	F-S strain (N-tropic)	F-B strain (NB-tropic)	C57MC virus (B-tropic)
B6	6.6 ± 6.6	$> 4 \times 10^6$	$4.4 \pm 0.3 \times 10^4$
B6.S	5.0 ± 5.0	$1.2 \pm 0.1 \times 10^7$	$1.7 \pm 0.1 \times 10^4$

Table 9
Relative sensitivities of congenic partners to different strains of Friend leukemia virus *in vivo* (exp. C61).

Host	Spleen focus-forming efficiency (FFU/ml)	
	F-S strain	F-B strain
B.6	0	0
B6.S	$2.5 \pm 0.7 \times 10^2$	$1.4 \pm 0.5 \times 10^4$

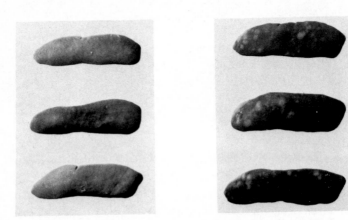

Fig. 5. Photograph of spleens taken from B6 (left) and B6.S (right) mice and fixed in Bouin's fluid 9 days after the mice received 5×10^3 FFU (as assayed in SIM mice) of Friend leukemia virus (F-S strain 28.9) intravenously. The failure to produce any spleen foci is characteristic of B6 mice. The foci on the spleens of B6.S mice show that these mice, which differ from B6 at a single gene locus, are susceptible to the virus.

Discussion

In the work we have described, the congenic partner strains SIM and SIM.R were shown to differ from one another at the Fv-1 locus, with the SIM strain carrying the allele Fv-1^n, and the SIM.R strain carrying the allele Fv-1^b (table 10). The evidence for this was: (1) The host mice showed a substantial difference in spleen focus response to infection by N-tropic FV but no difference in response to NB-tropic FV; (2) the embryo cell cultures prepared from SIM and SIM.R mice showed a substantial and reciprocal difference in sensitivity to infection by murine leukemia viruses of N-tropic or of B-tropic type, respectively, but little difference in response to NB-tropic virus; (3) resistance to infection with either N- or B-tropic virus was dominant over susceptibility (table 2) [19]; and (4) resistance was relative rather than absolute.

In both congenic partner strains, the alleles at the Fv-1 locus are on the genetic background of the SIM parental strain. There are no congenic partner strains differing at Fv-1 whose genetic background is that of the C57BL/6 parental strain.

Our data showed that the B6.S and B6 congenic partner strains do not differ at the Fv-1 locus. The evidence that they differed at another locus was: (1) The B6.S strain was susceptible to spleen focus formation by both N and NB-tropic strains of FV, while the B6 strain was resistant to both; (2) *in vitro*, there was no difference between B6.S and B6 mouse embryo cells in response to infection by any of the viruses; (3) susceptibility to infection by FV was dominant over resistance, and (4) resistance was absolute rather than relative.

It must be concluded that the B6.S and B6 strains differ at a locus other than Fv-1. The characteristics of this locus are not unlike those of Fv-2. However, until the locus is more definitely identified, we refer to it as Fv-U. The B6.S strain is highly sensitive to spleen focus-formation by FV; it may therefore be considered as Fv-U^s, and the B6 strain as Fv-U^r (table 10). Both

Table 10

Tentative genotypes of congenic strains and their partners which differ at loci controlling resistance and susceptibility to Friend leukemia virus.

	Fv-1	Fv-U
SIM	nn	ss
SIM.R	bb	ss
B6.S	bb	ss
B6	bb	rr

congenic partner strains share the C57BL/6 parental strain background; there are no congenic partner strains that differ at the Fv-U locus and share a SIM parental strain background.

It will be recalled that both in Tokyo and in Toronto, the F_1 hybrids between the FV susceptible and the resistant parental strains showed levels of susceptibility to FV which were intermediate [4-6], as measured with the spleen focus assay method. This indicates that, in both instances, 2 distinctly different genes were involved in control of spleen focus formation by FV, with susceptibility dominant at one locus and resistance dominant at the other. But Odaka has selected a recessive resistance allele and a dominant susceptibility allele, both apparently at the same locus, while we have selected a dominant resistance allele and a dominant susceptibility allele, at 2 different loci. Odaka was able to select for a recessive resistance allele presumably because he was using a cross-intercross breeding and selection scheme in order to transfer the resistance gene to the DDD background, while we were limited by our serial backcross scheme to the selection of dominant alleles only, for both susceptibility and resistance. A backcross system was used for transferring the susceptibility gene to the B6 background in both laboratories.

These observations seem to indicate that the locus which distinguishes Odaka's 2 pairs of congenic partners may be the same one that distinguishes our B6.S from B6. He has both susceptibility and resistance alleles on the B6 background, as we have, but he has both alleles on the DDD parental strain background as well.

The mechanism of action of Fv-1 on spleen focus formation is not understood at present. Steeves and Eckner [16,17] have presented evidence that the production of foci in the spleens of mice is dependent not only on a spleen focus-forming virus present in FV preparations (called SFFV) but also on another, non-focus-forming virus (called LLV) which acts as a helper for the focus-forming virus. SFFV appears to be defective [16,18] and many murine leukemia viruses seem to be capable of acting as helpers for it. At the Fv-1 locus, the host control of spleen focus response to FV preparations could thus theoretically be expressed through the control of the SFFV or the LLV, or both. It is known that the replication of non-focus-forming murine leukemia viruses is sustained in tissue culture but the focus-forming function of FV preparations is lost under these conditions [19]. Moreover, the Fv-1 locus influences the host range of a wide variety of murine non-focus-forming leukemia viruses *in vitro* [13]. It is therefore reasonable to suppose that the Fv-1 locus affects spleen focus formation *in vivo* mainly through its effect on the host range of the helper leukemia virus rather than on that of the spleen focus-forming virus. The helper virus might be necessary for replication and/or reinfection in order to produce macroscopically visible spleen foci.

Recently Kalnins and Weinroth in our department have found a decidedly greater number of budding type C particles in spleen cells from normal mice of the B6.S than of its B6 congenic partner strain [20]. These mice had never been deliberately infected with virus. We have obtained preliminary evidence that the development of lymphomas following a course of total body radiation was inhibited in SIM.R mice, although both SIM and B6 strain mice were susceptible. The present work thus indicates that these congenic mouse strains will be useful for studies on the mechanism of host control of resistance and susceptibility to infection with murine leukemia viruses not only of exogenous, but also of endogenous origin.

Summary

The Swiss-derived mouse strain SIM is highly susceptible to spleen focus formation by Friend leukemia virus (FV). The C57BL/6 (B6) strain is solidly resistant to spleen focus formation by this virus. Data from crosses between these strains were consistent with the hypothesis that the host response to the spleen focus-inducing action of FV is controlled at a single autosomal gene locus, the alleles for susceptibility and resistance behaving as codominants.

To investigate this locus, we produced 2 pairs of congenic strains of mice, the FV-resistant SIM.R strain congenic with the parental strain SIM, and the FV-susceptible B6.S strain congenic with the parental strain B6.

Genetic tests on these strains and their progeny indicated that the locus that distinguishes the SIM.R from the SIM strain is not identical with the locus that distinguishes the B6.S from the B6 strain.

The responses of SIM and SIM.R and of B6 and B6.S strains to murine leukemia viruses of known tropism were compared by the XC plaque assay method *in vitro* and by the spleen focus assay method *in vivo*. The results indicated that the SIM and SIM.R strains differ at the Fv-1 locus. B6 and B6.S mice were found to be identical to one another at Fv-1. However, both differed from the SIM and SIM.R strains in that susceptibility to FV was dominant and resistance was absolute. B6 and B6.S congenic mice therefore differ at another locus which has yet to be identified.

These congenic mouse strains should be useful for future studies on mechanisms of host resistance and susceptibility to exogenous and endogenous murine leukemia viruses.

References

[1] T. Odaka and T. Yamamoto, J. Exptl. Med. 32 (1962) 405.
[2] T. Odaka, J. Virol. 3 (1969) 543.
[3] A. Axelrad and R.A. Steeves, Virology 24 (1964) 543.
[4] A. Axelrad, Natl. Cancer Inst. Monograph. 22 (1965) 619.
[5] T. Odaka and T. Yamamoto, Jap. J. Exptl. Med. 35 (1965) 311.
[6] T. Odaka and T. Yamamoto, Jap. J. Exptl. Med. 36 (1966) 23.
[7] A. Axelrad and H. van der Gaag, Canad. Cancer Conf. 8 (1968) 313.
[8] T. Odaka, Intern. J. Cancer 6 (1970) 18.
[9] F. Lilly, Science 155 (1967) 461.
[10] F. Lilly, J. Natl. Cancer Inst. 45 (1970) 163.
[11] J.W. Hartley, R.P. Rowe and R.J. Huebner, J. Virol. 5 (1970) 221.
[12] W.P. Rowe, W.E. Pugh and J.W. Hartley, Virology 42 (1970) 1136.
[13] T. Pincus, J.W. Hartley and W.P. Rowe, J. Exptl. Med. 133 (1971) 1219.
[14] T. Pincus, W.P. Rowe and F. Lilly, J. Exptl. Med. 133 (1971) 1234.
[15] Discussion: Genetic factors in the Friend virus disease syndrome, Bethesda, 1971.
[16] R.A. Steeves and R.J. Eckner, J. Natl. Cancer Inst. 44 (1970) 587.
[17] R.J. Eckner and R.A. Steeves, Nature 229 (1971) 241.
[18] A.H. Fieldsteel, C. Kurahara and P.J. Dawson, Nature 223 (1969) 1274.
[19] M. Ware and A. Axelrad, unpublished results.
[20] V.I. Kalnins and H.J. Weinroth, unpublished results.

HUMAN HISTOCOMPATIBILITY SYSTEMS AND NEOPLASIA*

Roy L. WALFORD, Harold WATERS and George S. SMITH
*Department of Pathology, School of Medicine,
University of California at Los Angeles,
Los Angeles, Calif. 90024, U.S.A.*

Not long ago we expressed the view that the third phase of interest in human leukocyte isoantigens would be concerned in part with relations between HL-A types and disease susceptibilities [1]. Enough data have now been accumulated in a number of laboratories, particularly with regard to reticuloendothelial malignancies, that a provisional assessment of the situation can be made, and possible paths of further inquiry be suggested. The present report will be concerned chiefly with the HL-A system, and only casually with the ABO system, although both are known histocompatibility systems. Wiener [2] and Harris and Viza [3] recently discussed relations between erythrocyte group ABO and disease states. Their papers give sound advice about handling the kind of date-relationships that concern us here. One report is also available suggesting a disease correlation for Van Rood's Five-system [4].

Studies have been conducted of the HL-A pattern in Hodgkin's disease, lymphomas other than Hodgkin's, acute and chronic lymphatic leukemia, chronic myeloid leukemia, and a few other pertinent entities including systemic lupus erythematosus. Our first task will be to assemble the basic data for comparison. The data can be interpreted, albeit with reservation, to support our concept that relations might best be found between disease states and certain cross-reactive HL-A groups or families [5]. The suggestion of Harris and Viza [3] that HL-A complexity arose by gene duplication and sequential mutation, resulting therefore in "families" of cross-reacting antigens, would make such a group-relationship to disease theoretically attractive, if indeed it exists (and seductive if it doesn't exist).

There are convincing *a priori* probabilities why HL-A at least and perhaps other human histocompatibility systems, such as the ABO system [6,7] as well

*This study was supported by grants from the Jane Coffin Childs Memorial Fund for Medical Research, and the Blood Bank of San Bernardino-Riverside Counties.

255

as Van Rood's Five-system, which is not formally accepted as a (perhaps weak) histocompatibility system but does show wide tissue distribution [8], might correlate with disease states or susceptibilities in man. Chief among these are certain facts about the analogous mouse H-2 system and its influence upon disease and immunity [8,9]. These are well established in principle if not in all details, will not be exhaustively explored in the present essay, but will require mention in order to think constructively about the human situation.

A major hazard in correlative studies in humans is that of lumping etiologically different but histopathologically similar entities into the same category. Different H-2 alleles or linked factors in the mouse do correlate with susceptibilities to various mouse leukemia viruses [10-12]. Correspondingly in man, if the HL-A [2,12] genotype or the HL-A2 or 12 phenotypes are truly increased in childhood lymphatic leukemias, the real correlation might be with a particular human leukemia virus, i.e., with an etiologic agent. Correlation with the clinical entity "acute lymphatic leukemia" would depend, therefore, and among other parameters, upon what leukemia viruses were operating and in what proportions in the population under study. If it were possible to classify some human leukemias on the basis of virus associated antigens, a partial way around the impasse of heterogeneity might be found, and those correlations with the HL-A system which current data hint at would become clearer. In the meantime, subdivision of certain human disease states according to their age-specific incidence curves may prove to be quite useful, and will be discussed here in some detail.

While we ourselves have subscribed to the two-locus hypothesis about HL-A [13], we also believe [14], following the ideas of Batchelor et al. [15,16], that the hypothesis can be misleading. It tends to cause selection of typing sera for further study which fit into the framework of the hypothesis itself, therefore to a discarding of other antisera. An artificial situation can be created where important antigens are simply not detected. This tendency may already have obscured the earlier, more convincing relations found between HL-A and homograft survival. Ideas about a strict two-locus hypothesis for the HL-A system require overhauling, especially in view of recent reports by Klein [17] and Snell and associates [18,19] on the parallel H-2 system in the mouse. Antisera detecting so-called "public" antigens [17], and antisera made against "intermediate" alleles [18], if these exist in humans, would tend not to be selected for additional study. The findings of Amos and Yunis [20] with HL-A3 may indeed signify the presence of "intermediate" alleles in the human system. We have postulated the existence of HL-A factors for which there are no mutually exclusive opposites [21]. In the analogous mouse H-2 system these are known to exist. They apparently do not form part of a two-segregant-series arrangement [22,23].

HL-A types and reticuloendothelial malignancies

A word is first in order about statistical significance of data [2,3]. In studies of the sort under review, one generally tests the variation from normal incidence of, for example, 15 to 25 different HL-A specificities in a population with a particular disease. Now $p < 0.05$ means that for any particular event, that event would only be observed once or less if the series of events is repeated 20 times. The incidence of each HL-A specificity may be considered such an event. Therefore, if one is typing with 25 different specificities, one must in the initial series multiply any p-value by 25; if with 15 specificities, multiply by 15, and so on. Thus, if one is working with 25 different specificities, a p-value of 0.001 for any one must be multiplied by 25 to yield $p < 0.025$ for the corrected value. Hardly any of the data in the literature have been corrected in this fashion, and are therefore less significant than they seem by factors of from eightfold to 27-fold. This should not becloud the fact, however, that much of the reported data retains p-values substantially less than 0.05 even after correction. It is also true that once a specificity has shown significant variation in an initial series, then a fresh series, i.e., a confirmatory or non-confirmatory study referring to that particular specificity is not necessarily obliged to correct its p-value for the number of specificities.

In the present review, we shall in each instance for HL-A give the number of specificities along with the incidence figures, either known precisely or estimated from our knowledge of the particular laboratory. The p-values listed here will be left uncorrected.

Hodgkin's disease

Table 1 presents data from the world literature about certain HL-A types in Hodgkin's disease. In these and subsequent tables we include mainly those specificities for which a definite trend may exist or has been claimed, usually by more than one laboratory. The first report suggesting an atypical distribution of HL-A in Hodgkin's disease is Amiel's [24]. Among 41 patients typed for five specificities, 51% were 4c(+), compared to a normal population value of 27%. One may note that 4c is now thought to include HL-A5, R*(=4c*=W5), and CM*, which probably form a cross-reactive group [25]. W15 may also belong in this group according to Jeannet [26]. Both individual and accumulated data for the selected specificities are shown in table 1. The two populations studied by Thorsby *et al.* [27,28] were Canadian and Norwegian, and are listed separately. Among eight different populations studied, six

R.L. Walford et al.

Table 1
Hodgkin's disease.

Specificity	Number of patients	Frequency in patients*	Frequency in controls	Number of specificities	p-value[†] or χ^2	References
4c	78	0.51	0.26	5	$p < 0.001$	[24,70]
	127	0.37	0.26	13	$p < 0.025$	[30,31]
	44	0.16	0.27	18		[29]
	249	0.37	0.26		$p < 0.002$	
R*	127	0.32	0.12	13	$p < 0.005$	[30,31]
	98	0.33	0.18	19	$p < 0.002$	[36]
	23	0.26	0.19	22		[26]
	44	0.07	0.09	18		[29]
	50	0.06	0.12	23		[32]
	39	0.05	0.13	27		[25,28]
	78	0.16	0.26	27		[28]
	459	0.22	0.16		$p < 0.03$	
HL-A5	27	0.63	0.19	8	$p < 0.005$	[71]
	78	0.24	0.09	27		[28]
	39	0.15	0.08	27		[25,28]
	98	0.16	0.10	19		[36]
	127	0.13	0.09	13		[30,31]
	44	0.11	0.11	18		[29]
	50	0.10	0.12	23		[32]
	23	0.13	0.22	22		[26]
	486	0.15	0.12		$\chi^2 = 0.4$	
CM*	48	0.16	0.03	23	$p < 0.001$	[32]
	39	0	0.04	27		[25,28]
	87	0.09	0.04		$\chi^2 = 1.5$	
W15	23	0.40	0.12	22	$p < 0.005$	[26]
	44	0.23	0.10	18		[29]
	78	0.16	0.06	27		[28]
	39	0.21	0.20	27		[25,28]
	127	0.16	0.14	13		[30,31]
	98	0.12	0.12	19		[36]
	50	0.12	0.21	23		[32]
	459	0.17	0.14		$\chi^2 = 1.2$	

Table 1 (continued)

Specificity	Number of patients	Frequency in patients*	Frequency in controls	Number of specificities	p-value[†] or χ^2	References
HL-A1	27	0.59	0.38	8		[71]
	50	0.50	0.28	23		[32]
	23	0.44	0.27	22		[26]
	78	0.41	0.29	27		[28]
	98	0.37	0.33	19		[36]
	127	0.34	0.32	13		[30,31]
	39	0.31	0.28	27		[25,28]
	44	0.29	0.27	18		[29]
	486	0.38	0.30		$p < 0.015$	
HL-A8	50	0.44	0.22	23		[32]
	27	0.37	0.28	8		[71]
	98	0.25	0.24	19		[36]
	39	0.26	0.26	27		[25,28]
	78	0.23	0.16	27		[28]
	127	0.24	0.23	13		[30,31]
	23	0.22	0.18	22		[26]
	44	0.11	0.16	18		[29]
	486	0.26	0.22		$\chi^2 = 1.6$	
HL-A11	127	0.29	0.14	13	$p < 0.005$	[30,31]
	78	0.10	0.11	27		[28]
	98	0.08	0.12	19		[36]
	50	0.08	0.11	23		[32]
	44	0.04	0.06	18		[29]
	23	0.04	0.16	22		[26]
	39	0	0.11	27		[25,28]
	459	0.13	0.12		–	

*Frequency for total patients was calculated after reconversion to number of patients in each row, adding, and dividing by total number of patients.

†Values were calculated by the chi-square method and assuming total control population of 300 for the 4c and 400 for the remaining specificities.

revealed a statistically significant elevation (after correction for number of specificities) in at least one of these factors (or in the 4c "family"), except that of Coukell *et al.* [29], which nevertheless showed an uncorrected chi-square value of 3.4 for an increase in W15. The combined data on 4c for 249 patients yield a *p*-value <0.002, and this remains significant after multiplication by the five to 18 specificities tested for in the separate studies. Furthermore, the 4c data of Forbes and Morris [30,31] (*p* <0.025) need not necessarily be corrected in view of the earlier figures of Amiel [24], which established the trend. In addition, it can be emphasized that the initial report of Forbes and Morris [30] consisted first of a prospective study of 35 cases, followed by a "fresh" (see Wiener [2]) series of 75 patients, and that in their report the segregation of R* with HL-A was confirmed by a study of seven families in which one member had Hodgkin's disease. Their report is the most finished one to date concerning HL-A and disease states. In three of three Hodgkin's families which we have ourselves genotyped (unpublished), the afflicted person was 4c(+) in all instances and 4c segregated with HL-A in all families. From the total available evidence, we conclude that factors of the 4c family do in fact manifest an increased frequency in Hodgkin's disease, but that which factor is increased may vary in different studies, and therefore perhaps geographically.

Table 1 also gives data on three other HL-A specificities in Hodgkin's disease. Kissmeyer *et al.* [32] emphasized the possible association of HL-A1 and 8 with this disease, and the data from other laboratories, the report of Coukell *et al.* [29] again being the one exception, show the same trend. The overall data on HL-A1 and 8 in a total of 486 patients, however, are not statistically significant, particularly if corrected for the number of specificities tested, despite the "trend". We do note that the incidence of Hodgkin's disease as a fraction of all "lymphomas" in Japanese is 16.2%, and in Caucasians is 49.7% [33], and that HL-A1 and 8 are absent in Japanese [34]. Also, parenthetically and in anticipation of the next section, acute leukemia is less common in Negroes than Caucasians [35], and specificities HL-A2 and 12 constitute phenotypically 36 and 20% in blacks compared to 50 and 27% in Caucasians [34].

In a series of 85 cases of Hodgkin's disease Van Rood and Van Leeuwen [36] noted a decrease in 4a, and an excess of 4b (uncorrected χ^2 = 5.14). The majority of the HL-A antigens which seemed in their study to be decreased, although not individually to a statistically significant degree, were those "included" within 4a. The reality of 4a and 4b seems to us less in doubt than we [37] as well as others [38] thought a few years ago, and Van Rood's long insistence on the validity of this system, the first di-allelic human leukocyte system reported, might prove to have been correct. We think that 4a and 4b may be "public antigens" in the sense used by Klein [17], the components of which show extensive cross-reactions between one another. The position of 4a and 4b as public antigens might explain why, at least in Morris' series, better correlation using 4a and 4b alone was found for kidney graft rejection rates than using the 18 or so specificities of the established first and second segregant series of the HL-A system.

In Hodgkin's disease an increase (x^2 = 9.2) has also been noted in antigen 5a of the Five-system [36], which system is wholly independent of HL-A, but has a wide tissue distribution [4].

It is apparent from the above account that at least one and perhaps more than one family, group, or system of leukocyte specificities may display unexpected variation in incidence in Hodgkin's disease. It must be remembered that Hodgkin's disease can be histologically divided into the different types such as lymphocyte predominance, nodular sclerosing, mixed cellularity, and lymphocyte depletion. Further studies of HL-A distribution should take into account a more categorical histologic designation than has been done in most existing reports. Morris and Forbes [30] presented initial evidence that such might be fruitful.

Acute lymphatic leukemia

Our original study of the genotypes of 10 cases of ALL in children [39] indicated a great increase in the HL-A(2,12) genotype, and a decrease in HL-A1. An independent and earlier study by Thorsby *et al.* [40] showed a numerical but not statistically significant increase in the HL-A [2,12] genotype. Further cases from which numerical data are available are shown in table 2. The study of Kourilsky *et al.* [41] is not included in the table as the age range in their ALL patients was from four to 75 years; the "majority", however, were said to be children. A numerical increase in either HL-A2 or 12 and usually both has been found in most studies (table 2), but the overall results from 214 patients are significant only if left uncorrected ($p < 0.025$ and $p < 0.018$). There are, however, rather striking differences between the various studies, and the simple summation of all reported cases could be misleading. This aspect of the subject will be discussed later.

The finding of a decrease in HL-A1 in our own series [42] has not been confirmed by the overall data (table 2).

Lymphomas other than Hodgkin's disease

Data from Morris and Forbes [43] and Yunis [44] are given in table 3. While further studies are indicated, the existing data indicate that HL-A12 is significantly increased in frequency in at least certain types of lymphoma.

Table 2
Acute lymphatic leukemia in children.

Specificity	Number of patients	Frequency in patients	Frequency in controls*	Number of specificities	p-value or χ^2	References
HL-A2	28	0.68	0.58	27		[25,27]
	17	0.76	0.46	17		[72]
	17	0.53	0.42	27		[39]
	20	0.65	0.49	16		[73]
	26	0.54	0.48	22		[26]
	48	0.63	0.38	22		[74]
	58	0.45	0.49	16		[75]
	214	0.57	0.47		$p < 0.025$	
HL-A12	28	0.25	0.26	27		[25,27]
	17	0.18	0.27	17		[72]
	17	0.81	0.29	27		[39]
	20	0.30	0.27	16		[73]
	26	0.31	0.23	22		[26]
	48	0.38	0.17	22		[74]
	58	0.38	0.27	16		[74]
	214	0.36	0.25		$p < 0.018$	
HL-A (2, 12)	32	0.17	0.06			[39]
haplotypes	43	0.16	0.07			[25,27]
HL-A1	28	0.32	0.29	27		[25,27]
	17	0.25	0.25	17		[72]
	17	0	0.33	27		[39]
	20	0.35	0.25	16		[73]
	26	0.27	0.27	22		[26]
	43	0.39	0.38	22		[74]
	58	0.36	0.25	16		[75]
	209	0.29	0.28			
HL-A11	28	0.07	0.12	27		[25,27]
	17	0.18	0.12	17		[72]
	17	0.06	0.24	27		[39]
	20	0.20	0.12	16		[73]
	26	0	0.16	22		[26]
	43	0.37	0.38	22		[74]
	58	0.16	0.12	16		[75]
	209	0.16	0.18			

*Control values for references 73, 74, and 75 are not available and are therefore taken as the average frequencies of reaction of the higher quality antisera of the 1970 Workshop, except for the HL-A2 frequency of Batchelor's series (72) which is known to be 0.46.

Table 3
Lymphomas other than Hodgkin's disease.

Specificity	Number of patients	Frequency in patients	Frequency in controls	Number of specificities	p-value or χ^2	References
Follicular lymphoma						
HL-A12	56	0.63	0.32	13	$p < 0.0005$	[43]
Lymphosarcoma						
HL-A12	50	0.42	0.32	13	–	[43]
Reticulum cell sarcoma						
HL-A12	28	0.50	0.32	13	$p < 0.05$	[43]
All categories						
HL-A12	134	0.52	0.32	13		[43]
	43	0.44	0.26	–		[44]
	177	0.50	0.30		$p < 0.002$	

Chronic lymphatic and chronic myeloid leukemia

Numerical values are not currently available from the study of 44 cases of chronic lymphatic leukemia by Degos *et al.* [45], but no significant variation from normal was said to be found. Data from Jeannet [26] and Walford et al. [42] are shown in table 4, including only those specificities which one or the other of the two laboratories found at possible variance with expectation. The combined values are not far from normal.

Our earlier report of a great increase in FJH in chronic lymphatic leukemia was based upon the reactions of a single serum obtained from Dr. Thorsby. With a normal panel this Thorsby antiserum showed the expected FJH reactivity. Further study of our original plus additional CLL cases (not in remission) confirmed that the Thorsby-FJH serum does show an elevated reaction frequency with CLL cells, but certain other FJH anti-serums do not. Genotyping of four families, each with one member afflicted with chronic lymphatic leukemia, revealed that in three informative families the Thorsby-FJH serum reacted, with the exception of one person, only with the leukemic cells, and did not segregate as an HL-A specificity. A number of available HL-A typing sera may show this kind of reactivity with CLL cells. Examples are given in table 4. EV, which in normal populations appears included within HL-A9, was independent of HL-A in the one informative family tested. The reaction of antiserums Stitz, Rafter, and Laskey (see table 4) segregated with HL-A in one informative family having three children.

Table 4
Chronic lymphatic leukemia.

Specificity or serum*	Number of patients	Frequency in patients	Frequency in controls	Number of specificities	References
W15	10	0.35	0.12	22	[26]
	34	0.03	0.07	18	[42] †
	44	0.10	0.09		
HL-A9	10	0.50	0.21	22	[26]
	34	0.18	0.26	18	[42]
	44	0.25	0.24		
HL-A11	10	0	0.16	22	[26]
	34	0.18	0.24	18	[42]
	44	0.14	0.20		
HL-A5	10	0.12	0.22	22	[26]
	34	0.24	0.09	18	[42]
	44	0.21	0.16		
Stitz (HL-A12+)	34	0.67	0.34	–	[42]
Rafter (4c)	34	0.44	0.23	–	[42]
Laskey (R*)	34	0.40	0.06	–	[42]
EV (< HL-A9)	34	0.85	0.06	–	[42]
Thorsby-FJH (FJH)	34	0.50	0.04	–	[42]

*Specificities are given by HL-A or W designation and represent (for our own 34 cases) agreement between two or more known monospecific antiserums. Individual serums which show an increased reactivity with CLL cell populations are designated, except for the last row, by the donor's name, and the serum's specificity versus a normal panel is given in parenthesis. The last serum is an anti-FJH from Thorsby which shows the expected frequency with a normal panel but an increased frequency of reaction with CLL cells.
† Additional cases have been added to our original series of twenty-one patients.

In a series of 47 cases of chronic myeloid leukemia, Degos *et al.* [45], who were testing for 26 specificities, found an increase in HL-A3 ($p < 0.05$), and a decrease in HL-A12 ($p < 0.01$). These values are not significant when corrected, and the authors drew no definite conclusions. Pegrum *et al.* [46] reported an elevated incidence of HL-A3 in a rather miscellaneous collection of leukemias.

Systemic lupus erythematosus

While SLE is not itself a reticuloendothelial malignancy, it may be associated with an increased incidence of these diseases. Such an association holds for the LE-like malady of NZB mice, which appears quite similar in most respects to its human counterpart. Findings in human SLE are pertinent to the present survey.

Our observation of an increased incidence of LND-like antigens in this disease [5,47] accords with the independently conducted study of Grumet *et al.* [8,48]. Values for a total of 64 patients are given in table 5. W15 (=LND) is

Table 5
Systemic lupus erythematosus[†]

Specificity	Number of patients	Frequency in patients	Frequency in controls	Number of specificities	p-value or χ^2	References
W15	24	0.21	0.07	26		[47]
(=LND)	40	0.40	0.10	21		[48]
	64	0.33	0.08		$p < 0.0001$	
Thorsby-	15	0.47	0.08	26	$p < 0.0005$	[47]
LND-X	9	0.0	0.08	26		[47]
HL-A1	24	0.21	0.33	26		[47]
	40	0.32	0.27	21		[48]
	64	0.28	0.30		—	
HL-A8	24	0.30	0.26	26		[47]
	40	0.33	0.16	21		[48]
	64	0.32	0.16		$\chi^2 = 1.7$	

[†]The data from the 24 cases of Waters *et al.* [47] opposite the specificity designated as Thorsby-LND-X are divided into 15 patients with onset before and 9 after 25 years of age.

clearly increased in this combined series. We noted also that one anti-LND serum of Thorsby, shown recently to be detecting "broad" antigens [38], could be fractionated by selective absorption into several components, one of which, labelled Thorsby-LND-X, reacted with increased incidence with lymphocytes from SLE patients of a younger as opposed to an older age group.

Discussion

The existing data suggest the following tentative conclusions. In Hodgkin's disease there is an increase in frequency of the 4c family of specificities. Which of the specificities included within 4c (R*, HL-A5, CM*, and possibly W15 [25,26]) show an increase may vary from study to study. The finding of an increase in HL-A1 and 8 as emphasized in the series of Kissmeyer et al. [32] is not confirmed by the uncorrected p-values of the collected cases (table 1), nevertheless in all of eight studies some numerical increase in HL-A1 was found, and in seven of eight studies an increase in HL-A8. A trend might exist but be obscured by the heterogeneous nature of the cases within and between the different patient samples.

The above pattern, with the 4c family on the one hand and the HL-A1 and 8 combination possibly on the other, suggests that further subdivisions of the patient material might be worth looking into. Histopathologic type seems one obvious subdivision. Clinical course corresponds to a considerable degree with this categorization. Morris and Forbes [31] reported that the increase in R* in Hodgkin's disease was most striking in the nodular sclerosing form in males.

A segment of the age-specific distribution of Hodgkin's disease is illustrated in fig. 1. Two peaks exist, as expressed in the figure by the solid-line curve. This curve might well be the summation of two separate curves, as illustrated by the dotted lines, representing two etiologic or other subdivisions of Hodgkin's disease. A reexamination of existing data for HL-A types in Hodgkin's disease after subdivision into appropriate young and older groups might be fruitful.

For whatever reason, quite a number of diseases show more than one peak in age-specific incidence. Fig. 2, adapted from Dausset et al. [50] reveals a clearcut age-related subdivision of acute lymphatic leukemia among a population of 44 adult women, and two or even more peaks may exist for acute myeloid leukemia. The findings of Degos et al. [45] for chronic myeloid leukemia might also be worth reviewing by age distribution, for Ezdinli [51] reported that of 66 adult patients with chronic myeloid leukemia 43 possessed the Philadelphia chromosome and had an average age of 48 years; the 18 lacking this chromosome averaged 66 years. Some basis for an age-related subdivision of CML is suggested by these figures.

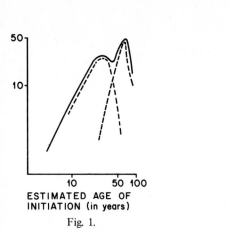

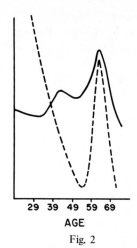

Fig. 1.   Fig. 2

Fig. 1. Relative age distribution of patients (males) with Hodgkin's disease (—). The shape of the curve could be derived from two (? etiologic) groups of clinicopathologically similar diseases but with different peak initiation ages (adapted from Burch [49]).

Fig. 2. Age related distribution of 120 cases of acute myeloid leukemia (—), and 44 cases of acute lymphatic leukemia (...), in adult women (adapted from Dausset *et al.* [50]).

Data from the mouse H-2 system and its relationship to susceptibility to different mouse leukemia viruses may be interpreted as supporting the approach suggested above. Lilly found that in appropriate homozygous inbred strains the H-2k genotype correlated with 100% susceptibility, and H-2b to only 26% susceptibility to Gross virus leukemia [10]. One notes also from his report that the latent period to development of the disease was 69 days in H-2k and 191 days in H-2b mice. The relationships are indeed more complex than this comparison implies, for the F_1-hybrids showed only a 9% total incidence and a 258-day latent period [10]. As noted by Tennant and Snell [52] in a study of the susceptibilities of congenic strains of mice to the B/T-L leukemic virus, different H-2 alleles predisposed not only to different overall incidences, but to different rates of development of leukemia. Thus precedence can be found in the mouse data for thinking that breakdown of certain reticuloendothelial malignancies in man according to known age-specific peak incidences might be informative in seeking correlation with HL-A types.

An association between HL-A and acute lymphatic leukemia in children is less convincing at present than for Hodgkin's disease. Most studies of childhood ALL do show a numerical increase in frequency for both HL-A2 and HL-A12, but the combined data for each specificity is only significant if uncorrected (table 2). What may be important is the magnitude of the differences between the various studies. If not wholly coincidental, these variations might reflect true regional differences in (etiologic) types of ALL, less striking than but reminiscent of the "clusters" of childhood leukemia reported in different localities [35]. If the patient population samples were of sufficient size, then the magnitude of differences between highest and lowest frequencies for a particular specificity among the various reports might be compared with similar values from the control populations. A significant increase in the figure derived from patients' data would mean that the series of ALL patients are not strictly comparable.

As pathologists, we are quite aware that "acute leukemia" is somewhat of a hodgepodge histologically, especially in adults. In children most acute leukemias are lymphatic. Cases with onset at about one-year or less of age should be excluded, however, because many are not lymphatic [53], and the exact diagnostic classification may be difficult. In fig. 3 the age-specific

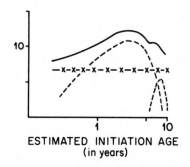

ESTIMATED INITIATION AGE
(in years)

Fig. 3. Relative age-specific mortality rates for acute lymphatic leukemia in children (——), myeloid and monocytic leukemias (x-x-x). The acute lymphatic leukemia curve may reflect two (? etiologic) subgroups of clinicopathologically similar diseases, but with different peak initiation ages (adapted from Burch [49]).

mortality rates for ALL in children are illustrated. The two peaks in the curve can be interpreted in the same manner as in figs. 1 and 2.

The kind of diagnostic problem illustrated above has parallels. Anti-EBV titers are elevated in all cases of Burkitt's lymphoma from Africa but in only half the cases elsewhere, so that the non-African Burkitt-like lymphomas diagnosed on histologic criteria are thought to represent a more heterogeneous group [54]. In addition, around 60% of patients with chronic lymphatic leukemia or lymphosarcoma manifest elevated anti-EBV titers, but patients with other reticuloendothelial malignancies do not [54]. Anti-EBV titers also tend to be elevated in nasopharyngeal carcinoma, but not in hypopharyngeal or oropharyngeal carcinoma [54]. It is known that in mice tumors of the same histologic type can be induced by different viruses, and conversely that tumors of different types can be induced under certain circumstances by the same virus [55].

The increased incidence of reactivity of a number of more or less standard anti-HL-A sera with cells of chronic lymphatic leukemia (table 4, and [42,56,57]) is of some interest. The subject has been reviewed by Schlesinger and Amos [57], who noted in leukemics a general tendency to over-reactivity with isoantibody. The point that we shall bring out here, however, is that this is not so with all but only with some isoantisera, and these may fall into two groups: those which seem related to an HL-A family, such as 4c, and those which react only with the leukemic cells, showing therefore no segregation in family studies. We agree with Harris and Viza [3] and with Dausset [58] that heightened incidence of reactivity of some anti-HL-A sera with leukemia cells might relate to tumor antigens, but other explanations are possible. Dausset speculated that leukemic antibodies independent of HL-A might occur due to chance immunization of the serum donor with leukemia-antigen-containing cells (polytransfused patient) [58]. However, many of the antisera in question are from post-partum women, while others result from planned immunization with cells from healthy individuals who have remained healthy. We are aware that cytotoxic antibodies reactive with Burkitt's lymphoma biopsy cells, leukemic lymphoblasts, and cultures of lymphoid cells can be found uniformly in sera of Burkitt patients and in up to 50% of children and 87 to 100% of adults [59]. These antibodies were not considered to be tumor-specific antigens. Using immunodiffusion technics, Greenspan *et al.* [60] found an antigen in human leukemic tissue not detected with "normal" sera but giving positive reactions with sera from laboratory personnel and family members who had had over six-months contact with mouse leukemia or human leukemic patients.

In line with the last possibility, we have tested the sera of 10 hematologists and selected laboratory personnel who have had extensive contact for one to many years with CLL patients. Against a seven-member panel of CLL cells and using our cytotoxicity test, these sera failed to manifest a single positive reaction. The increased incidence of reactivity of certain anti-HL-A serums with CLL cells may therefore not be simply on the basis of casual exposure to leukemia virus antigens. Nevertheless, the possibility remains. In mice antigen FMR is induced in the cell membrane by viruses of group B, and antigen G by viruses of group A [61].

Among still other possibilities, we note in studies of Rogentine and Gerber [62,63] that whereas the cells of long-term tissue cultures of human lymphoid cells reacted usually as expected with HL-A typing sera, some sera appeared hyper-reactive. Serums Pinquette and T-8 are both excellent anti-HL-A2 reagents but T-8 was found to react with substantially more cultures than did Pinquette [63]. When the normal lymphoid cells of the original tissue culture cell donors were compared with the cultured cells by careful absorption technics, the cultured cells sometimes contained as much as 12 to 44 times more antigen reactive with a particular anti-HL-A serum than fresh lymphoid cells from the same donor. Evidence of heightened expression of certain H-2 specificities in mouse leukemia also exists [64]. In the light of the above, the quantitative expression of certain HL-A and non-HL-A antigens (? thymic lymphocyte antigens) might be increased in CLL or other leukemic cells, which could explain why we have noted the increased reactivity so far only with certain anti-HL-A sera, and not with normal sera nor with sera from persons in clinical contact with CLL patients. In our hands all of eight antisera belonging to the 4c-family demonstrated an increased incidence of reaction with the CLL patients, whereas with other specificities the pattern was more variable, and one can generally type CLL cells satisfactorily if a number of antisera are employed for each specificity.

A possibility besides reaction with leukemia antigens, or with HL-A or even non-HL-A antigens showing increased expression in leukemic cells, would be expression of an antigen only in persons homozygous for a recessive allele. Susceptibility to the Gross leukemia virus in mice may be determined by a recessive trait [65], although this has not been shown to correlate with a serologically demonstrable specific antigen beyond the known H-2 correlations for this virus [65]. Schlesinger [66] has discussed this area, including possible determination of antigens by recessive genes, and gene interaction.

The above comments exemplify the problem arising in human studies from the necessity at present for pooling what are in many instances heterogeneous data. The use of age-specific disease rates, more attention to histologic classification, and certain additional laboratory investigations might assist in making the human pool less heterogeneous. In the mouse this has been partially accomplished by use of inbred strains and specified tumor viruses.

An inspection of the data shown in the tables, including those for lymphoma and SLE, suggests that in reticuloendothelial malignancies and related conditions the specificities of the 4c family, specificities HL-A2 and/or 12, and HL-A1 and 8 might be found to be variably increased, particularly with improved disease categorization. HL-A11 may be decreased in certain instances, as noted by Jeannet and Magnin [26] for all non-Hodgkin's reticuloendothelial diseases. It is interesting also to note that HL-A2 may be slighhtly increased in chronic glomerulonephritis [67], the HL-A(1,8) haplotype in asthma [25], and that HL-A(1,8) may also be rather frequently present in children rejecting parental kidney grafts [68]. The overall findings seem more than coincidental. They suggest an emerging but still obscure pattern relating the HL-A system, the main histocompatibility system in man, to certain disease susceptibilities and immune response capacities. In view of analogous data in a number of species of experimental animals [8,69], and particularly because of the constantly gathering parallels between serologic and other findings in HL-A and H-2, it would be highly surprising if the HL-A system did not have these effects. The main current problem seems to be to ferret out the information in such a non-homogeneous population as man, and without the advantage of knowing the etiologic agents involved. Several possible ways of attacking this problem have been suggested.

Summary and conclusion

In man the HL-A main histocompatibility system shows an as yet obscure but rather definite relationship with susceptibility to the development of reticulo-endothelial malignancy and other entities. Various specificities belonging to the 4c family reveal increased incidences of reaction among patients with Hodgkin's disease, and HL-A12 appears related to lymphomas other than Hodgkin's disease. HL-A12 and 2 are probably increased in acute lymphatic leukemia in children. W15(=LND) or a component thereof is increased in frequency among patients with systemic lupus erythematosus. Certain "families" or cross-reactive groups of HL-A specificities may thus be related to certain broad categories of disease. Subdivision of diseases according to peaks of age-specific incidence, where these exist, might be useful where a viral etiology is in question.

References

[1] R.L. Walford, The isoantigenic systems of human leukocytes: medical and biological significance. Series Haematologica (Munksgaard, Copenhagen, 1969) pp. 1-96.

[2] A.S. Wiener, Am. J. Human Genet. 22 (1970) 476-483.

[3] R. Harris and D. Viza, The HL-A polymorphism (in press, 1971).

[4] J.J. van Rood and J.G. Eernisse, Seminars in Hematol. 5 (1968) 187.

[5] R.L. Walford, Lancet ii (1970) 1226-1229.

[6] J. Dausset and F.T. Rapaport, Nature 209 (1966) 209.

[7] R. Ceppellini, E.S. Curtoni, P.L. Mattiuz, G. Leighes, M. Visetti and A. Colombi, Ann. N.Y. Acad. Sci. U.S. 129 (1966) 421.

[8] H.O. McDevitt and W.F. Bodmer, Am. J. Med. (in press, 1971).

[9] H.O. McDevitt and B. Benacerraf, Advan. Immunol. 11 (1969) 31.

[10] F. Lilly, Natl. Cancer Inst. Monograph 22 (1966) 631.

[11] J.R. Tennant and G.D. Snell, Natl. Cancer Inst. Monograph 22 (1966) 61-72.

[12] G.D. Snell, Folia Biol. 14 (1968) 335-358.

[13] J. Dausset, R.L. Walford, J. Colombani, L. Legrand, N. Feingold, A. Barge and F.T. Rapaport, Transpl. Proc. 1 (1969) 331.

[14] R.L. Walford, H. Waters and G.S. Smith, Fed. Proc. 29 (1970) 2011.

[15] J.R. Batchelor and A.R. Sanderson, Transpl. Proc. 2 (1970) 133.

[16] J.R. Batchelor and N. Selwood, In: P.I. Terasaki (ed.), Histocompatibility testing 1970 (Munksgaard, Copenhagen, 1970) p. 243.

[17] J. Klein, Nature 229 (1971) 635.

[18] G.D. Snell, P. Démant and M. Cherry, Transplantation 11 (1971) 210-237.

[19] P. Démant, G.D. Snell and M. Cherry, Transplantation 11 (1971) 242.

[20] B. Amos and E. Yunis, Science 165 (1969) 300-302.

[21] R.L. Walford, O. Wallace, E. Shanbrom and G.M. Troup, Vox Sanguinis 15 (1968) 338.

[22] E. Thorsby, Eur. J. Immunol. 1 (1971) 57.

[23] G. Snell, G. Cherry and P. Démant, Transpl. Proc. 3 (1971) 183.

[24] J.L. Amiel, In: E.S. Curtoni, P.L. Mattiuz and R.M. Tosi (eds.), Histocompatibility testing 1967 (Munksgaard, Copenhagen, 1967) p. 79.

[25] E. Thorsby, A. Engeset and S.O. Lie, Tissue Antigens (in press, 1971).

[26] M. Jeannet and C. Magnin, Transpl. Proc. 3 (1971) 1301.

[27] E. Thorsby and S.O. Lie, Transpl. Proc. 3 (1971) 1305.

[28] E. Thorsby, J. Falk, A. Engeset and D. Osoba, Transpl. Proc. 3 (1971) 1279.

[29] A. Coukell, J.G. Bodmer and W.F. Bodmer, Transpl. Proc. 3 (1971) 1287.

[30] J.F. Forbes and P.J. Morris, Lancet ii (1970) 849.

[31] P.J. Morris and J.F. Forbes, Transpl. Proc. 3 (1971) 1315.

[32] F. Kissmeyer-Nielsen, K.B. Jensen, G.B. Ferrara, K.E. Kjerbye and A. Svejgaard, Transpl. Proc. 3 (1971) 1287.

[33] R.E. Anderson, K. Ishida, Y. Li, T. Ishimaru and H. Nishiyama, Am. J. Pathol. 61 (1970) 85-97.

[34] E.D. Albert, M.R. Mickey, A.C. McNicolas and P.I. Terasaki, In: P.I. Terasaki (ed.), Histocompatibility testing 1970 (Munksgaard, Copenhagen, 1970) p. 221.

[35] L. Degos and J. Dausset, Sem. Hôp. 46 (1970) 309-317.

[36] J.J. van Rood and A. van Leeuwen, Transpl. Proc. 3 (1971) 1283.

[37] E. Shanbrom, E. Feingold, L. Shepherd and R.L. Walford, Blood 32 (1968) 402-411.

[38] F. Kissmeyer-Nielsen and E. Thorsby, Transpl. Rev. 4 (1970) 1-176.

[39] R.L. Walford, S. Finkelstein, R. Neerhout, P. Konrad and E. Shanbrom, Nature 225 (1970) 461-462.

[40] E. Thorsby, A. Bratlie and S.O. Lie, Scand. J. Haematol. 6 (1969) 409.

[41] F.M. Kourilsky, J. Dausset, N. Feingold, J.M. Dupuy and J. Bernard, In: J. Dausset, J. Hamburger and G. Mathé (eds.), Advance in transplantation (Munksgaard, Copenhagen, 1968) p. 515.

[42] R.L. Walford, E. Zeller, L. Combs and P. Konrad, Transpl. Proc. 3 (1971) 1297.

[43] P.J. Morris and J.F. Forbes, Transpl. Proc. 3 (1971) 1315.

[44] E. Yunis, Personal communication.

[45] L. Degos, Y. Drolet and J. Dausset, Transpl. Proc. 3 (1971) 1309.

[46] G.D. Pegrum, I.C. Balfour, C.A. Evans, and V.L. Middleton, Brit. J. Haematol. 19 (1970) 493.

[47] H. Waters, P. Konrad and R.L. Walford, Tissue Antigens 1 (1971) 68.

[48] F.C. Grumet, A. Coukell, J.G. Bodmer, W.F. Bodmer and H.O. McDevitt, New Eng. J. Med. (in press, 1971).

[49] P.R.J. Burch, An inquiry concerning growth, disease and ageing (Univ. Toronto Press, Toronto, 1969).

[50] J. Dausset, L. Degos, B. Estampe and J. Bernard, Nouv. Rev. Franç. Hematol. 10 (1970) 55-62.

[51] E.Z. Ezdinli, J.E. Sokal, L. Crosswhite and A.A. Sandberg, Ann. Int. Med. 72 (1970) 175.

[52] J.R. Tennant and G.D. Snell, J. Natl. Cancer Inst. 41 (1968) 597.

[53] H.J. Pluss, Schweiz. Med. Wochenschr. 100 (1970) 314-316.

[54] G. Klein, Israel J. Med. Sci. 7 (1971) 111-131.

[55] G. Klein, Transpl. Proc. (in press, 1971).

[56] R.L. Walford, *In:* R.T. Smith and M. Landy (eds.), Immune surveillance (Academic Press, New York, 1970) p. 60.

[57] M. Schlesinger and B. Amos, *In:* F.T. Rapaport and J. Dausset (eds.), Human transplantation (Grune and Stratton, New York, 1968) pp. 601-617.

[58] J. Dausset, Transpl. Proc. 3 (1971) 1139.

[59] R.B. Herberman and J.L. Fahey, Proc. Soc. Exptl. Biol. Med. 127 (1968) 938.

[60] I. Greenspan, E.R. Brown and S.O. Schwartz, Blood 21 (1963) 717.

[61] J.P. Levy, Transpl. Proc. (in press, 1971).

[62] G.N. Rogentine, jr. and P. Gerber, *In:* P.I. Terasaki (ed.), Histocompatibility testing 1970 (Munksgaard, Copenhagen, 1970) p. 333.

[63] G.N. Rogentine and P. Gerber, Transplantation 8 (1969) 28.

[64] R. Motta and M. Bruley, Transpl. Proc. 3 (1971) 1158.

[65] F. Lilly, Transpl. Proc. 3 (1971) 1239.

[66] M. Schlesinger, Progr. Exptl. Tumor Res. 13 (1970) 28-83.

[67] M.R. Mickey, M. Kreisler and P.I. Terasaki, *In:* P.I. Terasaki (ed.), Histocompatibility testing 1970 (Munksgaard, Copenhagen, 1970) p. 237.

[68] R.M. Mickey, M. Kreisler, E.D. Albert, N. Nanaka and P.I. Terasaki, Tissue Antigens 1 (1971) 57.

[69] H.O. McDevitt, Transpl. Proc. (in press, 1971).

[70] J.L. Amiel, Transpl. Proc. 3 (1971) 1270.

[71] J.D. Zervas, I.W. Delamore and M.C.G. Israëls, Lancet ii (1970) 634.

[72] J.R. Batchelor, J. Stuart and J.H. Edwards, Lancet (in press, 1971).

[73] R. Harris, unpublished observation.

[74] A. Sanderson, HL-A phenotypes in acute leukemia in children (in press, 1971).

[75] S.D. Lawler, P.T. Klouda, R.M. Hardisty and M.M. Till, Lancet (in press, 1971).

Part 6

MAMMARY TUMORIGENESIS IN MICE

HORMONAL FACTORS IN THE ORIGIN OF MAMMARY TUMORS

L.M. BOOT, G. RÖPCKE and H.G. KWA

The Netherlands Cancer Institute, Amsterdam, The Netherlands.

Professor Mühlbock was educated as a chemist and as a physician, specialized in gynecology. At that time this combination irrevocably led to an interest in the field of the sex hormones. When he came to the laboratory of the Netherlands Cancer Institute in 1946 as assistant of Dr. Korteweg, it was completely logical that his experience in gynecology and endocrinology would be applied to the study of the relation between hormones and breast cancer in mice.

Having been trained in plant physiology and phytopathology, it again stands to reason that when I came to this laboratory as student assistant, some 20 years ago, I was readily indoctrinated in his working hypothesis that hormones could induce tumors in their target organs by excessive growth stimulation, for short, in the principle of hormonal carcinogenesis. The following will show that the brain-washing performed by Prof. Mühlbock many years ago has been very effective.

As has been said many times before, in mammary gland carcinogenesis in mice a number of factors are involved: genetics, hormones, viral agents, and environmental factors, such as ionizing radiation, chemical carcinogens, etc.

In this paper I will restrict myself to the endocrine aspects for the reasons described above.

Estrogens and mammary cancer in mice

It has been known for a long time that estrogens are involved in the development of mammary tumors in mice. It has been shown by experiments in our institute that in animals infected with the mammary tumor virus (MTV) low estrogen doses are less effective than higher doses, provided that the latter are not toxic [1].

A second principle is that continuous treatment is much more effective than

275

discontinuous treatment, for instance with 5-day intervals [2]. In animals without the MTV but low tumor incidences are found after any type of estrogen treatment, with the exception of the C3Hf strain and its F_1 hybrids [1] in which quite a number of mammary tumors are found after continuous high dose estrogen treatment.

A few words on the way in which we treat our animals with estrogens are necessary. We have found that giving estrone in drinking water is a convenient method. The dosage is easy to vary and one can stop the treatment at will; moreover, the amount of labor involved is small as the waterbottles have to be refreshed only once a week.

The doses given are expressed in arbitrary units. One unit (U) is the dose which is just sufficient to maintain complete vaginal cornification in castrated female mice; the maximum dose which can be given this way is 16 U, or 2 mg per liter, which is the limit of solubility of this steroid in water. It is estimated that in the average normal female mouse the ovarian estrogen production is equivalent to 4 U in estrus and 0.25 U in diestrus.

The role of the pituitary

Some 15 years ago we were studying another model of hormonal carcinogenesis, that is the induction of granulosa-cell tumors in mice by their own gonadotropins, the so-called Biskind model. When an ovary is transplanted into the spleen of gonadectomized animals, it is subjected to excessive hormonal stimulation, because all estrogens produced by the graft are broken down in the liver and the feedback system pituitary-ovary, or in other words gonadotropins-estrogens is no longer functional, which leads to increased gonadotropin production, excessive stimulation of the ovary and ultimately the occurrence of ovarian tumors.

The relation of this model to mammary tumor formation may seem far-fetched at this point, but it happened that Prof. Mühlbock got the idea that if one implanted enough pituitaries or treated the animals with pituitary extracts long enough, one would ultimately produce ovarian tumors in normal female mice simply by means of the gonadotropin content of grafts and extracts. So we started to implant large numbers of pituitaries – up to 10 per day – in small groups of mice. Rather astonishing, at least at that time, was that we frequently obtained mammary tumors in the mice thus treated, also in strains free of the conventional MTV, and no ovarian tumors. On the basis of the knowledge at that time, it seemed logical to assume that the pituitary grafts had stimulated the ovaries to produce large amounts of estrogen, which would explain the occurrence of the mammary carcinomas. To prove this I was asked to have a look at the vaginal smears.

Untreated female mice have a 4-5-day estrous cycle due to increasing and decreasing ovarian estrogen production, with occasional spontaneous pseudo-pregnancies, that is periods of about 10 days of progesterone production through the influence of pituitary prolactin. The graft-bearing animals were expected to be in constant estrus, but instead we found them to be mainly in anestrus. In fact they showed a consecutive series of pseudopregnancies, interrupted at regular intervals by estrous peaks.

In a series of further experiments by Boot and Mühlbock, and Boot *et al.* [3-5] it could be proved beyond doubt that pituitary isografts in intact female mice produce prolactin, and none of the other pituitary hormones. In nearly all cases the grafts survive indefinitely.

The prolactin from the grafts has a double function: (a) mammotropic, acting directly on the mammary gland and (b) luteotropic, stimulating the ovarian corpora lutea to produce progesterone, which steroid also acts on the mammary gland. Estrogen levels appear to be more or less normal. The ultimate result is the induction of mammary tumors in all strains studied so far.

Eichwald-Silmser effect

In this model numerous variables can be introduced, such as age and sex of the donors, number and site of implantation and so on. The most favorable site of implantation appears to be the kidney, and generally pituitaries of males have a slightly better effect than those of female donors. However, one notable exception to this latter rule was observed. According to the transplantation rules of Snell [6] it was assumed that implants of hypophyses of F_2 hybrids into the parent F_1 hybrid would also prove to be fully active. The experiments were made on (C57BL x CBA)F_1 hybrids which were implanted subcutaneously with batches of 5 hypophyses of F_2 donors once a week for 4 weeks. The donors were 2-9 months old and the age of the recipient females was 4-6 weeks on the day of the first implantation. The tumor incidences found are given in table 1; the incidence is low in the animals receiving male donors, whereas the number found in the animals with female donors is up to expectation. The autopsy findings corresponded with these facts. In all animals with grafts of female donors the grafts could be recovered macroscopically at most implantation sites, often as quite large tissue masses. In the majority ($\pm 85\%$) of the hosts with grafts of male donors no grafted tissue could be found macroscopically at the sites of implantation, and in the remaining animals the number of grafts recovered was limited and these were mainly small. A number

Table 1
Incidence of mammary tumors in female (C57BL x CBA)F$_1$ mice implanted subcutaneously with 20 (4 x 5) hypophyses of F$_2$ hybrids.

		With tumor			Without tumor
Sex donors	No. animals	No.	Per cent	Av. age (days)	Av. age at death (days)
–	48	0	–	–	720
♀	28	17	61	580	583
♂	22	2	9	603	717

of whole-mount mammary gland preparations was studied. All animals with
implants of female donors showed the expected marked hyperplasia. In the
animals with grafts of male donors the results were much more variable. In
those in which surviving graft tissue could be recovered the usual type of
mammary gland hyperplasia was found; in the others various degrees of
involutionary changes were observed.

From the hormonal point of view the solution of the phenomena described
above was provided by the vaginal smear data from the (C57BL x CBA) F$_1$
hosts. Vaginal smears were taken from two animals each, implanted with female
or male hypophyses of F$_2$ donors, starting shortly after the last implantation
had been made. Those grafted with female hypophyses showed the usual
anestrous periods with but a few estrous peaks during the observation time of
one year. In the two animals implanted with male hypophyses initially the same
picture was observed, showing that the grafts had taken, but more or less
normal 4-5-day cycling occurred after an observation period of 60 days in one
animal and of 130 days in the second animal. On the basis of these results
vaginal smears were taken from another 8 animals of the two groups, starting
150 days after the last implantation of 5 hypophyses had taken place. Most
animals implanted with female hypophyses showed a nearly completely
continuous anestrus; a few still had some consecutive pseudopregnancies
interrupted by estrous periods, at least initially. From the 8 animals implanted
with male hypophyses 6 showed regular 4-5-day cycles interrupted by
occasional pseudopregnancies, like in untreated animals, whereas two animals
resumed the normal 4-5-day cycling only later in life during the observation
period of 220 days, both about 300 days after the last implantation. Before
that they had shown a more or less regular sequence of pseudopregnancies
interrupted by estrous phases. From the combined data it is concluded that
both female and male (C57BL x CBA)F$_2$ grafts in (C57BL x CBA)F$_1$ hosts do

take and produce prolactin. In the female host with female hypophyses the prolactin production increases in the lapse of time, parallel with the increase in size of the grafts, whereas in animals with male hypophyses the grafts are gradually rejected after a variable period of time in all cases in which vaginal smears were taken at or before about 300 days after the last implantation. In the few animals of the latter group, in which no vaginal smears were taken and in which viable grafted hypophyseal tissue was recovered at autopsy at an age of 550-700 days, the mammary glands did not show marked signs of involution.

The only logical explanation of the rejection of the grafts of male donors in the female host seems to be the so-called Eichwald-Silmser effect. As early as in 1955 Eichwald and Silmser [7] reported that skin grafts in mice regularly failed when the donor was male and the recipient female. By contrast, the other 3 combinations (male to male, female to female and female to male) almost always succeeded. This effect was more pronounced in the C57BL strain than in the A strain, and appeared to be due to the genotype of the host rather than that of the donor. Hauschka [8] and Snell [9] have suggested that rejection of tissues grafted from male donors to female hosts may be due to a sex-linked histocompatibility gene on the Y chromosome. Brocades Zaalberg [10] described the Eichwald-Silmser effect in skin graft experiments in the C57BL and CBA strain and their reciprocal hybrids; these two strains were originally derived from our institute. Complete graft rejection occurred in male to female grafts in strain C57BL, but no rejection occurred in the same combination in strain CBA. From experiments in which the F_1 hybrids were used as hosts, the hypothesis is derived that the absence of the sex effect in the CBA female seems to lie in the inability of the CBA female to react against the male-specific antigens. Later on numerous experiments have been performed in our institute with single pituitary isografts of F_1 donors in the left kidney of (C57BL x CBA)F_1 hybrids. In these experiments no indication for the occurrence of the Eichwald-Silmser effect was observed at any time.

Summarizing it is concluded that the Eichwald-Silmser effect can play a role in experiments with hypophyseal isografts in which male donors are used, but this seems to occur only very exceptionally.

Growth of pituitary isografts

As stated above, the pituitary isografts may increase in size markedly in the course of time. The phenomenon is strain or hybrid dependent, but estrogens play a role as well as shown by Boot *et al.* [11]. All further experiments to be discussed here were made again on (C57BL x CBA)F_1 hybrid mice which received single pituitary isografts of young adult (C57BL × CBA)F$_1$ donors in the left kidney at an age of ±6 weeks.

Without exogenous estrogen treatment the isografts grow markedly only in intact female hosts, some growth is observed in ovariectomized hosts (adrenal estrogens?). In intact or castrated male hosts the isografts show hardly any growth at ali, but a growth rate as found in intact females can be obtained by exogenous estrogen treatment of the male hosts, independent of the sex of the donors. Progesterone does not affect the growth rate of the pituitary grafts. Vaginal smear analysis in intact female animals with pituitary isografts has proved that increase of the size of the grafts goes parallel with an increase in the secretion rate of prolactin [12].

Progesterone and mammary cancer

Table 2 summarizes the most important results obtained thus far on the

Table 2

Mammary tumors in gonadectomized male (C57BL × CBA)F$_1$ mice with hypophyseal isografts.

		With tumor			Without tumor	Weight isograft
Treatment	No. animals	No.	Per cent	Av. age (days)	Av. age at death (days)	in mg at 300 days
–	49	0	0	–	618	2
16 U estrone	49	0	0	–	447	30
8 U estrone	50	9	18	409	447	30
16 U estrone discontinuous*	50	30	60	522	549	30
2 U estrone	42	23	55	481	514	40
0.1 U estrone	49	29	59	493	537	6
Progesterone (P)	42	12	29	558	583	2
P + 16 U estrone	52	48	92	379	373	30
P + 8 U estrone	48	37	77	336	366	30
P + 16 U estrone discontinuous *	50	49	98	356	424	25
P + 2 U estrone	42	42	100	271	–	35
P + 0.1 U estrone	47	47	100	306	–	10

*5-day intervals.

induction of mammary tumors with pituitary isografts in male mice. Pituitary isografts alone, in the absence of estrogen or progesterone do not induce mammary tumors in this hybrid. Intact females without graft also remain tumor-free (table 1). High-dose estrogen treatment (16 U and 8 U) is not very effective in this model, most probably because at these estrogen levels also the pituitary *in situ* starts growing, leading to deficiency of the normal pituitary hormones, exclusive prolactin, and ultimately to cachexia and death of the animals. Discontinuous and low-dose estrogen treatment, however, are effective, and this finding is exactly opposite to what was found in animals infected with the MTV. The lowest estrone level studied (0.1 U) itself hardly affects the mammary gland and the same is the case with discontinuous treatment. So we may conclude that, at least in this model, prolactin is the hormone which is primarily responsible for the tumor formation; the estrone acts by promoting the prolactin production of the grafts.

The second part of table 2 shows that progesterone greatly enhances the effect of the pituitary isografts and estrone at all dosage schedules. Even in the group without estrogen treatment the combined effect of low amounts of prolactin and progesterone leads to tumor formation in nearly 30% of the animals. The dose of progesterone given in these groups was 3 mg pellets implanted subcutaneously 3 times a week. Preliminary experiments have shown that 3 mg *once* a week is nearly as effective.

Comparison of the corresponding groups with and without progesterone shows that the growth of the isografts is neither inhibited nor stimulated by progesterone, so it appears that progesterone acts directly on the mammary gland in synergism with prolactin. Progesterone does have an effect on the pituitary *in situ*; it acts inhibitory on the enlargement with high estrone doses.

Quantitation of prolactin

Thus far the quantitative aspects of prolactin production have been dealt with only as related to the size of the grafts. By means of the radioimmunoassay of mouse prolactin developed in our institute by one of us (H.G.K.) it is possible now to measure the prolactin levels in the peripheral blood. It was shown that at each dose level of estrone the amount of prolactin measured increased with the lapse of time, and generally the higher estrone doses yielded higher prolactin levels. Basically there was no difference in the prolactin levels in animals receiving estrone alone or estrone and progesterone combined. The prolactin levels are not excessively high, and during the first 250 days of treatment are generally not much above those found in pseudopregnant animals. It appears again here that the continuity of stimulation is crucial in hormonal carcinogenesis.

Conclusion

It is well realized that the results of the experiments described above do not solve any problems of the virologists in their study on the relation between viruses and mammary gland carcinogenesis. By the various hormonal manipulations any hypothetical type of virus may have been induced, activated, derepressed or whatever one wishes to call it. On the other hand, the model discussed in this paper is closely related to other systems of hormonal carcinogenesis, such as the induction of thyroid tumors by an excess of pituitary thyroid stimulating hormone, and the induction of ovarian neoplasms by ovarian grafts in the spleen, in which system luteinizing hormone is the carcinogenic agent. As far as known, no viruses are involved in the latter two systems. So viral and hormonal carcinogenesis appear to exist side by side, and the mammary gland of the mouse appears to be the organ of choice to analyse their relationship.

References

[1] L.M. Boot and O. Mühlbock, Acta Unio Intern. Contra Cancrum 12 (1956) 569.
[2] O. Mühlbock and L.M. Boot, *In:* G.E.W. Wolstenholme and M. O'Connor, CIBA Foundation Symposium on Carcinogenesis. Mechanisms of action (J. and A. Churchill, London, 1959) p. 83.
[3] O. Mühlbock and L.M. Boot, Cancer Res. 19 (1959) 402.
[4] L.M. Boot, O. Mühlbock, G. Röpcke and W. van Ebbenhorst Tengbergen, Cancer Res. 22 (1962) 713.
[5] L.M. Boot and G. Röpcke, Cancer Res. 26 (1966) 1492.
[6] G.D. Snell, *In:* F. Homburger, The physiopathology of cancer (P.B. Hoeber, New York, 1959) p. 293.
[7] E.J. Eichwald and C.R. Silmser, Transpl. Bull. 2 (1955) 148.
[8] T.S. Hauschka, Transpl. Bull. 2 (1955) 154.
[9] G.D. Snell, Transpl. Bull. 3 (1956) 29.
[10] O. Brocades Zaalberg, Transpl. Bull. 6 (1959) 433.
[11] L.M. Boot, G. Röpcke and O. Mühlbock, Proceedings second international Congress Endocrinology, London, 1964 (Excerpta Medica Intern. Congress Series 83, 1965), p. 1058.
[12] L.M. Boot, Induction by prolactin of mammary tumours in mice (North-Holland Publishing Company, Amsterdam, 1969).

THE MOUSE MAMMARY TUMOR VIRUSES

Philomena HAGEMAN, Jero CALAFAT and J.H. DAAMS*

The Netherlands Cancer Institute, Amsterdam, The Netherlands

The mouse mammary tumor viruses belong to a group of viruses that are not too well studied. In some respects our knowledge about it is underdeveloped when compared to other tumor viruses, but it has some interesting aspects that also could be of some importance to other fields of virus research. One of the reasons of its arrears is the fact, that till now the virus has resisted the temptation to infect cells in tissue culture productively or to give a cytopathogenic effect [1,2]. It is possible to get virus production from cells derived from tumors, but in that case the tumors were already infected *in vivo* [3-5] and one cannot study the whole infection cycle or have a comparable uninfected cell.

The mouse mammary tumor virions were first described by Dmochowski in 1954 [6] and studied more in detail by Bernhard [7] who called them B particles. Unfortunately Huang *et al.* [8] have given this name later to the bullet-shaped particles of vesicular stomatitis virus.

B particles, like other RNA tumor viruses ripen at the membrane of the cells in which they are formed (fig. 1). Compared to others, the virus is rather fastidious, the cell of its choice is the epithelial cell of the mammary gland.

Occasionally some virus ripens in the epithelial cells of the epididymis [9], thymus [10], lung tumors [11] or even in a brain tumor [12].

The ripe virion has an eccentric electron dense nucleoid, surrounded by a nucleoid membrane and a large double membrane with spines (fig. 2). The spines can easily be seen if the preparations are negatively stained with phosphotungstate (fig. 3). The diameter of the virion is about 105 mµ. Some

*The authors are most grateful to Mrs. Rochelle Griffin for her help during the preparation of the manuscript and to Miss H. Eppenga, Mrs. L. van Heyde-Kleyne, T. van de Gronde and H. Lobbrecht for technical assistance.

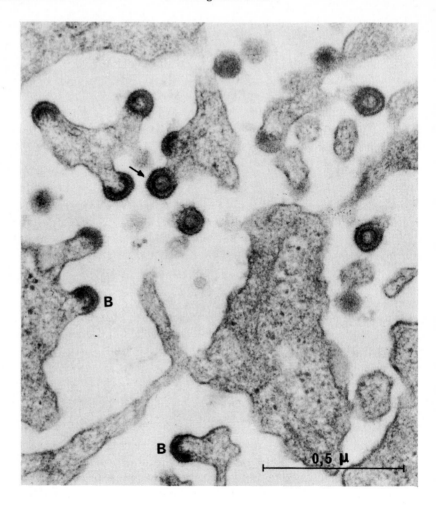

Fig. 1. Thin section of a mammary tumor of a C3H mouse. Budding B particles (B) at the plasma membrane, mostly on the microvilli, are present. The spines can already be seen at the surface of the budding particles (arrow).

Fig. 2. Thin section of a mammary tumor produced by MTV-O in BALB/c. Many B particles are present, some of them containing two or three nucleoids (arrows).

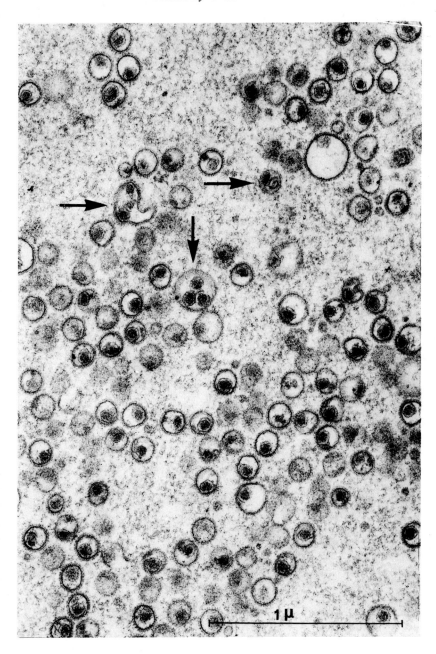

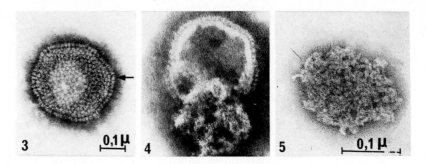

Figs. 3-5. B particles isolated from milk of C3H mice. Negative stain with phosphotungstic acid.
Fig. 3. Untreated B particle with spines at the surface (arrow). Magnification x 82,500.
Fig. 4. B particle after treatment with 0.1% sodium deoxycholate. The nucleoid is protruding from the envelope. Magnification x 177,500.
Fig. 5. B particle after treatment with 0.2% sodium deoxycholate. The nucleoid is free from the outer membranes and it has the appearance of a tangled thread. Magnification x 177,500.

particles contain more than one nucleoid (fig. 2), and Thomas *et al.* [*13*] described multinucleoid particles with as many as seven nucleoids.

The molecular weight of the B particle is ± 350 x 10^6 [14], it contains a large RNA of about 10 x 10^6 daltons [15] calculated from a sedimentation coefficient of 60-70. Other experiments and electron microscopic observations [17] indicate, however, that the RNA of MTV, like that of other oncornaviruses has an aggregate structure, consisting of a major 37 S RNA and smaller RNA molecules [14,16].

The exact mode of formation of the virus particle is only known through electron microscopy. The intracytoplasmic A particle is considered to be the precursor of the B particle. On many electron micrographs one gets the impression that the virus material is assembled immediately near the cell membrane (fig. 1). Yet when serial thin sections are made it can be seen that the buddings contain A particles. This requires a lot of careful work which was done by Imai and his coworkers [18]. Their results were confirmed by Gay *et al.* [19] who also demonstrated that B particles may contain cellular constituents like ribosomes.

From a biochemical point of view our ignorance about the formation of the MTV virion is still great. Labelled RNA precursors given to infected animals [15], cell lines, or tissue cultures producing B particles [5,20] give rise to labelled B particles, but nothing is known about the prestages of the virion.

Once formed, the virus particles are released into vesicles in the cell or through the plasma membrane, but preferably on the sides of the cell adjacent to the lumen. In this respect they are different from C particles that are also released between the cells [21].

The common budding place of the B particles are the microvilli of the mammary gland, many of the virions are released via the milk and infect the young mice. This was the first mode of transmission to be discovered [22-24] and maybe this caused the impression that it was the most important and general transmission route of MTV. Now that many more mouse strains and MTV strains are studied, it turns out that many mouse strains transmit MTV genetically with or without milk transmission. Examples of such a genetical transmission can be found in the mouse strains GR [25-27], C3Hf [28,29] and C3HA^{vy}fB[30]. One must keep in mind that the milk transmission might be an exception rather than a rule. Even the occurrence of B particles in the milk as we found in the mouse strain C3Hf does not mean that milk transmission takes place [31].

The structure of the B particle was studied by the various groups of Moore, Calafat and Almeida. Moore and his coworkers demonstrated that the particle during the budding process immediately gets other surface antigens than the plasma membrane [32]. They found a regular pattern in the arrangement of the spines on the B particle [33].

The group of Moore [34] could confirm earlier results of De Thé [35] about the presence of an ATPase in the viral membrane. Sarkar and Moore [36] studied the structure of the nucleoid of the B particle but the interpretation of the electron micrographs is different from those of Calafat [37].

After treatment with deoxycholate or Tween 80 and ether we could isolate viral nucleoids that look like an entangled thread (figs. 4 and 5). No clear helix-like structure of the thread can be seen, nor could Almeida see a regularity in the arrangement of the internal component of the MTV virion [38]. Sarkar and Moore [36] claim to have observed a helix-like structure in the nucleoid. This is shown but not conclusive in pictures of unripe virions, in which the nucleoid is not yet fully condensed. From their results they propose a helical model for the nucleoidcapsid of the oncogenic RNA viruses [39].

Many mouse strains harbor their own or even more than one MTV variant. Some of the more important and better studied variants are shown in table 1. The virus strains can be distinguished by their biological properties:
MTV-S (Standard MTV, the former Bittner strain) is very virulent.
MTV-L (Low-congenic MTV, the former nodule inducing virus) is very low

P. Hageman et al.

Table 1
MTV strains.

Virus strain	Natural host	Symptoms	Transmission in natural host	
			Milk	Egg or sperm
MTV-S	C3H	High tumorperc. at low age	+	−
MTV-L	C3Hf	Rather low tumorperc. at high age, nodule inducing virus	−	+
MTV-P	GR	High tumorperc. at low age, plaques, hormonedependent	+	+
MTV-X	O20	Induced by irradiation	+	+
MTV-O	BALB/c	After passage: high tumorperc. at low age	?	?

tumorigenic. Its name NIV is not so well chosen [40] because the other strains also cause nodules.

MTV-P (causing plaques, derived from the mouse strain GR, the former Mühlbock strain) causes a different type of tumor, unfortunately called plaque by Foulds [42].

MTV-O (overlooked) and MTV-X (found after irradiation of O20 mice with X-rays) are present in a hidden form in their hosts. [43].

It must be stressed that the genetical transmission is not a property of the virus concerned, but of the mouse strain. The GR mice or C3Hf mice transmit their virus as a gene, but when the virus is transmitted to other mouse strains, this property is lost [27,41]. Only transmission by the milk or artificially by giving an injection is possible in these strains. As far as they have been studied, these virus strains have morphologically indistinguishable virions [44]. Immunologically they have a strong cross reaction both in neutralization [45] and in double diffusion tests [46]. However, small differences exist [47,48] that are most clearly seen between MTV-S and MTV-L (fig. 6). The nature of these differences can be better understood via the scheme of the precipitation lines that appear in the double diffusion test when B particles are tested against antiserum made in rabbits (fig. 7). In the center well is anti-MTV, in the left well are B particles that are dissociated by shaking with ether. Several precipitation lines appear. By preparing separate nucleoid and membrane fractions and after studying the sensitivity for different enzymes [37] it was

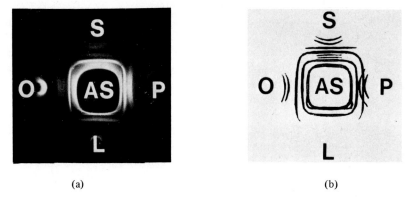

(a)   (b)

Fig. 6. (a) Immunodiffusion test of equal amounts of four strains of MTV (outer wells) and rabbit anti MTV-S serum (center well). MTV-L does not share all its antigens with MTV-S, MTV-P is slightly different, MTV-O and MTV-S cannot be distinguished. (b) Scheme of the precipitation lines in fig. 6a.

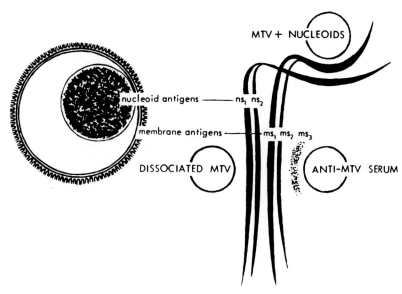

Fig. 7. Scheme of the antigenic structure of MTV.

possible to recognize some of the lines as derived from the membrane and others as nucleoid antigens. We can compare these nucleoid antigens with the group specific antigens of the mouse leukemia viruses, though the cross neutralization experiments of Blair [45] indicate that a group specific antigen is also present in the virus envelope. Other studies in this line were carried out by Nowinski et al. [49].

In fig. 6 a double diffusion test is shown in which an antiserum against MTV-S is used, the other wells contain purified B particles of the indicated strains in equal concentrations. MTV-L does not crossreact with all the antigens of MTV-S. Also MTV-P is slightly different.

A difference between the nucleoid antigens of MTV-P and MTV-S was found by Hilgers et al. [50]. He injected GR mice with MTV-P and could not find antibodies against the nucleoid antigens, whereas MTV-S evoked these antibodies. This proves a difference in the nucleoid antigens of MTV-S and MTV-P.

The total number of proteins of the B particle is larger than can be concluded from the immunodiffusion tests. Nowinski and Old [51] reported the separation of several proteins of the B particle after polyacrylamide gel electrophoresis.

At the University of Nijmegen (The Netherlands) in the laboratory for biochemistry, Gielkens and Salden, coworkers of Bloemendal, are studying the composition of the virion of Rauscher leukemia virus by gel electrophoresis. The pattern that is obtained when a RLV preparation and one of the MTV preparations are compared, is shown in fig. 8. The bands of the RLV material coincide with the results obtained by Schäfer et al. [52].

It is not surprising that purified B particles are highly antigenic to rabbits [46]. It is more remarkable that though the virions are formed by budding from the membrane of the mouse cell, they are also antigenic to mice [53], even to their own host. Hilgers et al. [50] found antibodies both against internal and membrane antigens of B particles in several strains of mice injected with virions. Müller et al. [54] even discovered spontaneously occurring antibodies in infected tumorbearing and tumorfree mice of different ages. In the GR strain in which the virus is already present at conception only antibodies against the membrane antigens of the virions were present.

The B particle can be considered as the infective form of MTV. It can be isolated from milk [14,15,30,55-58] or from mammary tumors [44,59] preferably by gradient centrifugation. A review about the purification procedures was given by Manning et al. [58]. The virions have a sedimentation coefficient of about 900-1000 S. The buoyant density is very dependent on the gradients that are used (1.16 g/cm^3 in citrate, lighter in Ficoll, heavier in CsCl). Another successful purification method was electrophoresis applied by Lyons and Moore [59].

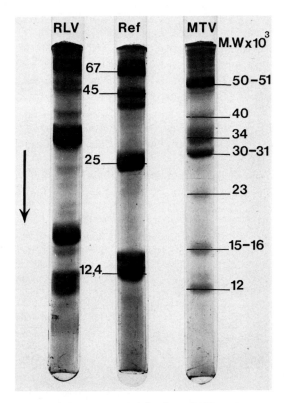

Fig. 8. Electrophoresis of Rauscher leukemia virus (RLV) and mammary tumor virus (MTV-S) in polyacrylamide gels. Highly purified RLV and MTV was degraded 90 sec at 100°C in the presence of 2% sodiumdodecylsulfate (SDS). The proteins were electrophoresed on a column composed of 12.5% acrylamide and 0.67% bisacrylamide containing 0.1% SDS. Protein staining was with Coomassie blue. The electrophoretic pattern was compared with reference proteins (center gel), from bottom to top: cytochrome C, MW 12,400, chymotrypsinogen A, MW 25,000, ovalbumin MW 45,000 and bovine serum albumin, MW 67,000. The approximate molecular weights of the polypeptides are indicated on the photograph. (Courtesy A. Gielkens and M. Salden, Laboratory for Biochemistry, University of Nijmegen.)

If such a purified preparation is injected into susceptible young female mice which are kept in the suitable hormonal conditions by breeding, force breeding or the administration of the appropriate hormones, the mice develop mammary tumors at 6-10 months, depending on the properties of the MTV strain and the test mouse strain.

The function of the B particle was less clear when virions of other strains than the common MTV-S were used, especially the low oncogenic variants. Mühlbock, Boot and Heston have done much work on these strains [60,61]. When tumor extracts or virions isolated from C3Hf mice (MTV-L) were injected into the BALB/c mouse strain which is very susceptible to MTV-S, no tumors were reported or only an occasional tumor occurred. These particles did not seem to be infectious at all. DeOme *et al.* [41] reported successful transmission of MTV-L to BALB/c by means of cell grafting. We have some doubts whether this virus is still a real MTV-L. Dmochowski and his coworkers found in several cases some activity of extracts from low oncogenic strains [e.g. 62].

B particles that we isolated from milk of the hybrid C3Hf x BALB/c caused a high percentage of tumors at a late age in BALB/c (table 2). As the virions were

Table 2
Infectivity of purified B particles from (C3Hf x BALB/c)F_1 milk tested in young BALB/c females.

Inoculum	Number of animals	Tumorperc.	Average tumor age (days)
10^{-1}	10	60%	484
10^{-2}	10	70%	510
10^{-3}	10	30%	558
Buffer	18	10%	432

$10^0 = \pm 100 \, \mu g$ virus/ml.

derived from the hybrid mouse, we cannot be sure that the virus is still a true MTV-L. However, the late appearance of the tumors caused by these virions points to a real MTV-L. The virions showed in immunodiffusion tests also the MTV-L pattern.

The recognition of the B particle as the infective entity of MTV was delayed a long time because both highly infective B particles of the MTV-S and hardly infective and barely tumorigenic particles of MTV-L were known. A review of the pros and cons was given by Moore [63]. Another difficulty was, that when after ultracentrifugation the various fractions of a density gradient were tested biologically, many fractions gave positive results, also other zones than the B particle band [64], but this zone contained most of the infectivity. It became established that B particles are very obstinate and could be present everywhere in the gradient. Results from CsCl gradients on which the virions are badly damaged, can hardly be considered to give a good idea about the infectivity of the B particle [65,66].

It is necessary to make this overly simple picture of MTV more complicated.

In several cases infectivity is reported in tissues or preparations where no B particles are found or could have been present. Moore *et al.* [67,68] concluded from experiments with Gradocol membranes and from irradiation and diffusion experiments the existence of an infective entity of about 30 mμ. This is much smaller than the B particle. Unfortunately, not much work seems to have been done upon this subject after his early and interesting experiments.

An even more puzzling situation exists in the blood of MTV bearing mice. Nandi and his coworkers [69,70] found biological activity of MTV in the blood, especially connected with the red blood cells. Recently he showed that the infectivity was present inside the red blood cell [71]. This R-MTV as he called it, to distinguish it from the already known M-MTV of the milk, had several characteristics that were different from M-MTV. A few will be mentioned here.

His R-MTV was not visible as B particles, it infected only syngeneic and allogeneic H-2 compatible hosts [72,73]. This was not confirmed by Hummel and Little [74], however. The R-MTV causes tumors in test animals carrying B particles, so it is a true form of MTV. In later experiments Nandi found that R-MTV was not neutralized by anti-B-particle serum [75]. From enzyme studies he concluded that R-MTV is a nucleoprotein of which the nucleic acid moiety is DNA or a DNA-RNA hybrid [76]. This idea is attractive, since the RNA dependent DNA polymerase activity is also reported to be inside the B particle [77].

Moore and his group [78] who did some experiments on MTV in the blood, do not want to assume an infective entity in the blood apart from the B particle, but wish to explain everything by the presence of a few B particles in the blood. In their experiments B particles indeed are found in the blood, maybe due to the fact that they often used tumor bearing mice as blood donors.

Two difficult points about this work on blood MTV need to be stressed. One is the fact that the electron microscope cannot always give the conclusive answer as to whether MTV virions are present or not. The biological test is far more sensitive. Between 10^9 and 10^{10} viral particles per ml must be present to be visible in the electron microscope. In titration studies of MTV-S in BALB/c mice we found a dilution endpoint of $\pm 10^{-9}$ - 10^{-10} g virus/ml. Giving a dose of 0.5 ml/animal and assuming a molecular weight of the particle of 350×10^6 [14], this corresponds with about 10^5 - 10^6 particles. The result agrees with the titration results for Rauscher leukemia virus in mice, where Boiron and coworkers found the same minimum infective dose [79].

Another drawback is the fact that blood MTV looses its infectivity very easily in a cell free system, and has not been purified. As Nandi has had to work with such an impure preparation, the results of his enzyme experiments are rather doubtful.

In our work on blood MTV, we found slightly different results from those of Nandi [80]. The most striking difference was that we found much more infectivity in the white blood cells than in the red ones, if the infectivity is compared on the basis of the number of cells. A representative experiment is given in table 3. The so-called white blood cells were obtained by spinning

Table 3
Infectivity of blood cells from MTV infected BALB/c males tested in young BALB/c females (500 μl/animal).

Inoculum cells per μl		Number of animals	Tumorperc.	Average tumor age (days)
Erythr.	Lymphoc.			
3×10^6	150	10	70	197
3×10^5	15	13	8	196
500	1100	12	75	188
50	110	11	90	196

down washed heparinized blood from young MTV infected BALB/c males on a density gradient of Isopaque and Ficoll [81]. The cells that are collected from the density interphase are lymphocytes. Experiments with the whole leukocyte population gave about the same result.

In this case the infectivity is mainly carried by the lymphocytes, the infectivity of the so-called red blood cell fraction may be explained by the few contaminating lymphocytes.

This result does not help us much to know more about the nature of the MTV activity in the white blood cells. Until now careful electron microscopic examination of the lymphocytes did not reveal any B particle or a particle that could be considered as a precursor of it. Bucciarelli et al. [82] found in one case intracytoplasmic A particles in lymph nodes of RIII mice. In the leukocytes viral antigens can be detected by immunofluorescence (fig. 9). This cell-bound virus activity, without the finding of the B particle but combined with the formation of at least some viral antigens is not restricted to the white blood cell fraction. Both thymus and spleen carry infectivity and viral antigens [83] but we did not succeed in separating this infectivity from the cells.

Fig. 9a. Immunofluorescence with anti MTV-S serum in lymphocytes of BALB/c mice infected with MTV-S.

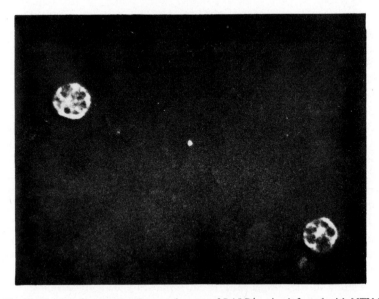

Fig. 9b. Immunofluorescence in granulocytes of BALB/c mice infected with MTV-S.

Some of our laboratory mouse strains carry a highly virulent MTV that causes a high percentage of tumors at a young age. Early occurrence of mammary carcinomas is not a frequent phenomenon in wild mice, or in human populations. Therefore the existence of latent or hidden viruses in mouse strains that were considered to be virus free is very interesting.

These strains are in fact carrying a tumor virus that waits for the right moment to appear. The BALB/c mouse strain was supposed to be MTV-free. Deringer [84] found 22% of mammary tumors at 17 months. It is a very sensitive test animal for MTV-S [31]. Yet occasionally MTV antigens were found in the mammary glands of old females. To test the biological activity, we used the mammary glands from 11-15 months old retired breeding females from our mouse colony. From pools of these mammary glands, cellfree homogenates and sham B-particle preparations were made. The zones from the density gradient in which B particles were supposed to be found, were examined by electron microscopy and injected into 3-week-old BALB/c females, that were force-bred later on. Table 4 shows that the injected animals had a high tumor percentage at a young age. The controls that were injected with buffer and force-bred had the common low tumor percentage at an old age, which is characteristic for the BALB/c mice.

Milk samples of the test mice carried MTV antigens, the milk of 27 controls did not (table 5). Many virus particles were found in the milk and the mammary tumors (fig. 2) of the mice injected with the mammary gland preparations (table 6). In the control animals, no B particles were found in the mammary tumors that occur at a late age, nor in the preneoplastic nodules, the mammary glands or the milk. Yet some virus is present in the mammary glands, for when sham B particle preparations were made some virus particles were observed (table 6).

These experiments do not explain through what kind of mechanism this hidden virus is manifested. It could be that the release of viral RNA is switched on at a late age [85], but it is also possible that other mechanisms inhibit the production of infectious virus particles at a younger age.

Maybe the virions are always present in a rather small amount, but when the equilibrium is disturbed in young animals in favor of the virus, the animals develop mammary tumors and then it is not necessary to assume a specific switching on of the virus.

Another example of the switching on of a virus, this time by irradiation, is the MTV-X in the mouse strain O20. This strain was considered to be free of MTV. After irradiation mammary tumors with infective B particles could be demonstrated in these mice [86]. In the supposedly MTV-free strain C57Black, also a hidden MTV, develops with aging [87]. The mechanism of this development of MTV is not yet clear.

Table 4
Preparations from mammary glands of old BALB/c mice tested in young BALB/c females.

Inoculum homogenate	Number of animals	Tumorperc.	Average tumor age (days)
10^{-1}	11	90	181
10^{-2}	10	60	228
'B particles'			
5×10^{-2}	10	90	198
5×10^{-3}	9	80	224
Buffer	37	16	453

Table 5
MTV antigens in milk of BALB/c mice (3rd lactation).

Inoculum		Positive	Negative
No. 454	homogenate		
	10^{-1}	4	3
	10^{-2}	3	7
	'B particles'		
	5×10^{-2}	5	1
	5×10^{-3}	5	3
No. 493	'B particles'		
	2×10^{-2}	6	1
	2×10^{-3}	3	1
Buffer		0	27

In preparation 493 a few and in preparation 454 no B particles could be observed by electron microscopic examination.

Table 6
B particles in BALB/c mice treated with homogenates of mammary glands of old BALB/c mice.

	Age donor (months)	Positive	Negative
Treated BALB/c			
Ma. tumor	5-6	10	0
Untreated BALB/c			
Ma. tumor	15-18	0	11
Nodules	8-11	0	2
Mammary glands	11-16	0	2
'B particle zone'	11-16	2*	2

*Only a small amount of B particles.

In any case the experiments indicate, that there are more tumor viruses present in mice (and men?) than meet the eye.

References

[1] E.Y. Lasfargues and D.H. Moore, *In:* W.H. Kirstner, Malignant transformation by viruses (Springer, Berlin, 1966) 44.

[2] J. Links and O. Tol, J. Gen. Virol. 5 (1969) 547.

[3] J.A. Sykes, J. Whitescarver and L. Briggs, J. Natl. Cancer Inst. 41 (1968) 1315.

[4] E.Y. Lasfarques, B. Kramarsky, N.H. Sarkar, J.C. Lasfarques and D.H. Moore, Cancer Res. 30 (1970) 1109.

[5] R.D. Cardiff, P.B. Blair and P. Nakayama, Proc. Natl. Acad. Sci. U.S. 59 (1968) 895.

[6] L. Dmochowski, J. Natl. Cancer Inst. 15 (1954) 785.

[7] W. Bernhard, A. Bauer, M. Guerin and C. Oberling, Bull. Ass. Franç. Etude Cancer 42 (1955) 163.

[8] A.S. Huang, J.W. Greenawalt and R.R. Wagner, Virology 30 (1966) 161.

[9] G.H. Smith, J. Natl. Cancer Inst. 36 (1966) 685.

[10] K.H. Hollmann and J.M. Verley, Z. Zellforsch. 78 (1967) 47.

[11] J. Calafat, J. Microscopie 8 (1969) 983.

[12] D.H. Moore, J. Charney, E.Y. Lasfarques, N.H. Sarkar, R.C. Rubin and R.P. Ames, Proc. Soc. Exptl. Biol. Med. 132 (1969) 125.

[13] J.A. Thomas, E. Hollande, M. Henry, M.C. Dutrillaux and M.C. Vilain, Compt. Rend. Acad. Sci. Paris 270 (1970) 2387.

[14] M.J. Lyons and D.H. Moore, J. Natl. Cancer Inst. 35 (1965) 549.

[15] P.H. Duesberg and P.B. Blair, Proc. Natl. Acad. Sci. U.S. 55 (1966) 1490.

[16] P.H. Duesberg and R.D. Cardiff, Virology 36 (1968) 696.

[17] N.H. Sarkar and D.H. Moore, J. Virol. 5 (1970) 230.

[18] T. Imai, H. Okano, A. Matsumoto and A. Horie, Cancer Res. 26 (1966) 443.

[19] F.W. Gay, J.K. Clarke and E. Dermott, J. Virology 5 (1970) 801.

[20] R.D. Cardiff and P.B. Blair, Intern. J. Cancer 5 (1970) 211.

[21] J. Calafat, J. Microscopie 7 (1968) 841.

[22] Staff of Roscoe B. Jackson Memorial Laboratory, Science 78 (1933) 465.

[23] R. Korteweg, Ned. T. Geneeskunde 79 (1935) 1482.

[24] J.J. Bittner, Science 84 (1936) 162.

[25] O. Mühlbock, Europ. J. Cancer 1 (1965) 123.

[26] G.H. Zeilmaker, Intern. J. Cancer 4 (1969) 261.

[27] O. Mühlbock and P. Bentvelzen, Perspectives Virol. 6 (1968) 75.

[28] D.R. Pitelka, H.A. Bern, S. Nandi and K.B. DeOme, J. Natl. Cancer Inst. 33 (1964) 867.

[29] I.E. Vellisto and F.B. Bang, J. Natl. Cancer Inst. 40 (1967) 1213.

[30] G. Vlahakis, W.E. Heston and G.H. Smith, Science 170 (1970) 185.

[31] P.C. Hageman, J. Links and P. Bentvelzen, J. Natl. Cancer Inst. 40 (1968) 1319.

[32] H. Tanaka and D.H. Moore, Virology 33 (1967) 197.

[33] N.H. Sarkar and D.H. Moore, *In:* P. Favard, Microscopie électronique 1970. Soc. Franç. Microsc. Electr. (Paris, 1970) Vol.III, biologie, 925.

[34] S.M. El-Fiky, N.H. Sarkar and D.H. Moore, *In:* P. Favard, Microscopie électronique 1970. Soc. Franç. Microsc. Electr. (Paris, 1970) Vol.III, biologie, 923.

[35] G. De Thé, J. Cell Biol. 31 (1966) 140 A.
[36] N.H. Sarkar and D.H. Moore, J. Microscopie 7 (1968) 539.
[37] J. Calafat and P. Hageman, Virology 38 (1969) 364.
[38] J.D. Almeida, A.P. Waterson and J.A. Drewe, J. Hygiene 65 (1967) 467.
[39] N.H. Sarkar, R.C. Nowinski and D.H. Moore, Virology 46 (1971) 1.
[40] S. Nandi and K.B. De Ome, J. Natl. Cancer Inst. 35 (1965) 299.
[41] K.B. DeOme, L. Young and S. Nandi, Proc. Am. Ass. Cancer Res. 8 (1967) 13.
[42] L. Foulds, J. Natl. Cancer Inst. 17 (1956) 701.
[43] P. Bentvelzen, J.H. Daams, P. Hageman and J. Calafat, Proc. Natl. Acad. Sci. U.S. 67 (1970) 377.
[44] J. Calafat and P. Hageman, Virology 36 (1968) 308.
[45] P.B. Blair, Proc. Soc. Exptl. Biol. Med. 103 (1960) 188.
[46] P.B. Blair, Cancer Res. 23 (1963) 381.
[47] P.B. Blair, Cancer Res. 30 (1970) 625.
[48] P.B. Blair, D.W. Weiss and G.H. Smith, Israel J. Med. Sci. 6 (1970) 611.
[49] R.C. Nowinski, L.J. Old, D.H. Moore, G. Geering and E.A. Boyse, Virology 31 (1967) 1.
[50] J. Hilgers, J.H. Daams and P. Bentvelzen, Israel J. Med. Sci. 7 (1971) 154.
[51] R.C. Nowinski and L.J. Old, Abstracts of papers presented at the second Tumor Virus Meeting, Cold Spring Harbor, New York (1970) 24.
[52] W. Schäfer, J. Lange, D.P. Bolognesi, F. Noronha, J.E. Post and C.G. Richard, Virology 44 (1971) 73.
[53] P. Blair, D.H. Lavrin, M. Dezfulian and D.W. Weiss, Cancer Res. 26 (1966) 647.
[54] M. Müller, P.C. Hageman and J.H. Daams, J. Natl. Cancer Inst. 47 (1971) 801.
[55] J.A. Sykes, C.E. Grey, J. Scanlon, L. Young and L. Dmochowski, Texas Rept. Biol. Med. 22 (1964) 609.
[56] W.T. Hall and W.F. Feller, J. Natl. Cancer Inst. 39 (1967) 1155.
[57] H.E. Bond and W.T. Hall, J. Natl. Cancer Inst. 43 (1969) 1073.
[58] J.S. Manning, A.J. Hackett, R.D. Cardiff, H.C. Mel and P.B. Blair, Virology 40 (1970) 912.
[59] M.J. Lyons and D.H. Moore, Nature 194 (1962) 1162.
[60] L.M. Boot and O. Mühlbock, Acta Unio Intern. Contra Cancrum 12 (1956) 569.
[61] W.E. Heston, Ann. N.Y. Acad. Sci. 71 (1958) 931.
[63] L. Dmochowski, C.E. Grey and J.A. Sykes, Acta Unio Intern. Contra Cancrum (1963) 276.
[64] D.H. Moore, N. Pillsbury and B.D. Pullinger, J. Natl. Cancer Inst. 43 (1969) 1263.
[65] G. Miroff and B.S. Magdoff-Fairchild, J. Natl. Cancer Inst. 34 (1965) 777.
[66] G. Miroff and H.V. Lamberson, Int. J. Cancer 5 (1970) 136.
[67] D.H. Moore, E.Y. Lasfarques, M.R. Murray, C.D. Haagensen and E.C. Pollard, Acta Union Intern. Contra Cancrum 15 (1959) 819.
[68] D.H. Moore, E.C. Pollard and C.D. Haagensen, Fed. Proc. 21 (1962) 942.
[69] S. Nandi, M. Handin and L. Young, J. Natl. Cancer Inst. 36 (1966) 803.
[70] S. Nandi, *In:* Carcinogenesis: A broad critique. Proceedings of the 20th Annual Symp. on Fundamental Cancer Res. (Williams and Wilkins, Baltimore (1967) 295.
[71] S. Nandi and S. Haslam, Cancer Res. 31 (1971) 479.
[72] S. Nandi, K.B. DeOme and M. Handin, J. Natl. Cancer Inst. 35 (1965) 309.
[73] S. Nandi, Proc. Natl. Acad. Sci. U.S. 58 (1967) 485.
[74] K.P. Hummel and C.C. Little, J. Natl. Cancer Inst. 30 (1963) 593.

[75] S. Nandi, S. Haslam and C. Helmick, Proc. Am. Ass. Cancer Res. 11 (1970) 59.
[76] S. Nandi, Nature (New Biology) 230 (1971) 146.
[77] S. Spiegelman, A. Burny, M.R. Das, J. Keydar, J. Schlom, M. Travnicek and K. Watson, Nature 228 (1970) 430.
[78] D.H. Moore, N.H. Sarkar and J. Charney, J. Natl. Cancer Inst. 44 (1970) 965.
[79] M. Boiron, J.P. Levy and J. Peries, Proc. Med. Virol. 9 (1967) 341.
[80] S. Nandi, D. Knox, K.B. DeOme, M. Handin, V.V. Finster and P.B. Picket, J. Natl. Cancer Inst. 36 (1966) 809.
[81] R. Harris and E.O. Ukaejiofo, Lancet II (1969) 327.
[82] E. Bucciarelli, G.B. Bolis and F. Squartini, Lav. Ist. Anat. Istol. Patol. 30 (1970) 57.
[83] J.H. Daams, *In:* L. Severi, Immunity and tolerance in oncogenesis. Proceedings of the 4th Perugia Quadrennial Int. Conf. on Cancer, 1969, Perugia (1970) 463.
[84] M.K. Deringer, J. Natl. Cancer Inst. 35 (1965) 1047.
[85] R.J. Huebner and G.J. Todaro, Proc. Natl. Acad. Sci. U.S. 64 (1969) 1087.
[86] A. Timmermans, P. Bentvelzen, P.C. Hageman and J. Calafat, J. Gen. Virol. 4 (1969) 619.
[87] P. Bentvelzen, this Symposium.

GENETIC ASPECTS IN THE GENESIS OF MAMMARY CANCER

Anna DUX
Department of Biology, The Netherlands Cancer Institute,
Amsterdam, The Netherlands

More than a year ago, while discussing the program of this symposium, it was decided not to deal so much with past achievements in the field of cancer research, but to focus attention on some actual problems. I have decided to adopt the same attitude in choosing the material for my paper. Rather than to analyse the past contribution of Professor Mühlbock and his co-workers in the field of mammary cancer genetics, I have concentrated mostly on the work actually going on and in which Professor Mühlbock is actively participating, and I have included in my report some preliminary results.

The establishment of inbred strains of mice has made it possible to prove that genetic factors play a role in the genesis of mammary cancer. Of all mouse strains investigated, the C57BL strain is considered as one of the most resistant strains to the inciting factors in the genesis of mammary cancer [1-7]. In our colony no mammary tumors have been found in untreated virgin females since 1931. The C57BL strain does not manifest the presence of the mammary tumor virus (MTV). When MTV is given to newborns of this strain by foster nursing on a MTV-carrying mother, the mammary tumor incidence rises only to 27% in force-bred females at the average age of 432 days.

The resistance of this strain to develop mammary tumors even when all inducing factors are present is remarkable. In a series of experiments this resistance was analysed.

In the first series the relation of the histocompatibility genes to the development of mammary cancer in mice was investigated. The relation between histocompatibility genes and the development of malignancy has already been considered for some time. First, a relation was sought between histocompatibility genes and the oncogenic virus effect. Such a relation has been found for mouse leukemia [8-14], but investigations with the mammary tumor virus have been less successful in this respect. Lilly [9] found no significant correlation between the H-2 histocompatibility locus and the development of cancer. Nandi [15] using another approach found that a special form of MTV, the so-called R-MTV or blood-MTV, is strain-specific and is related to certain alleles of the H-2 locus.

In our investigation the oncogenic influence of two variants of the mammary tumor virus has been analysed, *i.e.* C3H-MTV (Bittner virus) abundantly present in the C3H strain, transmitted by the mother's milk, causing mammary tumors in a high percentage early in life, and GR-MTV found in the GR strains, transmitted equally well by the mother's milk as by the sperm and the ovum at conception, causing mammary tumors in a high percentage at an early age, many of them being hormone-dependent [7,16-18].

The congenic resistant lines (CR lines) on the B10-background [19,20], kindly supplied by Dr. G. Snell, Bar-Harbor, used in this investigation are listed in table 1. These strains differ genetically from the background strain by one

Table 1
Mammary tumor incidence in C57BL/10ScSn strain and different CR lines.

Congenic resistant lines	Histocompatibility loci		Per cent mammary tumors in force-bred females with	
			C3H-MTV**	GR-MTV**
B10		$H-2^b$	25	
B10.A		$*H-2^a$	100	–
B10.D2		$*H-2^d$	100	50
B10.M		$*H-2^f$	90	43
B10.BR		$*H-2^k$	50	33
B10.AKM		$*H-2^m$	80	57
B10.D2(58N)	$*H-1^a$	$H-2^b$	22	50
B10.C(41N)	$*H-1^b$	$H-2^b$	0	55
B10.LP-a	$*H-3^b$	$H-2^b$	20	22
B10.C(47N)	$*H-7^b$	$H-2^b$	–	33
B10.D2(57N)	$*H-8^b$	$H-2^b$	7	43
B10.C(45N)	$*H-9^b$	$H-2^b$	23	–
B10.C(30NX)	$*H-13^b$	$H-2^b$	–	61

* Indicated are the alleles at which CR lines differ from the B10 strain.
** These are preliminary results, as the experiments are still in progress.
– Test not completed.

allele at the H-2 locus or by one allele at one of the weak histocompatibility loci. The susceptibility to MTV was measured by the percentage of mammary tumors appearing before the age of 12 months. In virus-free breeding females of the CR lines no mammary tumors have been found before the age of one year [21].

The first experiment was done with C3H-MTV. This virus was given to the newborns of the CR lines by foster nursing on ($\female$ C3H x $\male$ O20)F_1 females. To accelerate the appearance of mammary tumors the foster-nursed females of the CR lines were force-bred by removing newborns immediately after birth so that the females had pregnancies in rapid succession. The percentage of mammary tumors is given in tables 1 and 2.

Table 2
Average mammary tumor incidence in B10/CR-lines.

Allele H-2^b (and different other loci)	Alleles 2^d; 2^f; 2^k; 2^m
With GR-MTV	
44%	51%
With C3H-MTV	
14%	89%

It appears that the CR lines in which the H-2^b allele of the B10-strain is replaced by the alleles 2^a, 2^d, 2^f, 2^k and 2^m have a significantly higher incidence than the B10 strain and those CR lines which carry the H-2^b allele, but differ from the B10 strain at the weak histocompatibility loci H-1, H-3, H-8, or H-9.

Animals with the H-2^b allele are most resistant to the effect of C3H-MTV in contrast to animals with other H-2 alleles investigated so far. In the group of CR lines with other H-2 alleles than H-2^b the percentage of mammary tumors was 89, whereas the percentage in the group with the H-2^b allele but differing in weak histocompatibility genes was 14.

Similar experiments were carried out with GR-MTV given to newborn females of the CR lines by foster nursing them on ($\female$ GR x $\male$ O20)F_1 females throughout the entire lactation period. The results are given in table 1. No significant difference in the tumor percentage in the different CR lines could be found. Females carrying the H-2^b allele are as susceptible (average percentage = 44) as those carrying other alleles (average percentage = 51). Females carrying H-2 alleles other than H-2^b have a lower tumor percentage when given the GR-MTV than the C3H-MTV. Females with the H-2^b allele have a higher tumor incidence with GR-MTV than with C3H-MTV.

Another striking difference in biological behavior between the C3H-MTV and the GR-MTV has thus been found. The resistance of the B10 line is related to the H-2^b allele but this relation is only apparent with the C3H-MTV.

As all work in our Institute was done with the C57BL/LiA(= BL) line the question had to be answered whether that line also carries the H-2^b allele. Our BL strain was obtained in 1931 from Dr. Little and thus represents a very early branch on the genealogical tree. This line is separated from the C57BL/10 ScSn line (= B10) by about 200 generations. Only recently the histocompatibility loci have been tested in our line. From this extensive testing program [22] only some results are reported here. The direct transplantation of skin from the B10 line to our line showed only one acceptance out of 156 recipients; all other hosts have rejected the skin between 10 to 23 days. There was no acceptance in skin transplantation from our line to the B10 line; all mice rejected the skin grafts, the median survival time being 14,5 days. In the F1-test specific for H-2^b allele [23] our results were characterized by different proportions of takes and rejections with a considerable range of rejection time [22].

The conclusion was drawn that the BL line is different from the B10 line with respect to the H-2^b allele. The results were interpreted as due to a weak incompatibility. It was assumed that both alleles differ by one or maybe two specificities. Another argument in favor of a weak histo-incompatibility was the impossibility to induce humoral antibodies in the BL line against B10 antigens. Possibly there is another difference in one of the weak histocompatibility loci as was concluded from the comparison of the results of the F1 test and direct skin transplantation.

As the B10 line and our BL line seem to show a difference in the H-2^b allele, it had to be investigated whether this difference also influenced the responsiveness to C3H-MTV and GR-MTV. The results were clear cut, only 18% of the BL females foster nursed on a C3H mother had mammary tumors at the end of one year, whereas this incidence after foster nursing on a GR-mother was 62%. Our BL line is thus resistant to C3H-MTV, but susceptible to GR-MTV. The difference between the H-2^b allele in B10 and the H-2^b variant in our BL line apparently does not change the susceptibility to MTV. Both the B10 and BL lines respond equally to C3H-MTV and GR-MTV.

In a series of experiments the question was investigated where the effect of the genes responsible for the resistance to tumorigenesis is localized [24]. Mammary glands from the high-cancer strain C3H and the resistant strain BL were transplanted into the fat pads of completely mammectomized F1 hybrids between the two strains, carrying the MTV and receiving hormonal stimulation by hypophyseal isografts. In this way two mammary glands of different genetic constitution could develop in the same invironment. All conditions being equal, the possible difference in the susceptibility to develop a tumor must be ascribed to the transplanted organ. If both mammary glands retained the original degree of susceptibility after transplantation into the common host, one could conclude that this susceptibility is inherent to the transplanted tissue. Should the susceptibility, however, be different after the transplantation one would have to conclude that this characteristic depends on the host. In the studies with the C3H and the BL strains it was found that the susceptibility to tumor development was retained after transplantation into the F_1 hybrid. In 88% of the transplanted mammary glands from the C3H strain tumors developed, whereas of the BL strain only 8% of the glands showed tumors.

The susceptibility to tumor development is therefore determined at the level of the mammary gland tissue. No action of genetic factors through a general systemic mechanism could yet be demonstrated.

The question was then asked whether it was possible with genetic methods to develop a BL line with a mammary gland as susceptible as the gland of the C3H strain. In other words would it be possible to develop a BL line with the genes responsible for the high susceptibility to mammary tumor development. The first step was to look for easily detectable characteristics of a susceptible mammary gland, preferably in the morphology of the gland.

A study of the morphology of the C3H and the C57BL mammary glands showed several differences, from which gland size was chosen for selection [25]. The second C3H mammary gland is much larger than the corresponding BL gland. The size was measured by determining the circumference of the whole gland. The surface of the second mammary gland of adult BL females measured 44 to 118 mm^2 with an average of 88 mm^2, whereas in females of the C3H strain the surface of the corresponding gland was 170-268 mm^2 (average 217 mm^2). The C3H mammary gland is therefore average 2.7 times larger than the BL gland.

The selection procedure followed the scheme given by Snell for the development of co-isogenic lines [19]. Females of the BL strain were crossed with males from the C3H strain. In the F2-generation a selection was made according to the size of the second mammary gland. Females with the largest mammary gland were backcrossed with males of the BL strain. This backcross generation was bred *inter se* and again a selection was made for the largest second mammary gland. This system of backcross and *inter se* cross was repeated four times. After that brother x sister mating was done for 11 generations with continued selection for the largest size of the second mammary gland. The selection could only be done with females, no selection was possible with the males.

In the 6-11th generation of inbreeding the size of the second mammary gland was 158 mm^2 with a range from 86 to 270 mm^2.

A BL line was thus developed with a significantly larger mammary gland than that in the original BL strain. The size of the gland did not reach, however, that in the C3H strain. The new line was named: BIMA (Black-isogenic mammary gland). The line is now in its 34th inbred generation and the measurements of the size of mammary glands are being repeated.

The gene(s) responsible for the mammary gland size and other characteristic traits have not yet been determined. Reciprocal skin grafts, used to detect genetic differences at histocompatibility loci, were observed for 200 days. One out of 13 grafts (7,6%) from BIMA donors to BL recipients was rejected at 87 days, while 3 out of 8 BIMA hosts have rejected skin grafts from BL donors at 136-150 days. These results indicate a very weak incompatibility between these two strains, depending probably on a difference at one of the weak histocompatibility loci.

More interesting are the results of mammary tumor induction in all these strains. The incidence of spontaneous mammary tumors in breeding females of the BIM line was as low as in the BL strain, *i.e.* 4% and 2% respectively. After foster nursing BIMA females on C3H mothers the incidence of mammary tumors was significantly higher than in BL females foster nursed on C3H mothers (see table 3). The tumor incidence was raised from 27% to 78% and

Table 3
Mammary tumor incidence in force-bred females.

Strain	Tumor percentage	Average tumor age (in days)
With C3H-MTV		
C57BL	27	432
BIMA	78	256
With GR-MTV		
C57BL	62	310
BIMA	62	410

the average tumor age dropped from 432 days to 256 days. However, the high tumor incidence of the C3H strain was not reached. With the GR-MTV given in the same way, no difference was found between the BL strain and the BIMA line, although the average tumor age was higher in BIMA females.

Conclusion

The development of mammary cancer in mice is dependent on genetic factors.

The action of these factors is expressed at the level of the mammary gland tissue. The susceptibility of the mammary gland to the action of the inducing carcinogenic factors is one of the main features in the genesis of mammary carcinoma. The effect of the mammary tumor virus from the C3H strain, C3H-MTV, is related to the histocompatibility-2 locus. The presence or absence of the H-2^b allele determines the incidence of mammary tumors. Females with the H-2^b allele are resistant to tumor development. This only holds true for the C3H-MTV. Another variant of MTV, the GR-MTV, shows no such relation with the H-2^b allele. The different MTV's demonstrate the same variation in relation to the histocompatibility genes as was found earlier for different leukemia viruses.

Another point is that the influence of the H-2 alleles is not an all-or-none effect since intermediate dependence can be found. The difference of mammary tumor incidence in BL and BIMA lines, both carrying the H-2^b allele, however, clearly proves that other genes are also instrumental in the process of tumorigenesis.

The mechanism by which the histocompatibility alleles appear to govern mammary tumorigenesis or leukemogenesis, is as yet unknown. Histocompatibility genes might influence the penetration into, or the replication of virus in the target cells. It could be shown that C3H-MTV is slowly replicated in the C57BL strain contrary to the C3H strain; the C3H-MTV disappears in the C57BL strain after 2 or 3 generations [26-28]. Replication of MTV is also possible in the complete absence of susceptible mammary glands but then no tumors are formed elsewhere [29]. Thus, virus replication does not automatically lead to malignant transformation. It may appear that a certain differentiated cell state combined with histocompatibility gene action leads to neoplastic transformation.

The first recognizable and specific action of C3H-MTV is the formation of hyperplastic nodules in the mammary gland at an earlier age. Appearance of these hyperplastic nodules is in a certain way related to the histocompatibility-2-locus as shown by Nandi [15].

Another possibility is that the histocompatibility genes are of importance in the transformation of these hyperplastic nodules into true carcinomas. It could be shown that the ratio of the occurrence of nodules to the percentage of mammary cancer is strain specific and dependent on genetic factors [30]. These genetic factors have yet to be determined.

Much research has still to be done in order to understand fully the role of genetic factors in the origin of mammary cancer. I sincerely hope, that for several years to come, Professor Mühlbock will take active part in this research.

References

[1] R. Korteweg, Genetica 18 (1936) 350.
[2] R. Korteweg, Acta Unio Intern. Contra Cancrum 5 (1940) 78.
[3] W.S. Murray and C.C. Little, Am. J. Cancer 37 (1939) 536.
[4] O. Mühlbock, Adv. Cancer Res. 4 (1956) 371.
[5] O. Mühlbock and L.M. Boot, Cancer Res. 19 (1959) 402.
[6] W.E. Heston, J. Natl. Cancer Inst. 32 (1964) 947.
[7] P. Bentvelzen, Genetical control of the vertical transmission of the Mühlbock mammary tumor virus in the GR mouse strain (Amsterdam, Hollandia, 1968, Thesis Leiden).
[8] F. Lilly, E.A. Boyse and L.J. Old, Lancet ii (1964) 1207.
[9] F. Lilly, Natl. Cancer Inst. Monograph 22 (1966) 631.
[10] A. Axelrad, Natl. Cancer Inst. Monograph 22 (1966) 619.
[11] A. Axelrad, Can. Cancer Conf. 8 (1969) 313.
[12] J.R. Tennant, "Natural resistance to viral leukemogenesis", *In:* B. Roscoe, Jackson Memorial Laboratory, 34th Annual Report, (1962-1963) 30.
[13] J.R. Tennant and G.D. Snell, Natl. Cancer Inst. Monograph 22 (1966) 61.
[14] J.R. Tennant and G.D. Snell, J. Natl. Cancer Inst. 41 (1968) 597.
[15] S. Nandi, Proc. Natl. Acad. Sci. Wash. 58 (1967) 485.
[16] O. Mühlbock and P. Bentvelzen, Perspectives Virol. 6 (1968) 75.
[17] R. van Nie and P.J. Thung, Europ. J. Cancer 1 (1965) 41.
[18] R. van Nie and A. Dux, J. Natl. Cancer Inst. 46 (1971) 885.
[19] G.D. Snell, J. Natl. Cancer Inst. 21 (1958) 843.
[20] J.H. Stimpfling and A.E. Reichert, Transpl. Proc. 2 (1970) 39.
[21] O. Mühlbock and A. Dux, "Histocompatibility and mammary cancer in mice", Int. Symposium on histocompatibility (Praha, 1970, Karger, in press).
[22] A. Dux, D. Corduwener and O. Mühlbock, "Analysis of the difference at the H-2 locus between C57BL/LiA and C57BL/10ScSn strains", Int. Symposium on histocompatibility (Praha, 1970, Karger, in press).
[23] G.D. Snell and J.H. Stimpfling, "Genetics of tissue transplantation", *In:* E.L. Green (ed.), Biology of the laboratory mouse, sec. ed., (New York, McGraw-Hill, 1966) p. 457.
[24] A. Dux and O. Mühlbock, J. Natl. Cancer Inst. 6 (1968) 1259.
[25] O. Mühlbock, W. van Ebbenhorst Tengbergen and A. Dux, "Genetic studies of the susceptibility of the mouse mammary gland to MTV", unpublished. Reported at the 3rd MTV-conference in Houston, May 1970.
[26] H.B. Andervont, J. Natl. Cancer Inst. 5 (1945) 383.
[27] M.K. Deringer, W.E. Heston and H.B. Andervont, J. Natl. Cancer Inst. 5 (1945) 403.
[28] O. Mühlbock, Acta Unio Intern. Contra Cancrum 12 (1956) 665.
[29] A. Dux and O. Mühlbock, Proc. Soc. Exptl. Biol. Med. 115 (1964) 433.
[30] Th.G. van Rijssel, Acta Unio Intern. Contra Cancrum 12 (1956) 718.

HEREDITARY INFECTIONS WITH MAMMARY TUMOR VIRUSES IN MICE*

P. BENTVELZEN
Radiobiological Institute of the Organization for Health Research TNO, Rijswijk (Z.H.), The Netherlands

1. Introduction

The concept of genetic transmission of mammary tumor viruses which I have gradually developed found its origin in a discovery made by Professor Mühlbock with the GR strain. Mühlbock had developed several inbred mouse strains of European origin and one of them, the GR strain, produces a very high incidence of mammary tumors at an extremely early age. He tried to free this strain from its presumed mammary tumor virus by taking the young by cesarean section and foster nursing them on low-mammary-cancer strain females. With American high-mammary-cancer strains this procedure removes the classical mammary tumor virus (Bittner virus). To his surprise the result was a GR subline, which develops 100% mammary tumors at an early age. He accused his technicians of not taking the necessary precautions, but repetition of this experiment under strictly controlled conditions always gives the same result.

When Mühlbock [1] crossed the GR strain with several low-mammary-cancer strains, he observed no difference in tumor-incidences between the offsprings of the reciprocal matings. Such a difference is found in crosses between American high-mammary-cancer strains and low strains [2,3]. This has been the basis for the discovery of the milkfactor by Bittner [4], which proved to be a virus [5,6].

Mühlbock [1] discovered that the GR strain carried a mammary tumor virus (MTV) by (a) foster nursing of newborn mice of susceptible low-cancer-strains

*The author is much indebted to Doctors J.H. Daams, Philomena Hageman, Jero Calafat, A. Timmermans and O. Mühlbock for collaboration in several of the experiments reported in this paper and for making available new results from their own investigations. Gratefully acknowledged are Annemarie Amsen, J. Arend, J. Brinkhof, D. Aarssen and Rochelle Griffin for expert technical assistance and Mrs. E. Griffin for correcting the English version of the manuscript.

on GR females and (b) inoculation of cell-free extracts from GR mammary tumors into 4-week-old mice of such strains. In both cases he got a very high tumor incidence before one year of age and no tumors in the controls. He furthermore demonstrated that offspring of low-cancer females and GR males carries the virus. This indicates that the virus is effectively transmitted by the GR male.

The virus of the GR strain has the same electron-optic appearance as the standard mammary tumor virus discovered by Bittner [7]. There are, however, some immunological differences between both viral entities [see Hageman *et al.*, this Symposium]. It is also somewhat less virulent than the American MTV. The GR strain virus causes many neoplastic lesions in the mammary gland which have a peculiar histologic appearance, unfortunately called plaques by Foulds [8]. These tumors are strongly pregnancy-dependent but will finally progress to autonomous malignancies. I decided to regard the virus of the GR strain as quite a different virus strain and called it Mühlbock virus [9,10]. During an international conference on MTV, in an attempt to standardize nomenclature, it has been renamed MTV-P [11], which refers to the induction of the so-called plaques.

2. Male transmission of MTV-P in the GR strain

In 1963 I was assigned by Professor Mühlbock to study the male transmission of MTV-P in the GR strain whereby I gave much attention to the possible role of host genetic factors in this phenomenon. I had in mind the five following hypotheses:

(a) MTV-P has the capacity to be easily transmitted by the male in contrast to the standard virus (MTV-S).

(b) The GR male can produce so much MTV-P, that its female partner can become infected and transmit the virus to her offspring.

(c) The GR male produces so much virus that it can infect the offspring at conception.

(d) The GR strain would carry dominant susceptibility genes, which cause extreme sensitivity to the small amounts of virus being present in the semen.

(e) MTV-P is transmitted as a genetic factor of the GR host.

The last hypothesis has been my favorite one, although at times I was partial to the fourth.

With regard to the possibility that male transmission is solely controlled by the virus itself (hypothesis (a)), I observed that introduction of MTV-P into other mouse strains does not lead to male transmission of the virus by the new host [9]. This demonstrates the dependency on the GR host genome with regard to male transmission.

In relation to hypothesis (b), females of the low-mammary-cancer strains O20 and C57BL were mated to either intact or vasectomized GR males. After three matings the GR males were replaced by DBAf males. Ordinarily (O20 x DBAf)F$_1$ and (C57BL x DBAf)F$_1$ females do not get any mammary tumor before one year of age and at two years of age the incidence is still low. Introduction of MTV-P into these hybrids leads to a very high tumor incidence (approx. 90%) at 1 year. In our experiments only a few tumors developed at that age. An analysis demonstrated that C57BL females never got infected and O20 females in only 10% of the cases [9].

Hypothesis (c) (infection of zygotes by large amounts of virus in the GR semen) can be excluded on the basis of our genetic experiments (table 1). When

Table 1
Genetics of transmission of MTV-P by GR males.

♀		♂	Number of animals	Tumor % at 1 year
BALB/c	X	(BALB/c X GR)F$_1$	38	50
C3Hf	X	(C3Hf X GR)F$_1$	30	53
DBAf	X	(DBAf X GR)F$_1$	25	60
Af	X	(Af X GR)F$_1$	41	56
MAS	X	(MAS X GR)F$_1$	28	46
O20	X	(O20 X GR)F$_1$	88	50
TS	X	(TS X GR)F$_1$	33	46
C57BL	X	(C57BL X GR)F$_1$	78	49
O20	X	(RIII X GR)F$_1$	42	52
O20	X	(C3Hf X GR)F$_1$	17	60
O20	X	(C57BL X GR)F$_1$	59	51
BALB/c	X	(C3Hf X GR)F$_1$	115	64*
BALB/c	X	(DBAf X GR)F$_1$	32	66*
(O20 X DBAf)F$_1$	X	(C57BL X GR)F$_1$	37	51

*For an explanation of these high incidences see fig. 5.

low-cancer strain females are mated to GR males, about 100% tumors are found in the offspring and all mice will carry MTV-P (1). In case such females are mated to GR-hybrid males only about 50% is found. In the case of a large virus production, one would expect either 100% (dominance) or 0% (recessiveness). If the genetic complex that would control this presumed excessive virus production were semi-dominant, it would be very unlikely that in all these crosses 50% is found. In that case incidences might vary between 20 and 80%.

In the schematic representation of these crosses as given in table 2 it is remarkable that irrespective of what type of cross is made (*e.g.* backcross, triple cross, double hybrid), approximately 50% is found. This strongly indicates that a single mendelian factor controls male transmission of MTV-P in the GR strain.

In an analysis of crosses between the resistant C57BL and the GR strain more support for this single-gene postulate was found (table 3). In the second

Table 2
Schematic representation of the results in table 1.

			Tumor incidence at 1 yr (%)
Inbred strains	:	X, Y and Z all	0
		GR	100
F_1 Hybrids	:	(X × GR), (Y × GR) and (Z × GR)	100
First backcross	:	X × (X × GR) and so on	50
Triple cross hybrids	:	X × (Y × GR) and so on	50
Double hybrids	:	(X × Y) × (Z × GR) and so on	50

Table 3
Genetics of male transmission of MTV-P in crosses between the C57BL and GR mouse strains.

Cross	Number of animals	Tumor % at 1 yr
C57BL	28	0
GR	24	100
(C57BL × GR)F_1	41	100
{C57BL × (C57BL × GR)F_1}BC_1	78	49
[C57BL × {C57BL × (C57BL × GR)F_1}BC_1]BC_2	74	26

backcross to C57BL approximately 25% was found. Only half of the first backcross males, used to produce this second generation, were able to transmit the virus. About 50% of their offspring developed mammary tumors.

In all these experiments, the development of a tumor has been our criterium for the presence of MTV-P. In some experiments we tested females for the presence of virus by letting them nurse so-called virus-free but susceptible newborn mice. The results of these studies, being done on a much smaller scale than those with tumor incidences, are also in line with a single-gene postulate [ref. 9 and Zeilmaker, unpublished results].

These genetic studies have left us with hypothesis (d) (susceptibility gene) and (e) (genetic transmission). With regard to the latter, we observed that several organs of the GR strain contain mammary-tumor inducing activity whereas only a few organs have this activity when MTV-P is introduced into other mouse strains [12]. This finding is highly compatible with the idea that MTV-P is a part of the GR host genome. However, it is possible with some twisted reasoning to explain this on the basis of a susceptibility gene.

3. Eggborne transmission of MTV-P in GR strain females

I found that in GR females MTV-P is not only transmitted by the milk [9]. When GR females were mated to low-cancer strain males and the young taken by cesarean section followed by foster nursing on low-strain females, the young still contained MTV-P. Zeilmaker [13] took freshly fertilized eggs within seven hours after the mating of a GR female with a C57BL male and transferred them to so-called virus-free females, which were made pseudopregnant (fig. 1). The GR-hybrids procured this way proved still to contain the virus.

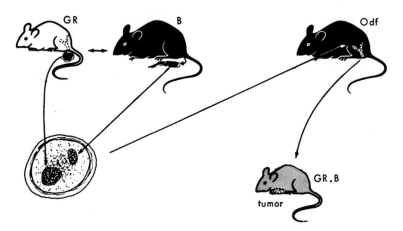

Fig. 1. Schematic representation of transfer of freshly fertilized (GR × C57BL)F_1 ova to pseudopregnant (O20 × DBAf)F_1 females.

In another experiment (fig. 2), freshly fertilized ova were taken from low-cancer strain females. These eggs were transplanted into the uteri of pseudopregnant GR females. The nipples of these GR females were extirpated to avoid milkborne infection in the young. After birth the young were given to

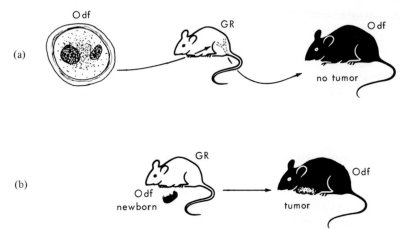

Fig. 2. (a) Schematic representation of transfer of freshly fertilized (O20 × DBAf)F₁ ova to pseudopregnant GR females. The young are foster nursed on (O20 × DBAf)F₁ females. (b) Foster nursing of newborn (O20 × DBAf)F₁ mice on GR females, leading to a high-mammary-cancer incidence.

so-called virus-free females for foster nursing. The hybrid (O20 × DBAf)F₁ is fairly susceptible to MTV-P given by the milk or by inoculations. In this experiment they did not develop any mammary tumor before one year, indicating that they are not infected with MTV-P.

These two experiments indicate that in GR females MTV-P is not transmitted through the placenta but by the ovum. If the virus is introduced into other mouse strains only milkborne transmission can be observed. Obviously, in case of transmission by the female sex cells, the GR host genome plays the determining role. I have done a single genetic experiment which gave results that were compatible with the idea that a single gene controls this mode of transmission by the ovum [9].

From some crosses between the GR and other mouse strains we procured the F₂ generation. Milkborne transmission of virus was prevented by immediately transferring the young, after birth, to foster mothers of low-mammary-cancer strains. Tumor incidences in these F₂'s were around 75% [9]. If different genes control eggborne and male transmission about 94% has to be expected. These results indicate that one and the same locus controls both modes of gameteborne transmission.

All these genetic data are strongly in favor of a genetic-transmission hypothesis but certainly do not disprove the susceptibility-gene postulate. Evidence for genetic transmission comes from our work with the low-oncogenic strain of MTV in the C3Hf strain.

4. Genetic transmission of MTV-L in the C3Hf mouse strain

When various high-mammary-cancer strains are freed from their MTV-S they are still able to develop mammary tumors but at a very late age. These tumors contain particles, which are similar to the virions of MTV-S (see for a review Hageman *et al.* [14]). Since no oncogenic activity could be retrieved from these tumors, several investigators in the mammary tumor field rejected these so-called B particles as mammary tumor virions. However, when Miss Hageman [14,15] demonstrated that highly purified B-particle preparations contain strong oncogenic activity, these sceptics were compelled to accept the B-particle as the MTV-S virion.

The B-particles in the late appearing tumors are now assumed to represent another less oncogenic variant of MTV [16,17]. Nandi [17] called it the nodule-inducing virus, which certainly is a misnomer. We renamed it MTV-L [11], referring to the low-oncogenic activity of this variant.

Initially we could demonstrate oncogenicity of MTV-L only in an indirect way: it acted as some kind of helper to small amounts of MTV-S, giving rise to a high incidence of tumors whereas MTV-S alone would induce only a few tumors in this case. At this conference Miss Hageman presented direct evidence for infectivity and oncogenicity of MTV-L.

DeOme *et al.* [18] made a quite different approach to demonstrate oncogenic activity of MTV-L (fig. 3). Mammary tissue of BALB/c mice, which are free from MTV-L, was transplanted into the hybrid (C3Hf x BALB)F$_1$ which carries the virus. After hormonal stimulation hyperplastic nodules appeared which proved to contain MTV-L and were capable of producing tumors. This experiment had been successfully repeated in Professor Mühlbock's laboratory by Dr. Zeilmaker. In one experiment DeOme [18] succeeded in infecting BALB/c mice with MTV-L by retransplantation of the infected BALB/c mammary tissue. The virus proved to be transmitted by the milk only in this strain.

A complication of this experiment is that BALB/c carries a latent MTV [see Hageman, this Symposium], which becomes manifest at a late age. However, this virus seems to be transmitted by the germ cells. The possibility is not excluded that the virus of DeOme in so-called MTV-L infected BALB/c mice is the product of recombination or phenotypic mixing of MTV-L and MTV-O, the virus indigenous to BALB/c mice. The remarkable virulence of this agent [Andervont, personal communication] would plead for this idea. Anyway, it is remarkable that MTV-L or "mixed" virus is transmitted through the milk in the BALB/c strain instead of the germ cells as it seems to do in the C3Hf strain [16,17] as may be concluded from the egg transplantation experiments of Boot

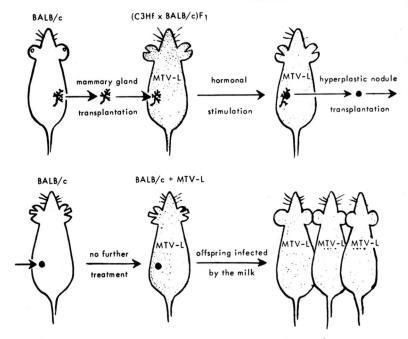

Fig. 3. Schematic representation of the experimental transfer of MTV-L from C3Hf to BALB/c mice.

and Mühlbock [19]. This situation remarkably parallels that of MTV-P in the GR strain.

In the case of MTV-L a susceptibility-gene hypothesis can be excluded. Hybrids of C3Hf and BALB/c do get earlier and more mammary tumors than C3Hf mice as found by Andervont and Dunn [20] and ourselves [11]. MTV-L seems to be much better replicated in this hybrid than in C3Hf [Hageman, personal communication]. It seems that the BALB/c strain contributes genes, which cause greater susceptibility as they do to several other MTV strains [11], whereas they do not cause transmission via the sex cells. The possibility that these tumors would be due to MTV-O can be excluded by the finding that the virus of (C3Hf x BALB/c)F$_1$ is immunologically identical to MTV-L [Hageman, this Symposium].

We may therefore conclude that the C3Hf strain carries genes, which control only transmission of an MTV. This genetic system is of a narrow specificity: only MTV-L is vertically transmitted this way in the C3Hf strain. The comparison of the situation in the GR strain and the analogous one in the C3Hf strain compels us to conclude that in both strains there is a hereditary infection with an MTV, *i.e.* the respective MTV strains are in some way transmitted as a genetic factor of the host.

5. "Repression" of MTV-L in some hybrids

Dr. Calafat observed that mammary tumors induced by extreme hormonal stimulation in hybrids of MTV-L carrying mouse strains with strains which do not carry this virus, such as O20 and C57BL, did not contain MTV virions (see [7,21]). These tumors also appear considerably later than in the MTV-L-carrying parental strains [21]. However, in 4 out of 11 tumors, originating in the F_2 generation of (C3Hf x O20), B-particles were found [11]. From this result may be concluded that in the F_1 MTV-L is still present but in some hidden form. Furthermore, that O20-strain genes can repress the electron-optic manifestation of MTV-L in the form of mature virions. It is very likely that such genes are also present in the C57BL strain.

In molecular biology repression is a term with a very restricted meaning. It is linked to the Jacob and Monod [22] model of the production of repressor molecules by a regulator gene which inhibits transcription of some genes. It is far from certain, whether such repressing systems exist in eukaryotic systems. However, we use the term repression in its restricted sense because we believe that classical types of repressor molecules are involved in the phenomenon described above.

6. Induction of MTV-X in the O20 mouse strain

The O20 mouse strain does not develop many mammary tumors spontaneously [23]. However, if extreme hormonal stimulation is given by means of pituitary isografts, many tumors will develop but at a much later age than in strains, which carry MTV-L. In these tumors no MTV virions have been observed despite extensive screening of many tumors [24]. Cell-free extracts of such tumors failed to induce mammary tumors in susceptible mice [21]. Only the occasional finding of MTV-specific antigens in the milk of old breeders [Hilgers and Nowinski, personal communication; Hageman, personal communication] indicates that a latent form of MTV is present in this strain.

X-irradiation combined with the administration of urethan in the drinking water leads to the early production of mammary tumors as found by Timmermans [24]. These tumors contained many B-particles and cell-free extracts were very effective in inducing mammary tumors in BALB/c mice [24]. The carcinogenic treatments described above obviously can activate an MTV, whose appearance is otherwise repressed. In view of the role of X-rays in the activation of the virus, but also because little is known about serological and biological properties of the virus, we have named this strain MTV-X [25].

Daams and Timmermans of the Netherlands Cancer Institute have studied serologically the release of MTV-X in O20 mice following irradiation. In young adult mice no MTV antigens could be detected, but such antigens appear between 3-6 days after radiation. The presence of viral antigens persists for several months now. The amount of viral antigens seems to be larger than when O20 mice are infected with MTV-S.

In the O20 strain there seems to be a system which represses the manifestation of its indigenous MTV-X. Most likely the same system (genes) also causes the repression of the manifestation of MTV-L in the hybrid with MTV-L-carrying mouse strains.

7. The induction of MTV-Y in the C57BL mouse strain

The C57BL mouse strain is even more resistant to mammary tumor development than the O20 strain [26]. It retains its resistance even when pituitary isografts are given [21,27]: approximately 20% will develop tumors at a late age.

As demonstrated by Boot and associates [28] whole body irradiation strongly increases mammary tumor development. I observed that mammary tumors can be induced at an early age in this strain when high doses of urethan are given.

Timmermans (see [28]) demonstrated that blood of irradiated C57BL females can induce many mammary tumors at an early age in susceptible hosts. He furthermore observed that the female offspring of irradiated C57BL females have a much higher tumor incidence than the controls. Another interesting observation by him is that irradiation of the spleen only also strongly promotes the development of mammary tumors in C57BL mice. All these data are strongly in favor of activation of a mammary tumor-inciting virus in C57BL mice by radiation.

Electron-microscopic examination failed to detect MTV virions in irradiation-induced mammary tumors of C57BL mice. I could not demonstrate mammary tumor-inducing activity of cell-free extracts from such tumors or extracts from spleens of irradiated animals. It is a good possibility, that an incomplete MTV becomes activated, which is involved in the genesis of the radiation-induced mammary tumors but cannot produce mature virions and which has therefore little infectivity. In this respect the observation of Hageman [this Symposium] that cell extracts of leukocytes from MTV-S-infected animals are considerably less infectious than whole cells has some relevance to the problem that no infectivity could be demonstrated of the presumed C57BL-strain MTV.

I have some serological evidence that indeed an agent may become activated which is related to the standard MTV. Daams [29,30] has found MTV-specific antigens in hemopoietic tissues of mice infected with MTV-S by means of indirect immunofluorescence with rabbit antisera to MTV-S. This has recently been confirmed by Hilgers [personal communication]. With Daams's antisera I could not detect MTV-specific antigens in untreated C57BL mice (fig. 4). However, X-irradiated or urethan-treated C57BL mice were positive in their spleens and bone marrow (fig. 4).

It is not very likely that the appearance of MTV antigens in irradiated C57BL mice is due to immunosuppression. I have given 20 female and male C57BL mice weekly inoculations with a very potent rabbit anti-mouse lymphocyte-serum. This serum is a very strong inhibitor of both cellular and humoral immune responses as determined by the rejection of foreign skin grafts and the production of anti-sheep erythrocyte antibodies. These treated C57BL mice did not show the presence of MTV antigens at one year of age. They did not develop any tumor at all, which brings us to the question whether immunological surveillance plays an important role in the inhibition of the spontaneous development of tumors.

The presumed MTV strain latently present in the C57BL strain has been christened by us MTV-Y because virtually nothing is known about its biologic properties [25].

8. The troublesome MTV-O in the BALB/c mouse strain

The BALB/c strain has been the golden standard of MTV-research. It was claimed to be MTV-free but extremely susceptible to infection with various MTV strains. In his immunofluorescence studies on the occurrence of MTV antigens in various tissues of infected animals, Daams was often bothered by the fact that this strain was never a nice negative control like the C57BL strain. The fluorescence was much less in ordinary BALB/c mice than in MTV-S-infected ones but still positive. To his relief he and his colleagues succeeded in isolating an MTV from BALB/c mice [see Hageman, this Symposium]. Also in some mammary tumors of the BALB/cCrgl subline a few MTV virions have

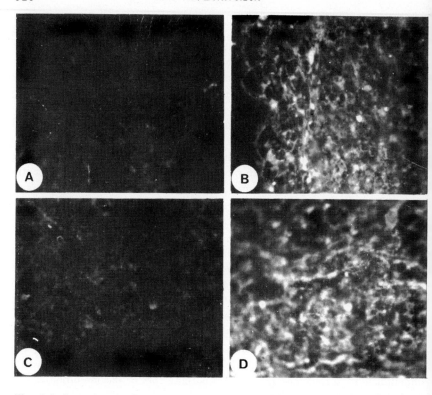

Fig. 4. Indirect immunofluorescence studies on the presence of MTV-antigens in the cytoplasm of aceton-fixed spleen cells. (A) C57BL female, 7 months old. (B) C3H female, 2 months old. (C) C57BL female, X-irradiated at 2 months of age (300 rad whole body), 8 months old. (D) C57BL female, X-irradiated (as above) + 0.15% urethan in drinking water, 3 months old.

been seen by Pillsbury and Moore [personal communication]. This virus, whose existence has been overlooked for so many years is called by us MTV-O [25].

So far I failed to retrieve oncogenic activity from late appearing mammary tumors in this strain. Only incidentally I did find such activity in hemopoietic tissues of BALB/c mice. There seems to be a mechanism in this strain, which inhibits considerably the maturation of MTV-O. It breaks down only during aging and even then the yield of particles is low, as can be concluded from the scarcity of B-particles in the late appearing tumors.

It is puzzling that when MTV-O is inoculated into young BALB/c mice, it proves to be highly virulent and virions are easily produced. In contrast, the BALB/c is highly susceptible to urethan-induction of mammary tumors which we believe to be due to the activation of a virus [25], but so far in these tumors no B particles have been observed by Calafat. At this time we are completely at a loss to explain the apparent inhibition of the maturation of indigenous MTV-O, but not of passaged MTV-O.

Since no MTV-O particles or antigens can be detected in the milk of young BALB/c females, the virus has to be transmitted by the sex cells. This idea is supported by our finding that germ-free BALB/c mice still carry MTV-O at a late age [25]. When other MTV strains are introduced into BALB/c mice, they are transmitted by the milk. Also in this case there seems to be a very close association between host genome and virus strain with regard to transmission by the gametes.

9. Switching on of mammary tumor viruses by age

Since I could not find any MTV in untreated C57BL mice, I was inclined to believe that the few tumors, which developed after strong hormonal stimulation, were due to the action of hormones only. However, I have always been unable to construct a nice theory on how these factors would bring out the neoplastic change.

To our surprise Daams and I found MTV antigens in the hemopoietic tissues of several aged C57BL mice (table 4). In the light of this finding it is reasonable to

Table 4
Switching on of MTV by age in C57BL mice.

Age	Number of mice tested	Number positive for MTV antigens	% positive
2 mth	9	0	0
1 yr	22	1	5
2 yr*	20	8	40
3 yr*	2	2	100

* Animals kindly provided by Dr. C.F. Hollander, Director of the Institute for Experimental Gerontology TNO, Rijswijk, Z.H., The Netherlands.

assume that the tumors mentioned above are due to the action of MTV-Y. The role of the hormones can be explained by (a) providing the substrate for the oncogenic action of MTV-Y, the mammary gland, and (b) stimulating DNA synthesis, which is necessary for the replication and transforming activities of the virus.

Daams has screened mice of twenty different strains and found all strains to be positive for the presence of an MTV. However, often young mice of these strains are negative. This demonstrates that aging plays an important role in the switch on of MTV in mice. In table 5 the results are presented of six strains

Table 5
Switching on of MTV in several mouse strains.

Strain	Presence of MTV antigens			Tumor % at 2 yr in force-bred females*
	2 mth	1 yr	2 yr	
BALB/c	+	+	+	30 (20)
C3Hf	+	+	+	37 (30)
MAS	±	+	+	11 (55)
O20	−	±	+	0 (27)
TS	−	±	+	0 (29)
C57BL	−	−	±	0 (32)

*Between parentheses the number of animals.

with which I have done many experiments. It has to be emphasized that these results are of a preliminary nature. Many more animals have to be screened and many more ages have to be taken into consideration. However, the picture emerges that there are three strains, which are switched on rather early: C3Hf, BALB/c and MAS. The three strains TS, O20 and C57BL are switched on only late in life. This corresponds well with the tumor incidences at two years of age in the various strains, strongly suggesting that in the various strains the endogenous MTV causes the so-called spontaneous tumors.

At an early age only some animals of the MAS strain are switched on. At a half year of age most of them are positive and all are positive at one year. Old MAS mice absorb much better anti-MTV antibodies from rabbit antisera to MTV-S than young mice, indicating an increase in the amount of antigen. Calafat failed to detect B-particles in MAS mammary tumors so far. It is possible that the MAS strain harbors only a defective MTV.

The O20 strain is switched on much earlier than the C57BL strain. This corresponds well with the greater susceptibility of the O20 strain to the induction of mammary tumors by pituitary isografts [21]. All these data demonstrate the ubiquity of MTV in mice. They also strongly suggest the all-viral etiology of this kind of neoplastic lesions.

10. Resistance to superinfection with MTV-S

Besides the correlation between the age of switching on of endogenous MTV and susceptibility to so-called spontaneous mammary carcinogenesis, there is a similar parallel with susceptibility to superinfection with MTV-S (table 6). It is

Table 6

Strain variation in susceptibility to MTV-S.

Strain	Indigenous MTV switched on	Tumor % at 1 yr[a]					
		Foster nursing[b]	Purified virus[c]				
			10^{-2}	10^{-3}	10^{-4}	10^{-5}	10^{-6}
BALB/c	+[d]	100 (36)	90 (10)	83 (30)	82 (50)	56 (27)	45 (22)
C3Hf	+	100 (24)	80 (20)	50 (16)	52 (21)	23 (13)	0 (31)
MAS	±	71 (21)	82 (28)	25 (36)	17 (36)	8 (37)	0 (38)
O20	−	25 (12)	28 (18)	0 (38)	0 (16)	0 (10)	0 (7)
TS	−	15 (33)	15 (16)	0 (22)	0 (19)	NT[e]	NT
C57BL	−	4 (25)	0 (15)	0 (29)	0 (17)	NT	NT

a All mice are force-bred. The number in parentheses indicates the number of mice used.
b The young have been transferred to a C3H female immediately after birth.
c Virus isolated according to Calafat and Hageman [15]. The stock solution contains 1 mg net weight of virus per ml. Four-week-old mice were inoculated intraperitoneally with 0.5 ml of a diluted preparation.
d BALB/c is switched on with regard to release of viral antigens but not of complete infectious virus.
e NT = not tested.

well known that the latter phenomenon is genetic in nature [see both Heston and Dux, this Symposium]. The observed parallel might mean that the same genes, which repress to a large extent the release of endogenous MTV also cause resistance to superinfection.

The parallel is much less striking in case of superinfection with MTV-P: the C57BL strain gets a surprisingly high incidence of tumors before one year of age, when MTV-P is introduced [Dux, this Symposium]. Nevertheless the incidence is still considerably lower than in BALB/cfGR and C3HfGR which also get their tumors much earlier. It may be expected that when graded dilutions of purified MTV-P are used, a similar pattern as in table 6 will be found.

The resistance of the C57BL strain to MTV-S I found to be associated with a poor production of infectious virus [31]. In the O20 strain this virus is so poorly replicated, that within a few generations of submating it will disappear from this strain [23]. The same has been observed by Mühlbock [26] for the C57BL strain. The laborious particle-counting by Hairstone *et al.* [32] in mammary tumors has demonstrated that susceptibility of a given mouse strain to MTV-S, as expressed by tumor incidence and tumor age, correlates well with the number of virions per tumor. This has been confirmed by Hageman, who did not count the virus particles under the electron microscope but isolated virus from the tumors and estimated the amount of virus by determining the turbidity of the virusband in a spectrophotometer.

In oncornavirology there is no indication, whatsoever, that virion production *per se* is necessary for neoplastic conversion. We have interpreted in the past the correlation between virion production and susceptibility to infection to be that the viral genome must be replicated considerably before transformation can take place. In the light of the recent findings on the replication of oncornaviruses, it is safer to state that a considerable amount of viral RNA has to be produced before neoplastic transformation will occur.

The C3Hf strain is somewhat less susceptible to MTV-S than BALB/c. Andervont [33] exposed newborn mice of the C3H strain for only a short time to MTV-S infected mothers and thereafter to so-called virus-free foster mothers. In this way the virus disappeared within five generations of submating from the C3H strain, whereas in the BALB/c strain it remained there at full strength despite this manipulation. The results can be explained by the BALB/c being more susceptible and replicating the virus much better.

Nandi and DeOme [34] stated that adult C3Hf mice were completely refractory to MTV-S and that this would be due to the presence of MTV-L. We could not confirm this strong resistance. It is not very likely that MTV-L would be responsible for the lesser susceptibility of C3Hf mice to MTV-S since a similar interference may be expected in BALB/c mice with their MTV-O.

C3Hf mice are also somewhat less susceptible to MTV-P [9]. This may be reflected in the earlier tumor age of $(BALB/c \times GR)F_1$ as compared to (C3Hf $\times$ GR)F_1 (fig. 5). In the cross BALB/c $\times$ (C3Hf $\times$ GR) F_1 approximately 50% of the animals developed tumors in the same age-range as $(BALB/c \times GR)F_1$. A few tumors appear after ten months. That is comparable to the yield of tumors at that age in the hybrids of BALB/c with C3Hf.

This distribution can only be explained in my opinion on the basis of a single locus. The BALB/c strain would carry the allele Ms^1, which causes great susceptibility to MTV-P (and also to MTV-S and other strains). The C3Hf strain would carry the allele Ms^2, which causes a much lesser susceptibility to MTV-P and the O20 and C57BL strains Ms^+, which is responsible for relative resistance. The strain GR would carry Ms^E, which would cause extreme susceptibility to

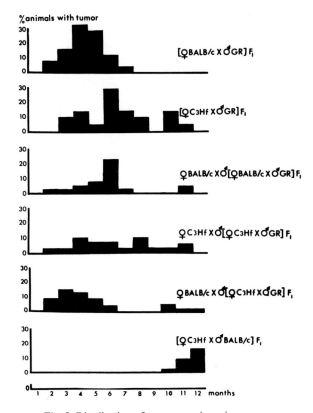

Fig. 5. Distribution of tumor ages in various crosses.

carcinogenesis by MTV-P by controlling its transmission and subsequent release. The cross BALB/c × (C3Hf × GR)F$_1$ can be symbolized by Ms^1/Ms^1 × Ms^2/Ms^E. In the offspring one may expect 50% Ms^1/Ms^2 (comparable to C3Hf × BALB/c), of which only some will get a tumor before one year of age, and 50% Ms^1/Ms^E (comparable to BALB/c × GR), which will get MTV-P induced tumors at an early age. This interpretation implies that the same locus, which controls transmission of MTV-P, also controls susceptibility to superinfection.

The genetic resistance to the development of mammary tumors under influence of an administered MTV is not solely explained by this locus. Genetic analysis demonstrates that at least two genes control resistance to MTV-S in the C57BL strain, although the number of resistance genes does not seem to be large [see both Heston and Dux, this Symposium]. In the case of MTV-S, the histocompatibility-locus-2 plays an important role [see Dux, this Symposium]. A possible explanation for this is influencing the penetration of the virus into the cell or preventing the alteration at the cell surface which leads to neoplasia.

11. Susceptibility to urethan-carcinogenesis in the mammary gland

Another correlation observed by us is between susceptibility to spontaneous and MTV-S induced mammary carcinogenesis on the one hand and to urethan on the other (table 7). A similar correlation in susceptibility to spontaneous

Table 7
Strain variation in susceptibility to urethan-induction of mammary tumors.

		Tumor % at 1 yr[a]		
Strain	Spontaneous tumor % at 2 yr[a]	0.05% urethan drinking water	30 mg i.p. injection at 4 wk	4 × 15 mg i.p. injection[b]
BALB/c	30 (20)	53 (30)	64 (22)	44 (27)
C3Hf	37 (30)	78 (32)	50 (18)	32 (19)
MAS	11 (55)	32 (22)	5 (22)	6 (17)
O20	0 (27)	0 (14)	13 (15)	10 (20)
TS	0 (29)	10 (31)	12 (16)	25 (24)
C57BL	0 (32)	0 (24)	0 (19)	15 (20)

[a] Animals force-bred. The number in parentheses indicates the number of mice used.
[b] Injections with weekly intervals beginning at four weeks of age.

carcinogenesis and urethan-induction has been observed by us [35] in the pulmonary tumor system in mice. In the mammary tumor system it has to be concluded that genes which control release of indigenous virus also control susceptibility to urethan-carcinogenesis. This strongly suggests that urethan acts as an accelerator of viral processes. In the O20 strain we found [24] that urethan activates the appearance of MTV-X and in the C57BL strain the appearance of MTV-specific antigens *(vide supra)*.

It can be theorized, that in strains in which virus is released rather easily, the further release of virus under influence of urethan will not be very difficult either. It is worthwhile to investigate genetic resistance to other carcinogenic compounds and the eventual appearance of MTV antigens under influence of these drugs in strains such as O20 and C57BL.

12. Germinal provirus hypotheses

In order to explain the genetic control of gamete-born transmission of some MTV-strains and the induction of others by urethan or radiation, we have developed the model (fig. 6) that in every mouse would be present, in one of its

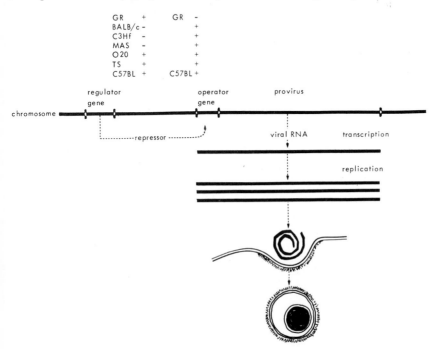

Fig. 6. Provirus model for vertical transmission of MTV in several inbred mouse strains. A DNA copy of viral RNA is integrated into a chromosome. Ordinarily transcription is repressed. After derepression the released messenger becomes viral RNA. Above the regulator and operator gene is indicated which strain is normal (+) or mutated (–).

chromosomes, a DNA copy of MTV-RNA. Transcription of this copy would be inhibited by a classical repressor molecule produced by a regulator gene. Due to germinal mutations in the regulator gene as in the C3Hf strain or in the operator gene as in the GR strain, transcription could take place leading to a continuous virus release. The same repressor would cause resistance to superinfection. That in C3Hf the regulator gene would be mutated follows from the rather recessive nature of virus release as detectable in crosses with "wild type" O20 and C57BL. Since release of MTV-P is not influenced by the presence of genes from these "wild type" strains we postulated an operator gene mutation in the GR. That the repressor would still be produced in this strain was concluded from the inability of the GR to replicate MTV-S [11].

Temporary derepression by radiation or injection of carcinogenic drugs would lead to release of some viral RNA, which can replicate rather independently from the germinal provirus. The effect of aging can be explained by somatic mutations in the controlling genes, giving rise to continuous transcription. Strain-differences in the onset of virus release are not satisfactorily explained this way, however.

I still favor this model as the most economic one. Since according to Duesberg and Cardiff [36] the MTV genome is an aggregate of some RNA molecules, it is conceivable that not one single provirus would exist, but that there are separate "proviral chromosomes", each coding a different RNA molecule. These "proviral chromosomes" can either be linked to each other (fig. 7a) or randomly distributed throughout the genome (fig. 7b).

Another alternative hypothesis as suggested by Vigier is that only one "proviral chromosome" is present in the host genome (fig. 8). This would carry all the specific information as for example MTV-L in the C3Hf strain and for MTV-P in the GR mouse strain. This "proviral chromosome" or protovirus

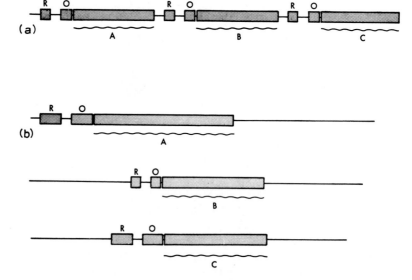

Fig. 7. "Proviral chromosomes" hypothesis for vertical transmission of MTV. (a) Linkage of "proviral chromosomes". (b) Random distribution in the host genome.

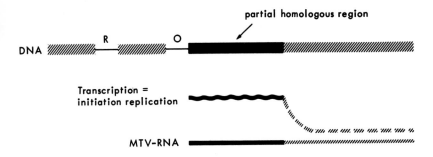

Fig. 8. Modified protovirus hypothesis for vertical transmission of MTV. A small homologous piece of DNA (proviral chromosome or protovirus) is integrated into a chromosome. After transcription coupling of messenger RNA and other viral RNA takes place.

would eventually be transcribed and the released RNA coupled to other RNA molecules, which are present independently from the host genome. This would give rise to a complete viral genome. This sophisticated hypothesis, somewhat resembling Temin's protovirus hypothesis, is inspired by the finding of Harel *et al.* [37] of partial homology between the RNA of leukemia viruses and the DNA of their respective natural hosts. In the case of our original provirus postulate full homology has to be expected. In view of the many difficulties with DNA-RNA hybridization in eukaryotic systems [see Spiegelman, panel discussion at this Symposium], I still regard it much too early to reject the original provirus or "proviral chromosomes" hypotheses and to accept the Vigier idea.

At the present stage, I have more confidence in mapping the various viral markers in the host genome in order to elucidate the genetic structure of the germinal provirus or protovirus. So far, the only results I have are crossing-over between the presumed regulator gene of C3Hf and operator ·gene of the GR strain in one case and between the regulator gene of C3Hf and a virulence marker of MTV-X in the O20 strain. With new immunological markers of the various MTV strains and new marker genes in the mouse, future studies along these lines seem to be highly promising.

13. Comparison of the germinal and somatic proviruses

The provirus for vertical transmission (germinal provirus) is often confused [38-40] with that for replication and transforming activities of oncornaviruses as hypothesized by Temin [41]. The provirus in the germ line is present from the very beginning in a species [see also Gilden, this Symposium]. It does not need a RNA-instructed DNA polymerase for its continuity. I have never observed the replacement of one germinal provirus by another after introduction of another virus strain in the MTV-system. As far as I know it has not been found in any other oncornavirus system either. Therefore, there is a very stable relationship between germinal provirus and host genome.

The discovery of the RNA-instructed DNA polymerase in many oncornaviruses [see both Montagnier and Temin, this Symposium] strongly supports Temin's idea that a DNA copy is made of the vira RNA. It is not certain, whether this copy (somatic provirus) is integrated into one of the host cell's chromosomes. It is possible that it is present as some kind of microchromosome, which is replicated to some extent under the control of the cellular genome. Another possibility is integration into nonchromosomal structures. But for simplicity's sake let's assume that the somatic provirus is integrated into a chromosome. The problem then rises as to whether the germinal provirus hypothesis is compatible with that of a somatic provirus. A solution to this problem is given in fig. 9.

Ordinarily, transcription of the germinal provirus is repressed due to the neighborhood of a regulator gene. Due to a momentary derepression following carcinogenic stimulation, some viral RNA has been produced by the germinal provirus. The repression system is restored soon again. The RNA-instructed DNA polymerase and related enzymatic machinery make a DNA copy of this viral RNA and the new somatic provirus then becomes integrated at a different site (*e.g.* another chromosome). At that new site the repressor has considerably less influence because the new provirus is at a greater distance from the regulator gene. Therefore continued transcription of this provirus can take place, which finally may lead to neoplastic transformation if enough viral information for this has accumulated in the cell. It must be pointed out that comparable thoughts have been developed by Temin in his protovirus theory (this Symposium).

In cases where due to germinal mutations spontaneous transcription of the germinal provirus will occur, no RNA-instructed DNA polymerase is needed for neoplastic conversion. However, one must keep in mind that these are abnormal situations. The thus released viruses are capable of tumor induction in other mouse strains for which the mentioned enzymes are necessary.

In case of superinfection, the viruses bypass the germinal proviruses. A somatic provirus is being made, which can be transcribed continuously. However, the repressor associated with the germinal provirus has some influence upon this new somatic provirus. In strains in which much repressor is produced such as O20 and C57BL, viral RNA production and therefore virion production is strongly interfered with but not completely inhibited.

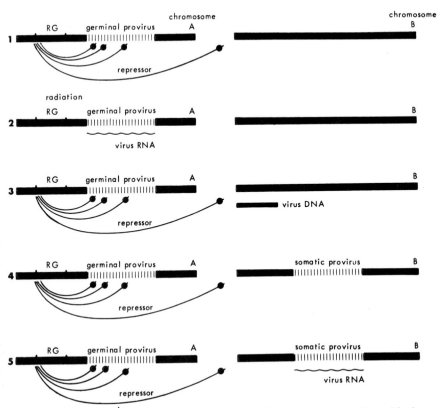

Fig. 9. Combination of the germinal provirus theory for vertical transmission with the somatic provirus theory for virus replication and neoplastic transformation. After derepression virus RNA is released by the germinal provirus. A DNA copy is made, which then becomes integrated into another chromosome. Because repressor molecules usually do not reach the somatic provirus continuous transcription (release of virus RNA) can take place.

14. General considerations

Ambitious cancer researchers often cannot resist the temptation to extrapolate their findings in a specialized field to a general theory of carcinogenesis. But the ideas as developed in the preceding pages are not extremely original in the framework of general theories on the interaction between viruses and host genome in oncogenesis.

In 1953, in his classical review of lysogeny, Lwoff [42] suggested that in neoplasia, lysogeny would have its animal counterpart. In 1960 in his concluding remarks at a conference about oncogenic viruses, Lwoff [43] worked out this idea in a more detailed form. Neoplasia could arise either after the integration of the genomes of administered viruses or by the induction of genetically transmitted viruses following the administration of carcinogenic drugs. Support for this idea comes from the finding, that several carcinogenic drugs are also inducing agents in lysogenic bacteria [42,43]. Similar thoughts have been developed by Gross [44] in his book on oncogenic viruses.

With regard to the oncornaviruses, already in 1963 Moore [45] suggested that MTV-L would be transmitted as a genetic factor of the host. Law [46] suggested the same in 1966 for the Gross leukemia virus in AKR mice. In 1968 we first published [9,10] our model of DNA provirus in the germ line as presented in fig. 6. We implied that this model might also hold true for the murine leukemia viruses and some other oncornaviruses. In the same year Payne and Chubb [38] published their findings on the mendelian inheritance of a group-specific antigen of the avian tumor viruses in some inbred chicken strains. They also favored a hypothesis related to lysogeny.

A year later Huebner and Todaro [47] presented their widely publicized oncogene theory, which has many features in common with the provirus theory that I have developed. The oncogene theory is not based upon extensive genetic analyses as in my studies or those of Payne, Weiss of Hanafusa [this Symposium]. Besides that this theory has been launched as a universal theory for carcinogenesis, it has some noteworthy transgressions compared to our initial theory: (a) the ubiquity of the oncogene, (b) the role of the oncogene in embryonic development, (c) switching on of the oncogene by age, and (d) the frequent defectiveness of the products of the oncogene.

In the mouse mammary tumor system we have since then confirmed the ubiquity of MTV (and presumably MTV-provirus) and the switching on by age. There are some meager indications that also defective mammary tumor viruses exist. It may be recommended that such defective agents be called viroids, which according to Altenburg [48] would play an important role in the genesis of many tumors. Since the oncornaviruses have many unvirus-like properties it might even be considered to call them all viroids.

I am not sure whether the germinal provirus for MTV would play any role in embryogenesis. Huebner's postulate [49] is mainly based on tolerance to various group-specific antigens of the C-type oncornaviruses in species they belong to. So far, we have little evidence for tolerance to group-specific antigens in the mouse mammary tumor system [50]. One has to take into account, however, that the mammary gland is an organ with the main development taking place after puberty. It seems possible that the MTV germinal provirus is involved in postnatal development of the mouse mammary gland. Some meager support for this idea comes from the observation of Ben-David *et al.* [51] that infection with MTV-S leads to a more rapid development of the mammary gland after hormonal stimulation.

It is very obvious that mammary tumors in mice are not caused by Huebner's oncogene. The viruses which are known to induce mammary tumors in mice are morphologically distinct from the C-type particles, which are associated with the oncogene. So far we have not found any common antigen in B and C type particles. This is not the only reason, however, that I am sceptical of the idea that all tumors would be induced by one and the same oncogene.

In table 8 are given incidences of tumors in various organs of the inbred

Table 8

Strain variation in susceptibility to spontaneous carcinogenesis of various organs.[a]

Strain	Mammary tumors	Pulmonary tumors	Lymphoreticular neoplasms	Hepatomas	Uterus tumors	Ovarian tumors	Skin papillomas	Sarcomas
Af	1	57	15	6	0	0	0	0
AKR	0	0	94	0	0	0	0	0
AKR/ FuA	6	70	39	0	3	3	0	0
A2$_G$	0	76	10	4	7	5	0	0
C57BL	1	8	25	0	0	0	0	0
CBA	5	13	11	20	9	47	0	0
C3Hf	35	10	30	3	3	4	0	0
DBAf	9	11	7	4	14	3	0	0
GR	75	17	12	0	0	0	6	0
LTf	4	10	19	4	2	2	6	15
LIS	0	19	10	0	0	0	0	0
MAS	3	51	23	5	2	2	0	0
O20	2	48	10	0	0	0	0	0
P[b]	0	64	3	0	3	0	0	0
TSI	0	15	41	0	0	0	0	0
TSII[c]	0	48	40	0	0	0	0	33
STS	0	25	8	0	0	0	0	0
WLLf	1	8	5	1	2	4	0	10

[a] Only tumor % in breeding females are reported here. Animals were permitted to live their span. When the animals were in bad shape, they were killed and autopsied.
[b] A congenic line to C57BL carrying some DBA-strain genes.
[c] Separated early during the development of the TSI line.

mouse strains in the breeding colony of Professor Mühlbock. (These data have been compiled by Miss W. van Ebbenhorst Tengbergen.) The results strongly suggest that susceptibility to spontaneous tumor-development differs from organ to organ. In other words separate genes cause susceptibility for oncogenesis in the different organs. In case the various genes (oncogenes) cause cancer in their target organ by releasing a virus (or viroid), it is not impossible that several of these agents have common properties such as group-specific antigens. Especially a "proviral chromosome" hypothesis or protovirus concept is very helpful in this respect. RNA molecules, which determine organ-specificity, after being released by the organ-specific oncogene may be coupled to another RNA molecule, which controls group-specific properties. In this respect it is interesting that from BALB/c mice can be retrieved several different leukemia viruses as found by Salaman [52]. In my laboratory it has been found that ND2 mice harbor both a virus causing lymphatic leukemia, which is related to the Gross virus from AKR mice, and an erythroblastosis inducing virus, which is related to the Friend and Rauscher agents [Brinkhof, unpublished results].

The finding of group-specific antigens of the leukemia-sarcoma virus groups in various tumors may not always be interpreted, however, as evidence for the etiologic role of the factor, which produces these antigens. For instance MTV-S can replicate in several other tissues than the mammary gland and produce group-specific antigens but not cause a tumor in them. The virus can also be present in tumors, of which it is known that they are produced by other agents.

An alternative to the poly-oncogene hypothesis worked out above is that a single oncogene is responsible for neoplastic conversion in many tissues but that separate expression genes cause organ-specific switching on of this oncogene.

The protovirus theory of Temin is discussed at this conference. An essential difference with the concepts developed by us for the MTV proviruses is that only a small homologous part of the viral genome would be present in the host genome. (This idea is comparable to the Vigier hypothesis presented in fig. 8.) Furthermore, that due to somatic mutation, release of viral RNA takes place, which can lead to the establishment of a new provirus or after recombination with other RNA molecules giving rise to new viruses.

The somatic mutation hypothesis is not very acceptable because it fails to explain the strain differences in susceptibility to both spontaneous and chemically-induced carcinogenesis in lungs and mammary glands of mice. In addition, the release of so much MTV antigens in irradiated O20 mice, in contrast to superinfection with MTV-S, is not compatible with a somatic mutation postulate either.

Here I want to express sincere gratitude to Professor Mühlbock with whom I have worked for several years on the problems outlined above. In the years I have been in his laboratory, he taught me patience, which is certainly important in the mammary tumor virus field. After all it proved to be rewarding as may become obvious from the preceding pages. Professor Mühlbock has been tolerant to all my new ideas, which seemed outrageous to many of my colleagues. Of course, quite a few did not hold true and Professor Mühlbock has been very instrumental in disproving some of them. But several concepts remain to be disproven yet. I am furthermore very grateful to him, because from his great wealth of experimental data on the interaction between genetic and viral factors in murine mammary carcinogenesis, I could borrow many which nicely fitted into my schemes. Some of his newest data made clear that some of my schemes were too simplistic.

I regard it a privilege to have been a student of Professor Mühlbock.

15. Conclusions and summary

The various experimental data described above strongly suggest that every mouse carries genetic information for the production of a mammary tumor virus. In one case single-genic inheritance of transmission by the sex cells could be established. The genes controlling such transmission do not achieve this by causing extreme susceptibility to small amounts of vegetative virus being present in or around the gametes. The transmission by the sex cells is specific for the MTV strain, which is indigenous to a given mouse strain. All these data strongly suggest genetic transmission of MTV strains in the mouse strain they naturally belong to.

In some mouse strains virus is released at a young age. This property proves in some strains to be a recessive trait as tested in crosses with strains in which virus release is switched on late in life. In one case early virus release proves to be a dominant character. There is a very good correlation in the age at which virus release is switched on and susceptibility to spontaneous mammary carcinogenesis. In strains which release virus only late in life treatment with urethan or irradiation leads to the production of viral antigens. These data strongly support an all-viral etiology of mammary cancer in mice, irrespective of the initial stimulus.

There is a striking correlation between the rate of release of indigenous MTV and susceptibility to superinfection with MTV, associated with the rate of virion production.

All these findings have led to the hypothesis that a repressor molecule

P. Bentvelzen

ordinarily inhibits the transcription of a germinal provirus (DNA copy) being present in one of the chromosomes. This repressor would also cause resistance to superinfection by interference with the replication. Germinal mutations in regulator or operator genes would lead to release of viral RNA. Temporary abrogation of repression by radiation or carcinogenic chemicals would have the same result as does aging.

The germinal provirus is different from the somatic provirus, which will be established after infection for replication and oncogenic activities of the oncornaviruses. The germinal provirus does not need an RNA-instructed DNA polymerase for its continuity. It is theorized that after release of viral RNA by the germinal provirus a somatic provirus will be produced and inserted into the host genome at a site which is less accessible to the repressor of the germinal provirus. In this way continuous release of viral RNA can take place, finally leading to neoplastic transformation.

References

[1] O. Mühlbock, European J. Cancer 1 (1965) 123.
[2] Staff Jackson Laboratory, Science 78 (1933) 465.
[3] R. Korteweg, Ned. Tijdschr. Geneesk. 78 (1934) 240.
[4] J.J. Bittner, Science 84 (1936) 162.
[5] M.B. Visscher, R.G. Green and J.J. Bittner, Proc. Soc. Exptl. Biol. Med. 49 (1942) 94.
[6] W.R. Bryan, H. Kahler, M.B. Shimkin and H.B. Andervont, J. Natl. Cancer Inst. 2 (1942) 451.
[7] O. Mühlbock and P. Bentvelzen, Perspectives Virol. 6 (1968) 75.
[8] L. Foulds, J. Natl. Cancer Inst. 17 (1956) 701.
[9] P. Bentvelzen, Genetical control of the vertical transmission of the Mühlbock mammary tumor virus in the GR mouse strain. (Hollandia, Amsterdam, 1968).
[10] P. Bentvelzen, A. Timmermans, J.H. Daams and A. van der Gugten, Bibliotheca Haematol. 31 (1968) 101.
[11] P. Bentvelzen and J.H. Daams, J. Natl. Cancer Inst. 43 (1969) 1025.
[12] P. Bentvelzen and J.H. Daams, European J. Cancer 6 (1970) 273.
[13] G.H. Zeilmaker, Intern. J. Cancer 4 (1969) 261.
[14] P.C. Hageman, J. Links and P. Bentvelzen, J. Natl. Cancer Inst. 40 (1968) 1319.
[15] J. Calafat and P. Hageman, Virology 36 (1968) 308.
[16] D.R. Pitelka, H.A. Bern, S. Nandi and K.B. DeOme, J. Natl. Cancer Inst. 33 (1964) 867.
[17] S. Nandi, Canadian Cancer Conf. 6 (1966) 69.
[18] K.B. DeOme, L. Young and S. Nandi, Proc. Am. Ass. Cancer Res. 8 (1967) 13.
[19] L.M. Boot and O. Mühlbock, Acta Unio Intern. Contra Cancrum 12 (1956) 569.
[20] H.B. Andervont and T.B. Dunn, J. Natl. Cancer Inst. 14 (1953) 317.
[21] L.M. Boot, Verhandel. Koninkl. Ned. Akad. Wetenschap, Afd. Natuurk., 2nd series, vol. LVIII, 3 (North-Holland, Amsterdam, 1969).

[22] F. Jacob and J. Monod, J. Mol. Biol. 3 (1961) 318.

[23] O. Mühlbock and T.G. van Rijssel, J. Natl. Cancer Inst. 18 (1954) 73.

[24] A. Timmermans, P. Bentvelzen, P.C. Hageman and J. Calafat, J. Gen. Virol. 4 (1969) 619.

[25] P. Bentvelzen, J.H. Daams, P.C. Hageman and J. Calafat, Proc. Natl. Acad. Sci. U.S. 67 (1970) 377.

[26] O. Mühlbock, Acta Unio Intern. Contra Cancrum 12 (1956) 665.

[27] W.E. Heston, J. Natl. Cancer Inst. 32 (1964) 947.

[28] L.M. Boot, P. Bentvelzen, J. Calafat, G. Röpcke and A. Timmermans, Proc. Xth Intern. Cancer Congress, Houston, 1970, in press.

[29] J.H. Daams, J. Calafat, E.Y. Lasfargues, B. Kramarsky and P. Bentvelzen, Virology 41 (1970) 184.

[30] J.H. Daams, *In:* L. Severi, Immunity and tolerance in oncogenesis (Div. of Cancer Research, Univ. of Perugia, 1970) p. 463.

[31] P. Bentvelzen, J. Natl. Cancer Inst. 41 (1968) 757.

[32] M.A. Hairstone, J.B. Sheffield and D.H. Moore, J. Natl. Cancer Inst. 33 (1964) 825.

[33] H.B. Andervont, J. Natl. Cancer Inst. 10 (1949) 201.

[34] S. Nandi and K.B. DeOme, J. Natl. Cancer Inst. 35 (1965) 299.

[35] P. Bentvelzen and G. Szalay, *In:* L. Severi, Lung tumors in animals (Div. of Cancer Research, Univ. of Perugia, 1966) p. 835.

[36] P.H. Duesberg and R.D. Cardiff, Virology 36 (1968) 696.

[37] L. Harel, J. Harel and J. Huppert, Biochem. Biophys. Res. Commun. 28 (1967) 44.

[38] L.N. Payne and R.C. Chubb, J. Gen. Virol. 3 (1968) 379.

[39] S. Spiegelman, A. Burny, M.R. Das, J. Keydar, J. Schlom, M. Travnicek and K. Watson, Nature 227 (1970) 1029.

[40] R.C. Nowinski, L.J. Old, N.H. Sarkar and D.H. Moore, Virology 42 (1970) 1152.

[41] H.M. Temin, Virology 20 (1963) 577.

[42] A. Lwoff, Bacteriol. Rev. 17 (1953) 269.

[43] A. Lwoff, Cancer Res. 20 (1960) 820.

[44] L. Gross, Oncogenic viruses (Pergamon Press, New York, 1961).

[45] D.H. Moore, Nature 198 (1963) 429.

[46] L.W. Law, Natl. Cancer Inst. Monograph 22 (1966) 267.

[47] R.J. Huebner and G.J. Todaro, Proc. Natl. Acad. Sci. U.S. 64 (1969) 1087.

[48] E. Altenburg, Am. Naturalist 80 (1946) 559.

[49] R.J. Huebner, G.J. Kelloff, P.S. Sarma, W.T. Lane, H.C. Turner, R.V. Gilden, S. Oroszlan, H. Meier, D.D. Myers and R.L. Peters, Proc. Natl. Acad. Sci. U.S. 67 (1970) 366.

[50] J. Hilgers, J.H. Daams and P. Bentvelzen, Israel J. Med. Sci. 7 (1971) 154.

[51] M. Ben-David, W.E. Heston and D. Rodbard, J. Natl. Cancer Inst. 42 (1969) 207.

[52] M.H. Salaman and J. Flocks, British Empire Cancer Campaign for Research 42 (1964) 192.

Part 7

THE FOURTH WASSINK LECTURE

THE VALUE OF EXPERIMENTAL CANCER RESEARCH FOR THE UNDERSTANDING OF THE HUMAN DISEASE

O. MÜHLBOCK

Antoni van Leeuwenhoekhuis,
The Netherlands Cancer Institute, Amsterdam,
The Netherlands

I consider it a privilege to be invited to deliver the Wassink Lecture. The Wassink Lecture was instituted by the Governing Board of the Netherlands Cancer Institute in honor of Dr. W.F. Wassink, who has so greatly influenced, as no other man, the development of the clinic of the Antoni van Leeuwenhoek-huis (The Netherlands Cancer Institute) in the first 40 years of its existence.

Dr. W.F. Wassink worked from 1913 until 1959, with only a short interruption, in the clinic of the Netherlands Cancer Institute. As a surgeon Dr. Wassink was in the first place interested in clinical problems, but he also always had a special interest in experimental cancer research. He was of the opinion that no distinct borderline can be established between clinical and experimental research. Therefore it is logical that in a cancer institute the clinic and the laboratory must form a unity. The promotion of this unity is one of the major tasks with which we are confronted daily. When Dr. Wassink retired in 1959, the Wassink Lecture Fund was founded to promote "synthetic considerations over the results of clinical and experimental research".

Communication is one of the main problems in bringing the results of experimental work to the attention of clinicians or to make the experimenta-lists aware of the human problems. Complicated terminology and many abbreviations demand a concentrated effort from both sides for mutual understanding.

Having once been a clinician myself and having worked the last 25 years in the field of experimental cancer research I thought it especially valuable on this occasion to contemplate how much experimental research has contributed to the understanding of the human disease.

The interest of our group was concentrated upon mammary cancer the last 25 years. It is this type of cancer which I will discuss today.

It is well established that several factors play a role in the genesis of mammary carcinomas. One of these is the genetic constitution of the bearer of this tumor. The first genetic observations have been made by clinicians as is often the case with fundamental discoveries in medicine. They reported that mammary cancer was more frequent in certain families than could be expected on a random basis.

The famous and often cited example is the Broca family. Broca was a well-known French surgeon who published his family tree in 1866 which shows an extraordinary frequency of mammary carcinoma over 4 generations. His great-grandmother died in 1788 with a mammary carcinoma. She had four daughters, of which two died with mammary carcinomas and the other two with cancer of the liver. One of the daughters with the liver cancer had four daughters, again two of these had mammary cancer. One of these daughters with mammary cancer had five daughters of which three died with mammary cancer. One out of three women of the fourth generation had also a mammary carcinoma. One very striking fact that has frequently been observed is that in such families the age at which the cancer appeared was much earlier in subsequent generation than in the preceding ones.

Since Broca's publication many family histories have been reported in which breast cancer was abnormally frequent [1].

Great interest in the possibility of breast cancer as a familial disease was aroused by observations in mice at the beginning of the century that in certain colonies more animals died with mammary cancer than in others. At that time the laws of Mendel were rediscovered and therefore everyone was convinced that breast cancer is a hereditary disease, which follows mendelian rules. In conflict with these laws, the predisposition for mammary cancer in mice is more often dependent upon the mother than the father as reported by Leo Loeb and his assistant Miss Lathrop in 1918. One group of geneticists (Maud Slye) was convinced that the predisposition of this cancer of the mouse is recessive whereas others (Little, Clara Lynch) were convinced that it would be dominant. This problem was insolvable at that time because necessary inbred mouse strains needed 10 more years to be developed.

The observations of the experimental workers aroused new interest of the clinicians into this problem. Among the first clinicians who started a systematic and extensive investigation of the occurrence of mammary tumors in the families of breast cancer patients were Dr. Wassink and Mrs. Wassink [2,3]. They have studied several hundreds of patients and their families: mothers, sisters, grandmothers and first cousins. They observed a marked increase in breast cancer in the female relatives of women with this tumor. Wassink concluded that the tumor incidence is highest with sisters of a patient, followed by mothers and aunts and is less in grandmothers and cousins. Accordingly, a woman, whose mother or sister developed a breast tumor has approximately a

2-fold greater risk of also contracting this disease. However, there is no evidence that the relatives of breast cancer patients have an increased risk of cancer at other sites. Wassink's conclusions have repeatedly been confirmed.

Familial factors in the genesis of a disease are not necessarily genetic. The possibility of environmental factors must also be considered. This idea has been nurtured by laboratory investigations too.

When the first inbred strains were developed, it was found that there were strains in which the females have a high incidence of mammary tumors and others which developed no tumors. These strains were suitable for the study of the genetic factors in the genesis of mammary tumors. Korteweg [4] in the Netherlands Cancer Institute did the first experiments in this direction. He had two strains at his disposal, one with a high incidence (DBA) and one with a low incidence (C57BL). When Korteweg wanted to make a cross between these two strains, he was faced with a practical difficulty. One can cross in two ways. Firstly ♀ high x ♂ low and secondly ♀ low x ♂ high. The first cross gave very poor results because of the high intra-uterine mortality. Korteweg then asked geneticists for advice. They told him, that it is not necessary to make the crosses in both directions, since all F1-hybrids are genetically identical. Korteweg did not follow this advice and made the cross in both directions. By doing this he made an unexpected discovery. Only when the mother belongs to the high cancer strain, the F1-hybrids had also a high mammary tumor percentage whereas when the mother belonged to the non-cancer strain, the offspring also has no tumors. It had to be concluded therefore, that an extrachromosomal factor determines the breast tumor incidence. This factor is transmitted from mother to offspring. The same observation was made in the United States at the same time by Little and his co-workers at the Jackson Laboratory [5]. A few years later Bittner found that this factor is transmitted with the mother's milk. If the young of a high cancer line are transferred immediately after birth to a foster mother of the low cancer line, the young do not develop breast cancer [6].

Later on it became established that this milkfactor is a virus. In honor of the late Dr. Bittner it is called the Bittner virus.

Although in the beginning nothing was known about this milk factor, the statisticians took this finding as a lead for further investigations into the human disease. Is there a milk factor in humans too?

An indication against the existence of a "human milk factor" is that in populations or social groups where breast feeding is least practiced the highest rates of breast cancer are found. An even clearer indication against it was that mammary tumor incidence was the same among the paternal as among the maternal grandmothers. This was also found for paternal aunts as compared to the maternal ones.

The conclusion of the statisticians, therefore, was, that there is no evidenc(for a milk factor causing human breast cancer [7].

A new discovery in our laboratory, however, gave a new lead to th(statisticians. The experimental work on the genesis of mammary cancer wa almost exclusively done with inbred strains of mice developed in the Unitec States. As the development of a new inbred strain is very tedious anc time-consuming, only very few investigators and laboratories could pursuε development of new strains. Therefore the strains which have been developed. very often have common ancestors. It was a possibility that the milk factor waς a speciality of American mouse strains. I thought it worthwhile to develop so-called European inbred strains in the Netherlands Cancer Institute. Several of these new strains had ancestors, which − as far as could be ascertained − had no relations with American mice. One of these strains showed a very high incidence of mammary tumors at an early age [8]. This strain called GR harbors a milk factor, but crosses with non-cancer strains showed that this factor was not only transmitted by the mother's milk but also with the sperm of the father. Consequently it was also found that transmission takes place with the ovum. In this strain the mammary tumor agent is thus transmitted at conception. The viral genome is incorporated into the sex-cells of the parents.

The statisticians have to take a fresh look at their pedigree-charts in view of our results with the GR strain. That such paternal transmission can take place shows the family-tree of a patient seen by Dr. Cleton in our clinic. In this tree it is apparent that a high incidence of mammary cancer is only found in the family of the patient's father.

The consequence is that in all future statistical studies the family-tree of the father must also be taken into consideration.

There is still another variant of the mammary tumor virus found in mice: NIV, the nodule inducing virus, intensively studied by the group of DeOme and Nandi in Berkeley and by us [9,10]. This NIV is present in certain mouse strains, usually in a low concentration. It is also transmitted with the genome at conception. This virus induces nodules which are precancerous stages in the mouse mammary gland, and it has a very low carcinogenic potential. Mammary tumors induced by this virus appear very late in life in a low percentage.

It has been a painstaking work to prove the oncogenicity of this virus. DeOme and his collaborators could demonstrate this only in a rather indirect way. They seldom achieved cell-free transmission of this agent. In our laboratory we finally succeeded to transfer this virus after passage in a susceptible host and to induce tumors with it.

Tumor virology usually occupies itself with viruses with an explosive effect which induce tumors very early. It is sometimes more realistic, however, to study slow acting viruses which induce tumors late in the life of an animal. In women breast cancer often develops at a high age. Assuming a viral etiology for these tumors, they must have arisen under influence of an agent comparable to NIV.

Still unexplained is the great variation in breast cancer incidence in different areas of the world. Especially striking is the low incidence of mammary cancer in Japanese women as compared to European or American women.

When the milk factor was discovered by biologic experiments nothing was known about the nature of this agent. It is now firmly established that it is a RNA virus. But it took almost 20 years of laboratory work to develop methods for its isolation and recognition. Biophysical procedure such as density gradient centrifugation and especially electron-microscopic techniques had to be perfected. The development of these techniques had to be combined with biological tests, which are very time-consuming. The mammary tumor virus is abundant in tumors of certain mouse strains. With this knowledge at hand and the methods available, breast cancer tissues from women have been investigated with the electron microscope [11], and indeed a few particles have been found, which were similar to the mouse virus. One must realize that the search with an electron microscope can cover only a very minute area of a tumor. Unless there is a tremendous production of virus particles in the cell, it is very unlikely that one can find a virus. Another way would be to make an extract but these extracts proved only occasionally to contain a virus particle.

From the mouse-experiments it was known that the milk contains the virus. Therefore, a search has been made in human milk, which can be obtained in abundance [12,13].

The methods developed over the last 20 years for the isolation of the Bittner virus from mouse milk could not be applied directly to human milk since the latter is quite different in composition. After modification of the technique milk specimen from women in the general population were processed and indeed in a few samples virus particles could be isolated which are morphologically identical with the mouse mammary tumor virus. Furthermore milk from Parsi women in Bombay was investigated. These women belong to a caste which is comparatively inbred for 12 centuries through interfamilial marriages. The breast cancer incidence in these Parsi women is 5 times higher than in other women from Bombay. The number of positive samples were higher in these women. The positive samples were still higher in women with at least one member of the family with breast cancer. The highest proportion of positive samples was found in patients with breast cancer.

These are highly important findings, which have to be followed up. This will by no means be an easy task. First it is necessary to test more samplings of milk from women of various categories and communities and to establish a good correlation between a high incidence of these virus-like particles in the milk and the individual risk of breast cancer.

It is out of the question that the same experiments can be done in human beings as those in mice like infection of new-borns with virus containing materials in order to establish a causal relationship between these particles and the development of breast cancer. It will be necessary to produce extensive circumstantial evidence before these particles can be implicated in the origin of the human disease.

Since it is so extremely difficult to find virus particles with the electron microscope in human breast cancer, other tools for the study have to be developed. An immunological approach of a possible human breast cancer virus seems to be highly promising. Antisera to purified human virus particles may be used to see whether virus-specific antigens are present in those tumors or milk samples, in which no particles could be detected. In view of our findings that the mouse virus can replicate in other tissues than the milk gland, it is worthwhile to look for the presence of viral antigens in other human tissues. In this way a correlation might be found between tumor incidences in certain families and the occurrence of such antigens.

In addition it will be interesting to look for a cross reaction between the mouse virus and the human particles. Since it is at the moment much easier to prepare antisera to the mouse virus, the screening program outlined above could eventually be done with these antisera in case of a cross reaction. There are indeed some indications for common antigenicity of the mouse and human particles [14].

The Bittner virus was incubated with sera taken from women who have breast cancer or, as a control, normal women. The tumorigenicity of the treated virus was then assayed. It was claimed that a statistically significant neutralization of the murine virus by the sera of the cancer patients occurred, but the number of data were very limited.

More and more evidence is accumulating that similar to other viruses, the mammary tumor virus may be present in many perfectly healthy hosts either as such or in some masked form. They are like harmless parasites, but may be triggered into action by various stimuli and then change from harmless into carcinogenic agents.

Experiments in our laboratory have recently shown that X-rays and urethan may act as such triggers in mouse strains in which virus particles never previously were found [15]. After such treatments mammary tumors develop containing numerous virus particles that have a strong carcinogenic activity.

It is at the moment difficult to envisage how the insight, that breast cancer may be caused by a virus, will contribute to therapy. This is especially difficult if the virus is genetically transmitted because then one never will get rid of the virus. New roads must be found to keep such transmitted viruses under control. It is obvious that much experimental work has to be done before this problem is solved.

Even if we assume that a virus plays a role in the development of mammary cancer it is certain that other factors are essential too. The conclusion that cancer is a multifactorial event is one of the major achievements of experimental work in the laboratory. One of the most important factors in the genesis of breast cancer are hormones. Again the clinic gave the first indication: never has a breast cancer been reported in a person with undeveloped mammary glands. The experience that castration is a powerful inhibitor for breast cancer development has pointed to the ovary as the primary endocrine organ concerned.

This observation in humans received still more emphasis, when it was found that in mice oestrogenic hormones can cause mammary cancer. In the course of the years numerous studies in women have been performed on oestrogens, steroid metabolism and excretion patterns in an effort to relate these to the aetiology of breast cancer. Another aim was to determine indices of prognostic value or to find an indication of the treatment to be followed. All these studies have given only a few results, leaving the situation more or less in a deadlock [16].

New laboratory results can lead to a fresh attempt. Investigations, in which our laboratory had a leading part, have pointed to the role of prolactin, the lactogenic hormone produced by the anterior pituitary lobe as a major factor in the genesis of breast cancer. Oestrogenic hormones are essential in that they induce the hypophysis to produce prolactin via an effect on the hypothalamus. The hypothalamus produces a factor which inhibits the hypophysis to produce prolactin. This inhibitor is suppressed by oestrogenic hormones. Prolactin is produced and the growth of the mammary gland is stimulated. The picture as we have developed in recent years is as follows: prolactin is the dominant factor in the hormonal genesis of mammary cancer. Oestrogenic hormones act mainly as inciter for prolactin production and progesterone is active only in the presence of prolactin.

In view of these new discoveries in the laboratory about the primary role of prolactin in the genesis of breast cancer in mice as compared to the secondary role of the ovarian steroids, an analysis of the relation between prolactin and human breast cancer seems to be of utmost importance. The first problem is to prove the existence of prolactin in humans as a separate entity from the growth hormone. Evidence is accumulating that also in man prolactin exists. The next step then is to work out an assay method for human prolactin. Investigations in our laboratory have led to radio-immunoassay methods for prolactin of various species which are so sensitive that they can determine very small amounts in blood samples [17,18]. With such a method it may be possible to study the role of prolactin to human breast cancer.

In the analysis of anamnestic material from patients with breast cancer special attention has been paid to the period from the menarche till the first pregnancy. Women who have had a child after the age of 25 years have more breast cancer than women who gave birth before that age [19]. It is assumed that in the first menstruation periods certain deviations in the metabolism and the excretion pattern of the steroids can be found which might be correlated with the risk for the development of a breast cancer.

Another assumption could also be that the essential factor in the origin of mammary cancer is the hormonal stimulation of mammary growth associated with each menstrual cycle. This stimulation is not followed by a "physiological" secretory stage of the mammary gland, but ends abruptly during the "unphysiological" menstruation period, followed by the immediate return to the subsequent cycle. This would imply that endocrine disorders should not necessarily occur in the history of patients suffering from cancer of the breast [20].

From animal experimentation it has been absolutely proven that genetic factors play an important role in the development of mammary cancer. The question then arises, where is this genetic factor localized? One could imagine that the gene or the gene-complex is responsible for an abnormal hormonal production. Although we have studied this intensively we have never found a good indication for it. More likely is that the susceptibility of the target organ e.g., the mammary gland is of importance. This was experimentally tested in our laboratory and it could be demonstrated by means of technically very difficult mammary gland transplantations that genetic susceptibility is localized in the mammary gland itself [21].

Genes may control susceptibility of the mammary gland to hormonal action, to the virus or endow capacity to transform from a normal to a malignant cell. All these possibilities need to be studied in the coming years. We have directed our attention in the last years to the histocompatibility genes. These genes show an enormous species variability. Many genes are concerned with coding for histocompatibility antigens. The biological function of these genes is not yet known. It has been suggested that because the histocompatibility genes are distributed throughout the genome they act as a sort of monitor device for the intactness of the genetic material.

Cells which do not fit into the pattern because of somatic variation could then trigger the immunological machinery. This has been termed "immunological surveillance" [22]. Other elimination processes may be involved as well. Another possible function of these genes could be an influence on the infectivity or oncogenicity of the oncogenic viruses. The study of these H-genes has been made possible by the pioneer work of George Snell, who developed a whole system of so-called congenic resistant lines which differ from the original strain by a change of only one allele. Our first results with these strains have indicated that resistance to the development of mammary cancer is related to the histocompatibility genes H-2^b [23]. The mechanism of this H-2^b associated resistance is not yet clear.

In man exists a comparable histocompatibility system. In view of our results with mice it is worthwhile to look for a correlation between histocompatibility genes and the development of breast cancer in women. If such correlation exists this would help screening women early in their lives for those who have a high risk of contracting breast cancer. These women could be kept under close observation.

All these investigations which try to elucidate the causal factors in the genesis of mammary cancer are of eminent significance for the prevention of breast cancer. Without doubt prevention of the disease is the solution of the problem. This is, however, still a prospect in the future.

Today and in the years to come, the treatment of breast cancer remains a challenge to the physician. The treatment with surgical and radiological means gives satisfactory results in a great number of patients. But there are other patients in whom these procedures fail. What has the laboratory done so far and what can it do in the future to help the clinician to device new forms of treatment?

The laboratory investigations in this respect once more have been prompted by clinical observations. Already in 1896 it was demonstrated by Bateson in Glasgow that ovariectomy is beneficial in certain cases of breast cancer. An enormous amount of work has been done to elucidate the basis of this observation in animal models. According to the classical definition malignant tumors are autonomous, that means independent from causative factors. However, in the case of breast cancer there are some tumors which are dependent on steroid hormones, mostly estrogens. The ablation of the organs that produce oestrogens had some success but it proved to be impossible to eliminate all oestrogens. New investigations made it probable that the tumor cells themselves can produce steroid hormones or their precursors. Another question is if prolactin is not the hormone which is also essential for the growth of a mammary tumor. In certain animal models indeed mammary tumors proved to be dependent on prolactin for their growth [24]. If this should be true for women also a new hopeful tool could be developed which already proved to be effective in animal experiments.

Antibodies to prolactin producing cells or chemical inhibitors of prolactin production may counteract the harmful effects of this hormone on breast cancer. These exciting laboratory results may lead to a new treatment of this disease in women. Unfortunately it has also been found in the laboratory that such hormone-dependent tumors can change irreversibly to autonomous malignancies. This change has been termed "progression". Progression is a characteristic of all tumor cells. Progression is one of the factors which explains why hormone therapy in the end so often failed. We do not know the factors which cause the progression and we do not know any means yet to prevent progression.

It appears here as in other oncological investigations that there is an enormous variation in cancer cells which makes each classification almost impossible. Each cancer cell seems to have some inviduality which moreover is never constant but always changing under the influence of many factors. The capacity of the cancer cell to adapt to different environments, is an expression of the plasticity of living material which is the basis for the further existence of life. This plasticity makes investigations in oncology so extremely complicated.

I have illustrated in the field of research with mammary carcinoma how fruitful has been the intellectual exchange between clinicians and laboratory workers. I hope that also in the future this close cooperation is favored in the Netherlands Cancer Institute. Only then progress in an area as complex as cancer research can be achieved.

References

[1] P.L.M.M. Taminiau, Bijdrage tot de kennis van het familiair en hereditair voorkomen van carcinoom (Thesis Utrecht, 1926).
[2] W.F. Wassink and C.Ph. Wassink-van Raamsdonk, Ned. T. Geneesk. 67 (1923) 326.
[3] W.F. Wassink, Genetica 17 (1935) 103.
[4] R. Korteweg, Ned. T. Geneesk. 77 (1933) 4038.
[5] Staff Jackson Memorial Laboratory, Science 78 (1933) 465.
[6] J.J. Bittner, Science 84 (1935) 162.
[7] M.T. Macklin, J. Natl. Cancer Inst. 22 (1959) 927.
[8] O. Mühlbock, Europ. J. Cancer 1 (1965) 123.
[9] D.R. Pitelka, H.A. Bern, S. Nandi, et al., J. Natl. Cancer Inst. 33 (1964) 867.
[10] Ph.C. Hageman, this Symposium.
[11] L. Dmochowski, G. Seman and H.S. Gallager, Cancer 24 (1969) 1241.
[12] H.C. Chopra and W.F. Feller, Texas Rep. Biol. Med. 27 (1969) 945.
[13] D.H. Moore, J. Charney, B. Kramarsky, et al., Nature 229 (1971) 611.
[14] J. Charney and D.H. Moore, Nature 229 (1971) 627.

[15] A. Timmermans, P. Bentvelzen, Ph.C. Hageman and J. Calafat, J. Gen. Virol. 4 (1969) 619.

[16] L.M. Boot, Intern. J. Cancer 5 (1970) 167.

[17] H.G. Kwa, A.A. van der Gugten and F. Verhofstad, Europ. J. Cancer 5 (1969) 559.

[18] H.G. Kwa, A.A. van der Gugten and F. Verhofstad, Europ. J. Cancer 5 (1969) 571.

[19] P. Cole and B. MacMahon, Lancet 1 (1969) 604.

[20] O. Mühlbock, Adv. Cancer Res. 4 (1956) 371.

[21] A. Dux and O. Mühlbock, Intern. J. Cancer 1 (1966) 5.

[22] M. Burnet, Immunological surveillance (Oxford, Pergamon, 1970).

[23] O. Mühlbock and A. Dux, Histocompatibility genes and mammary cancer in mice, Proceed. Int. Symposium on Histocompatibility genes, Praha 1970. (Basel, S. Karger, 1971).

[24] O.H. Pearson and H. Nasr, Role of steroid hormones in the pathogenesis and treatment of breast cancer. Workshop on "Estrogens and mammary cancer" (Buffalo, 1970).

Part 8

DNA, RNA AND VIRAL CARCINOGENESIS

THE PROTOVIRUS HYPOTHESIS AND CANCER*

Howard M, TEMIN

McArdle Laboratory, University of Wisconsin, Madison, Wis. 53706, U.S.A.

In inviting me to this conference, the organizers suggested that by now I would be "fed up with speaking over and over again about the DNA copy of viral RNA". They asked me to give "the very last paper at the symposium" and "to speculate about carcinogenesis".

There are three major classes of theories of carcinogenesis: viral, mutational, and embryonic or differentiative. In classical viral theory, a tumor virus enters an organism from the outside, either by vertical or horizontal transmission. The virus causes the tumor without itself being altered. In classical mutational theory, genetic change occurring in a classical genetic element — that is, a gene or chromosome — causes the neoplasia. In classical embryonic or differentiative theories, there is no change in the information in the cellular DNA in neoplastic transformation. There is activation and deactivation of genes leading to neoplastic transformation.

At present we know of a number of related viruses, the Rous viruses or RNA tumor viruses, that differ greatly in their oncogenicity. I shall use a discussion of possible mechanisms of carcinogenesis by these viruses to show that some present ways to look at viral carcinogenesis encompass all of these classical theories of carcinogenesis. Many of the ideas I shall present are more extensively documented in a recent review in *Annual Review of Microbiology* [1] which should be consulted for literature references.

My general conclusion is that only viruses like Rous sarcoma virus (RSV) and murine sarcoma virus (MSV) are tumor viruses in the strict sense of containing in the virion genes for neoplastic transformation. RNA leukemia viruses (RLV) and mammary tumor virus (MTV) are considered not to have

*The work in my laboratory is supported by Public Health Service research grant CA 07175 from the National Cancer Institute. I hold Research Career Development Award 10K 3-CA 8185 from the National Cancer Institute. I thank my colleagues for helpful comments.

351

such genes, but to be more like non-viral carcinogens in their mechanism of neoplastic transformation; that is, RLV and MTV increase the probability of a misevolution of cellular genetic elements, the protoviruses, which replicate DNA to DNA, and DNA to RNA to DNA [2,3].

Neoplastic transformation by Rous Sarcoma virus (RSV)

I have divided the life cycle of an RNA sarcoma virus in a sensitive cell, for example Rous sarcoma virus in sensitive chicken cells, into 8 steps (table 1) [1].

Table 1
Life cycle of RNA sarcoma virus in sensitive cells.

1. Initial events
2. Formation of provirus
3. Activation of virus-specified RNA and protein synthesis
4. Synthesis of virus-specified RNAs
5. Synthesis of virus-specified proteins
6. Formation of virions
7. Replication of provirus
8. Neoplastic transformation

(1) Initial events: the RSV virion attaches to and enters the cell. It is uncoated so that the virion core enzymes are exposed, and the core is transported to the cell nucleus[1]. (2) Formation of provirus: DNA is synthesized with the viral RNA as a template. The DNA is integrated at a specific[1] site in the host chromosome, forming an integrated DNA provirus. (3) Activation of virus-specified RNA and protein synthesis: RNA synthesis, using the provirus DNA as template, begins. This virus-specified RNA is processed and transported to the cytoplasm. Virus-specified RNA-directed protein synthesis begins. (4) Further synthesis of virus-specified RNA: a modified[1] cellular polymerase transcribes RNA from the provirus DNA. This RNA is processed and transported to the cytoplasm by modified[1] cellular machinery. (This step differs from step 3 in that, since viral syntheses have already started, modified cellular machinery is involved.) (5) Further synthesis of virus-specified proteins: virus-specified RNA directs the synthesis of virus-specified proteins. Viral

---

[1] Many of the specific mechanisms given for these steps are not now supported by experimental evidence.

glycoproteins are made. (6) Formation of virions: membranes of the infected cell are modified by inclusion of virion envelope components. Virion cores are formed. Virions are formed and released by budding from the cell plasma membranes. (7) Replication of provirus: the provirus is replicated with the rest of the cellular chromosomes and is passed to daughter cells at mitosis. (8) Neoplastic transformation: the infected cell is altered by virus-specified proteins. These proteins are not essential for virus replication and are not structural components of the virion[1].

All of these steps, with the exception of 6, formation of virions, appear to be necessary for the establishment and maintenance of neoplastic transformation. RSV is such an efficient carcinogenic agent because (a) the virion contains the machinery for step 1, initial events, and step 2, formation of the provirus; (b) viral syntheses, steps 4 and 5, are specifically and efficiently activated, step 3, by the first cell division after formation of the provirus; and (c) the genome of RSV controls both the nature of the virion and of the neoplastic transformation (fig. 1).

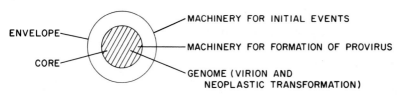

Fig. 1. Diagrammatic representation of a virion of an RSV.

(a) *Virion machinery.* Virion components, probably glycoproteins in the envelope, appear to control viral entrance into cells [4]. Other virion components including RNA- and RNA-DNA hybrid-directed DNA polymerase, DNA endo- and exonucleases, DNA ligase, and nucleotide kinase, are probably located in the virion core [5]. This enzymatic machinery is sufficient to transfer viral information from RNA to DNA integrated in a specific site in the cell genome. The necessity for some of these enzymes for infection is suggested by the experiments with RSVa [6]. The specificity of the site of integration of the DNA provirus is suggested by the results of superinfection experiments and of genetic crosses [7-9].

(b) *Activation.* If stationary cells are exposed to RSV, the cells are infected and provirus is formed, but viral syntheses do not begin. The infected stationary cells do not produce virus, are not converted in morphology, and do not contain virion antigens. All of these processes start after mitosis. The mechanism of this activation is not known. However, it may be related to the activation by cell division of some types of differentiation in embryogenesis [10].

(c) *Genome of RSV.* The RSV genome controls the envelope components and probably codes for the proteins involved. The RSV genome also controls the enzymatic machinery of the virion, though not necessarily by coding for the enzymes. RSV*a* does not appear to have a DNA polymerase when produced by cells which are infected with no other avian tumor virus [6]. It is also non-infectious. However, an infectious particle with the genome of RSV*a* is produced by a cell infected with RSV*a* and avian RLV. The infectivity of this particle implies the presence in virions of a DNA polymerase along with the genome of RSV*a*. Therefore, the avian tumor virus genome controls the presence of DNA polymerase in an avian tumor virus virion.

Similarly, there are genes in RSV that control the shape of converted cells and determine whether or not conversion itself is temperature sensitive [11-15].

The combination of these three properties, virion machinery, activation, and genes for transformation, is important. For example, in the absence of the linkage of the genes controlling neoplastic transformation and the rest of the viral genome, the specific activation of the viral genome would not activate neoplastic transformation. The neoplastic transformation would then remain latent until activated by normal cellular processes.

The difference between RSV and other carcinogens, except MSV (see next section), relates to the efficiency of formation and activation of the genes for neoplastic transformation. It is not now known whether or not there are in addition qualitative differences between the genes for neoplastic transformation in a cell transformed by RSV and in a cell transformed by a chemical or physical carcinogen.

Neoplastic transformation by murine sarcoma virus (MSV)

Some stocks of MSV appear to be a mixture of two types of virions, and these stocks are more accurately called MSV-MLV (see for example [16]). One virus type has the genome of a murine leukemia virus encapsidated in the envelope and other virion proteins specified by the murine leukemia virus (fig. 3). The second type has the genome of MSV encapsidated in the envelope and other virion proteins specified by a murine leukemia virus. A single virion containing the MSV genome is then similar to RSV as concerns neoplastic transformation (fig. 2). The non-genome portions, supplied by phenotypic mixing with a murine leukemia virus, are presumably like those of RSV, that is, the machinery necessary to insert viral information into a specific place in the cell genome. (However, at present no information exists about sites for integration of the MSV genome.)

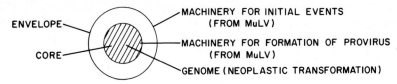

Fig. 2. Diagrammatic representation of a virion of MSV.

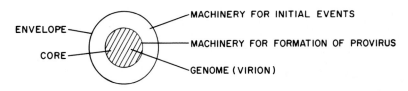

Fig. 3. Diagrammatic representation of a virion of an RLV.

The MSV genome is activated by the first cell division after the formation of the provirus, analogously to RSV [17]. Further, the MSV genome probably contains genes controlling neoplastic transformation. (As yet, there is no critical evidence for this supposition.) In this model, MSV has genes only for neoplastic transformation and controls part of the mechanism for activation. Therefore, a cell transformed by MSV alone cannot produce any new transforming virus. It is the combination of the MSV genome in a murine leukemia virus virion that is an efficient transforming agent.

RSV and MSV are maintained only by experimental passage. They are not wild-type viruses, although viruses like them may arise "spontaneously".

Neoplastic transformation by RNA leukemia/leukosis viruses (RLV)

Laboratory strains of RLV appear to differ from wild-type RLVs, probably because of the selection of variant RLV or the creation of new viruses (see below). A good example of a laboratory strain of RLV is avian myeloblastosis virus, which causes myeloblastosis in chickens. This virus is a mixture of a transforming virus and some viruses which do not transform cells in culture and are a myeloblastogenic (myeloblastosis associated viruses) [18]. In the terms used here avian myeloblastosis virus is a mixture of RLV and a virus with transforming properties with some characteristics of RLV and some of RSV. A similar finding is reported for strain R avian (erythroblastosis) virus [19].

Wild-type RLVs are very inefficient oncogenic agents. Their virions have all of the machinery necessary to insert the viral information into a specific place in the cell genome (fig. 3). This machinery appears to include the same enzymes as are present in virions of RSV. RLV viral syntheses are also activated by the first cell division after formation of the provirus. However, the RLV genome does not appear to contain genes controlling neoplastic transformation. Therefore, this activation merely leads to production of RLV and does not lead to neoplastic transformation. For neoplastic transformation, there must still be formation and activation of genes controlling neoplastic transformation. This process is more frequent in cells infected with RLV than in uninfected cells, which is why RLV causes tumors.

If there is phenotypic mixing between RLV and the RNA transcribed from genes controlling neoplastic transformation, a virus like murine sarcoma virus may result. If there is recombination between RLV and the genes controlling neoplastic transformation, an RSV may result. A similar recombinational process was proposed by Altaner and Temin [20] to explain the variation of avian RSV after passage through rat cells. The process of formation of an RSV from an RLV can be reversed. If in an RSV there is inactivation of the genes controlling neoplastic transformation, an RLV results [21-24].

This hypothesis of neoplastic transformation in cells infected with RLV states that there is more frequent formation and/or activation of genes controlling neoplastic transformation in cells infected with RLV than in uninfected cells. A number of possibilities exist to explain this increase.

One possibility is that the RLV itself undergoes some change, either genetic or epigenetic during neoplastic transformation. Although RLVs can undergo genetic changes, either by mutation or recombination, the RLV isolated from transformed cells is not usually different from the RLV isolated from untransformed cells or from the RLV used for the original infection [see Huebner, this Symposium]. Therefore, a genetic change in RLV does not appear as a constant correlate of neoplastic transformation in RLV-infected cells. An epigenetic change of RLV leading to neoplastic transformation could be activation of genes for neoplastic transformation carried in an RLV genome, or a new site for integration of the RLV provirus. It is unlikely that an RLV genome carries such information for neoplastic transformation. Since this information is so rarely expressed (transformation by RLV is extremely rare on the basis of the total number of cells infected for many generations, and the low frequency of disease per infected animal), it would not be selected for and would disappear in normal evolutionary processes. An alternative site in the genome of nontransformed and transformed cells for integration of the RLV provirus is a possible hypothesis to explain neoplastic transformation in RLV-infected cells. However, RLV probably has no requirement for excision of the DNA provirus from cellular DNA, since information is transferred from the

DNA provirus by transcription to RNA. The neoplastic transformation would, therefore, represent an additional integration in a usually forbidden site. Since RLV-infected cells are continually producing virus, and the cellular DNA seems to contain only a very small number of proviruses [25], there must be strong restrictions against additional integration. This hypothesis of transformation as a result of integration of the RLV provirus in a previously forbidden site could be tested by experiments involving nucleic acid hybridization on the location of provirus in RLV-infected transformed and untransformed cells. A more general form of this hypothesis is considered below. (A similar site-specific hypothesis might be applied to transformation by SV40 [Defendi, personal communication]). Although this mechanism is epigenetic for the RLV, it is genetic for the cell.

A second possibility to explain more frequent formation and/or activation of genes for neoplastic transformation in cells infected with RLV than in uninfected cells is that as a result of the RLV infection there is an increased probability of a genetic or epigenetic change in the cells leading to neoplastic transformation. One type of theory states that the genes for neoplastic transformation exist in all cells that can undergo neoplastic transformation. The neoplastic transformation occurs when there is an epigenetic shift in the regulation of these genes. (A recent version of this theory [26] also states that the genes for neoplastic transformation are in the provirus of an RNA tumor virus. However, why this linkage occurs is not clear in the theory.) If these genes have no other function than causing neoplastic transformation, they would be selected against. Clearly, genes for childhood neoplasia would have a large negative selective advantage. I cannot imagine a positive selective advantage for neoplasia after the reproductive age. Therefore, there must be some selective advantage for these genes to counteract the selective disadvantage of the occurrence of neoplasia. (This advantage would not be a heterozygous advantage, since the genomes of all cells would include the same genes for neoplasia.) Furthermore, this selective advantage would have to be such that it could not be separated from neoplasia by mutation or recombination. Neoplastic transformation is a partial escape from the usual controls of differentiation and cell multiplication. But because neoplastic cells arise from normal cells, one cannot say that the same genes control both a normal process and the neoplasia [27]. It is necessary to have an additional explanation for the double manifestation of such genes, normal and neoplastic, and why the neoplastic manifestation has not been selected against. I cannot provide a reasonable explanation. Therefore, I do not think that RLV-infection could increase the "differentiation" of a cell into a cancer cell by epigenetic means.

However, as I have described in detail elsewhere in the protovirus hypothesis [2,3], we can postulate in all cells genes affecting cell multiplication and movement, which are located in regions of the genome involved in frequent genetic exchanges using DNA to RNA to DNA information transfers, as well as the usual DNA to DNA transfers (fig. 4). In this protovirus hypothesis, the

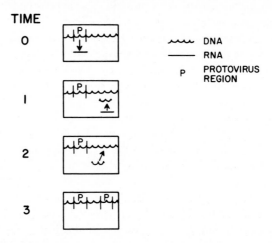

Fig. 4. A possible step in protovirus evolution. One cell is shown at different times. At time 0, RNA is transcribed from the protovirus region of DNA. At time 1, DNA is transcribed from this RNA. At time 2, this DNA is integrated into the cell DNA. At time 3, the cell has two regions of protovirus DNA. Other types of transfer could lead to duplications at other places in the cell genome and could transfer information from one cell to another. If RNA was transcribed from regions between two protoviruses, new sequences would result.

protovirus is an episome in its normal manifestation. Some abnormal genetic events leading to a stable extra-cellular phase of the protovirus would lead to the formation of a Rous virus. Therefore, RLVs would have some homology with these normal cellular genes, having originated from them. Some rare genetic event or series of events involving either RLV nucleic acids or enzymes and protovirus nucleic acids or enzymes might lead to the formation of the genes for neoplastic transformation. These new genes would then need to be activated before transformation occurred (a two-stage process). This model differs slightly from the model of a change in the site of RLV provirus integration discussed above, in that it involves further changes in the cell DNA. This model will be further generalized in the discussion of non-RNA tumor virus carcinogens.

I have less detailed knowledge of mammary tumor virus (MTV). Chickens are not infected with this type of virus, for obvious reasons – they are only honorary mammals. However, it seems to me that a discussion similar to that for RLV could be applied to MTV. The major additional point raised by MTV is the difference in frequency of spontaneous occurrence of MTV and of neoplasia in different strains of mice [see Bentvelzen, this Symposium]. (Of course, this is paralleled by the different incidences of other neoplasias and of RLVs in strains of mice.) Since protovirus changes are postulated to be part of a cell's normal development, they also will be under genetic control. Therefore, these differences between strains of mice could relate to differences in the frequencies of protovirus transfers, for example, more frequent transfers in high tumor strains, or to the existence in the germ-lines of high tumor strains of protoviruses already partially altered along the way to neoplasia. If an RNA tumor virus was formed from protoviruses, and then infected germ-line cells, an inherited provirus would be formed.

The major point of this article is that there is no reason to think of viruses like RLV and MTV as tumor viruses in the sense that RSV or MSV are tumor viruses. In the present terms, the mechanism of neoplastic transformation by RLV and MTV may not be different from the mechanism of neoplastic transformation by non-viral carcinogens. Further, it appears that viruses which replicate RNA to DNA to RNA and have an RNA-directed DNA polymerase in their virions, which I have called Rous viruses [28], differ widely in their oncogenicity. I have already discussed the oncogenic ones. In addition to these there are variant RLVs which appear aleukemogenic and Rous viruses like visna and primate or feline syncytium-forming virus which are rarely or never oncogenic. The hypotheses suggested above for neoplastic transformation in cells infected with RLV require for neoplastic transformation some rare events involving interaction of viral nucleic acids or enzymes with cellular genetic elements. Therefore, there might be a correlation between the extent of replication of Rous viruses and their oncogenicity. The more latent ones might be less oncogenic. When an event is rare, as is neoplastic transformation by RLV, a small decrease in rate might prevent its occurrence.

Neoplastic transformation by non-viral carcinogens

The same type of argument can be applied to non-viral carcinogens. With these carcinogens there is no possibility of integration of the carcinogen since they are not information-carrying nucleic acids. Therefore, by the same reasoning used before, I would discard an epigenetic effect of non-viral carcinogens and say they have some genetic effect. The same genetic hypothesis used for RLV could then apply.

If in all cells there are genes affecting cell multiplication and movement, which are located in regions of the genome involved in frequent genetic exchanges using DNA to RNA to DNA information transfers, as well as the usual DNA to DNA transfers, the non-viral carcinogens could interact with these genes to produce oncogenic altered protoviruses. Once these oncogenic altered protoviruses – that is, the genes for neoplastic transformation – were formed, they would have to be activated by normal cellular processes. The specific RNA tumor virus activation would not apply. This requirement for activation after the formation of the genes for neoplastic transformation might be a partial explanation for the two stages seen in chemical carcinogenesis [29]. Since the processes of neoplastic transformation by RLV and non-viral carcinogens may be similar, synergism between them is not surprising [see Huebner, this Symposium].

In this model, the establishment of genes for neoplastic transformation in the genome of an untransformed cell is similar for all carcinogens. A DNA copy of an RNA, either the genome of an RSV or of an altered protovirus, is integrated in some site in the cell genome, with or without concurrent genetic alteration. The activation of this information is similar for RSV and other carcinogens in that cellular controls are involved in both activations. However, in the case of RSV, the RSV provirus is so situated that it becomes activated by the first cell division after the establishment of the genes for neoplastic transformation, that is the formation of provirus. Maintenance of neoplastic transformation requires in all cases replication of the genes for neoplastic transformation and expression of the products of these genes. There is no reason to think that these processes are not the same for all carcinogens, involving cell machinery and being susceptible to control by cellular processes. RSV would differ only in having genes that are less subject to control by cellular processes.

Other theories of neoplastic transformation

Now we can contrast the protovirus theory of this paper to the classical theories of carcinogenesis. Classical viral theory is similar to that described here for experimental RSV, MSV, RLV and MTV infections. Classical mutational theory is also related to the protovirus theory. However, in the protovirus theory, the site of the genetic changes leading to neoplastic transformation is a normal, but non-classical genetic element with some viral properties.

Classical embryonic and differentiation theories are, however, quite different from the protovirus theory. In these classical theories, in the oncogene theory, and in theories involving embryonic arrest, dedifferentiation or Jacob-Monod cycles, there is no change in the information in the cellular DNA in neoplastic transformation. However, since the protovirus theory states that some aspects of differentiation and embryogenesis also involve changes in the information in the cellular DNA, neoplastic transformation becomes a special case of this type of differentiation.

Not many data are available now that can be used to distinguish among these theories of carcinogenesis. I shall briefly mention systems where such data might be developed, and what kind of data might be most useful.

First, it is clear that we need to continue to study the model systems, especially RSV and MSV which have tissue culture assays, to test the present ideas about these viruses. With the new general respect for RNA tumor viruses as a legitimate subject for study, such data should be available soon.

Second, we need to work with systems which can be used to test for the existence of protoviruses. At first I had hopes that the finding of RNA-directed DNA polymerase activity in uninfected cells would be helpful in this respect. However, the nearly universal occurrence of this activity makes me wonder about its significance [20,31,32, etc.]. Some kind of genetic data will be needed. The best hope for that appears to be the studies on interactions of RSV and chicken cells started by Payne and Chubb and by Weiss (see their articles in this Symposium), and also carried out by Hanafusa and Vogt and their co-workers [33,34], and studies on interactions of RNA tumor viruses and heterologous cells [20,35]. The clonal distribution of susceptibility to RSV(O) seen by Weiss [36] may be relevant. Other possible systems are gene amplification in Xenopus [37] and transfer of immunological specificity by RNA [38].

Third, we shall need refinements of nucleic acid hybridization so that small changes in cellular DNA, on the order of 1 part in 10^5, can be reliably measured. Larger differences may already have been seen in antibody-forming cells [39,40]. Sequencing of the amino acids of the viral antigens and enzymes might also be useful.

Summary

Table 2 presents a summary of the models discussed in this article. The various RNA tumor viruses are distinguished on the basis of what information is contained in their genomes. RLV is not considered to be a tumor virus in the sense of having information for neoplastic transformation in its genome. RLV and non-viral carcinogens may cause neoplastic transformation by increasing

the probability of genetic changes in natural genetic elements called protoviruses.

Table 2

| Virus | Information in genome | | Activation of genome by first cell division after formation of provirus |
	Virion[a]	Neoplastic transformation[b]	
RSV	+	+	+
MSV	0	+	+
RLV	+	0	+
Protovirus	0	0	0
Altered protovirus	0	+	0

[a] Control of initial events and formation of provirus.
[b] Control of cell morphology, serum requirements, membrane structure, etc.

References

[1] H.M. Temin, Ann. Rev. Microbiol. 25 (1971) 609.
[2] H.M. Temin, Perspectives Biol. Med. 14 (1970) 11.
[3] H.M. Temin, J. Natl. Cancer Inst. 46 (1971) 111.
[4] P.K. Vogt and R. Ishizaki, Virology 26 (1965) 664.
[5] S. Mizutani and H.M. Temin, J. Virol. 8 (1971) 409.
[6] H. Hanafusa and T. Hanafusa, Virology 43 (1971) 313.
[7] H.M. Temin, Virology 13 (1961) 158.
[8] L.N. Payne and R.D. Chubb, J. Gen. Virol. 3 (1968) 379.
[9] R.A. Weiss and L.N. Payne, Virology 45 (1971) 508.
[10] H. Holtzer and J. Abbott, Results Prob. Cell Diff. 1 (1968) 1.
[11] H.M. Temin, Virology 10 (1960) 182.
[12] G.S. Martin, Nature 227 (1970) 1021.
[13] J.M. Biquard and P. Vigier, Compt. Rend. Acad. Sci., Paris 271 (1970) 2430.
[14] R.R. Friis, K. Toyoshima and P.K. Vogt, Virology 43 (1971) 375.
[15] H.M. Temin, Proc. Xth Int. Cancer Congress (1970) in press.
[16] S.A. Aaronson and W.P. Rowe, Virology 42 (1970) 9.
[17] R. Murray and H.M. Temin, Int. J. Cancer 5 (1970) 320.
[18] R.E. Smith and C. Moscovici, Cancer Res. 29 (1969) 1356.
[19] R. Ishizaki and T. Shimizu, Cancer Res. 30 (1970) 2827.
[20] C. Altaner and H.M. Temin, Virology 40 (1970) 118.
[21] A. Goldé, Virology 40 (1970) 1022.
[22] T. Graf, H. Bauer, H. Gelderblom and D.P. Bolognesi, Virology 43 (1971) 427.
[23] H. Hanafusa, Current Topics Microbiol. Immunol. 51 (1970) 114.
[24] K. Toyoshima, R.R. Friis and P.K. Vogt, Virology 42 (1970) 163.
[25] M.A. Baluda and D.P. Nayak, Proc. Natl. Acad. Sci. U.S. 66 (1970) 329.

[26] R.J. Huebner and G.J. Todaro, Proc. Natl. Acad. Sci. U.S. 64 (1968) 1087.

[27] R.J. Huebner *et al.* Ann. N.Y. Acad. Sci. 181 (1971) 246.

[28] H.M. Temin, *In:* L.G. Silvestri (ed.), The biology of oncogenic viruses, Proc. of 2nd Lepetit Colloq., Paris, Nov. 1970 (North-Holland, Amsterdam) p. 176.

[29] I. Berenblum, Adv. Cancer Res. 2 (1954) 129.

[30] R. Gallo, S.S. Yang and R.C. Ting, Nature 228 (1970) 927.

[31] E.M. Scolnick, S.A. Aaronson G.J. Todaro and W.P. Parks, Nature 229 (1971) 318.

[32] P.E. Penner, L.H. Cohen and L.A. Loeb, Biochem. Biophys. Res. Commun. 42 (1971) 1228.

[33] H. Hanafusa and T. Hanafusa, Virology 43 (1971) 313.

[34] P.K. Vogt and R.R. Friis, Virology 43 (1971) 223.

[35] S.A. Aaronson, Nature 230 (1971) 445.

[36] R.A. Weiss, J. Gen. Virol. 5 (1969) 511.

[37] G.P. Tocchini-Valentini and M. Crippa, *In:* G. Silvestri (ed.), The biology of oncogenic viruses, Proc. of 2nd Lepetit Colloq., Paris, Nov. 1970 (North-Holland, Amsterdam), p. 237.

[38] C. Bell and S. Dray, Science 171 (1971) 199.

[39] J.R. Little and H.A. Donahue, Proc. Natl. Acad. Sci. U.S. 67 (1970) 1299.

[40] R.G. Krueger and B.J. McCarthy, Biochem. Biophys. Res. Commun. 41 (1970) 944.

Part 9

PANEL DISCUSSION

CHAIRMAN: H.S. KAPLAN

Part I. Invited participants: P. Bentvelzen, R.J. Huebner, F. Jacob and H.M. Temin

R.A. Weiss: From the sort of data I presented earlier it appears that there is a virus-like activity in normal cells. Now occasionally if you treat these cells with chemical carcinogens or X-rays you can activate a replicating virion which does not seem to be a transforming virus. So maybe Dr. Temin can add another row to his last slide saying that a protovirus can go into a virion. Now if you infect these cells, instead of treating them with non-viral carcinogens, with other tumor viruses you regularly rescue such a virion in nearly every cell. This seems to me to be something much more akin to complementation and activation, and would seem in this case to speak against a mutational hypothesis.

H.M. Temin: This gets fairly complicated and I think perhaps illustrates the development that still has to take place. We really know very few characteristics of these viruses and we have to be careful because we have one characteristic, say one antigen or one envelope, to assume that the entire information of the virus is present. What I think is that in the chicken there are two quite separate events. Originally there may exist some genetic information for part of a virus which one may call the protovirus or the defective provirus, and this portion of the virus genetic material is making RNA, and this RNA, like that of MSV, appears to be able to phenotypically mix with the proteins of the Rous virus or the other viruses. This will undoubtedly require some special sequences of secondary structure and so this type of RNA can be very efficiently rescued. That is what Dr. Hanafusa has called Chf. In addition there appears to be a much rarer phenomenon which is the creation of RAV-O or RAV-60, which is not merely this kind of complementation or phenotypic mixing, but requires then the production by some means or other of the entire information for an overt virus. This is a very rare event as far as one can tell at the present time. It appears that chemical carcinogens may increase the frequency, but it is still an extremely low frequency. One can wonder here if this is some kind of recombination process as we have discussed for Rous virus growing in rat cells, or Aaronson has described for mouse viruses in human cells, which eventually lead to a genetic change. So there are two processes concerned. It is only as we get more genetic markers, and perhaps more precise methods of looking to the nucleic acids that it will be possible to say just how much of the viral genome is concerned in all these processes.

J. Hilgers: Dr. Temin, I would like you to consider the results obtained with MTV. The mammary cell has a complete reproductive cycle of MTV and can be transformed by this virus, whereas the lymphoid cell, which has only a restricted synthesis of MTV, i.e. only synthesis of the group-specific antigen, can probably not be transformed by MTV. Could you on this basis favor the hypothesis of activation of genes in cellular genomes?

H.M. Temin: Of course we know with Rous virus that there are all kinds of controls in different cells, whether virus is produced or not, but I was trying not to describe that. So the picture that I am trying to talk about is very simplified, just about the genetic information. In addition there are going to be all kinds of controls over this — all the differentiated processes of the cells affect these. I do not think that this would tell us much about which of these genetic models is correct.

H.S. Kaplan: Along the same line as Dr. Hilgers brought up, I think that a similar objection can be raised to your notion that the RLV category does not contain the information for neoplastic transformation, whereas the sarcoma viruses do. It seems to me that you are testing *in vitro* in both the MSV and RSV systems against fibroblasts which are in fact the target cells for the neoplastic transformation by sarcoma virus, but systems for growing lymphoid cells, which are susceptible target cells for the action of leukemia viruses, are notoriously lacking. Your statement that you do not get tumors for a long time in the chicken, I think, is perhaps open to serious debate. There are systems in which you can get leukemia in five or six days in the mouse, and it is clear that although these are tumor cells, they nonetheless are dependent on a particular environment for their evolution to a fully autonomous state. They are, however, transformed cells. I think therefore that unless you are looking to the correct target cell system, you are not able to make a statement about whether the virus does or does not carry the information for the neoplastic transformation.

H.M. Temin: I think the best system to look at is that of avian myeloblastosis which Baluda originally described with chicken embryonic cells of the reticulo-endothelial system, in which he found transformation by AMV. He showed just the phenomena that Dr. Kaplan was talking about, that this transformation was cell dependent. It is clear that for MSV to transform, one needs a cell in a particular epigenetic state. Whatever that is and why that is, is not clear. Perhaps it involves sites of integration or the interaction of the virus-specific product with other cellular products. However, when the Baluda system was analyzed later on by Moscovici, he found that there were two types of viruses in the AMV, the majority component could not transform in this system, while a minority component was the transforming virus – it is not clear whether it is defective but perhaps it is. So it is clear that viruses which we usually call RNA-leukemia viruses are not what I have been talking about here, that the viruses that we are working with are more like an RSV, but they might be under a stricter kind of control of differentiation than RSV. But what I was trying to say is that there is this other class which appears to be much less so. Of course, as I indicated, one can say it is only a statistical argument as to whether or not these viruses still have the genes, and this requires, as Dr. Kaplan indicated, development of more kinds of systems and better genetic kinds of markers, so we could perhaps do genetic complementation and ask whether these additional genes exist.

F. Jacob: I have not so much a question as a comment to make, which may seem to have relevance to the protovirus hypothesis. I am thinking of some results recently reported by Dan Brown from Baltimore on the situation of DNA which makes the ribosomal RNA in Xenopus. He has done a beautiful series of experiments which show that there are approximately 200 or 300 tandem genes, which repeat the ribosomal RNA in the DNA, so that there is the 28S, the 18S and repeat 28 and 18S, and in between is what they call the "spacer" which is not transcribed. Now they find that in one species the spacer is the same, but when they go from one species to another, which is *Laevis muelleri*, they find that the 28S and 18S are absolutely identical as far as hybridization is concerned but that the spacers are different. So clearly you cannot evolve the 300 system and identical change, you have to start at some stage of the life cycle from one unit which contains the two rRNAs plus the spacer, and then amplify them. It does not say anything about whether the multiplication is DNA or viral RNA, but it does clearly say that something that you call the protovirus is necessary to explain such a result.

J. Svoboda: We usually work under conditions in which we superinfect a cell which already contains some specific genome or protovirus or something like this, which exerts certain functions or has the ability to exert functions similar to the virus we are introducing. Now I think the very important point for further development of the mechanism of the interaction of the viruses with the genome, would be to find a suitable system for studying the persistent integration of the virus in the cell. The work discussed by Dr. Temin and others has been done only on the chicken cell. In every case the cells already had a number of protoviruses or some other stages in virus development present there. So, they really can never distinguish between what they are adding and what was already there. The other system which could be used effectively, particularly for studying the integration of the viral genome in the cell, is the heterologous cell again. This enables really the permanent fixation of the virus genome in the cell, and, in addition it probably could distinguish between the contribution of foreign tumor virus genomes and the cellular functions because as Dr. Huebner has shown, there are clearcut antigenic differences between the expression of genomes in different cellular species.

H.M. Temin: May I just comment to say that approximately two years ago when I was discussing early forms of these ideas with Sidney Brenner, he said if I could infect an *E.coli* with Rous virus and give it to him, at the end of a week he would solve all these problems and perhaps that still is the best approach.

R.J. Huebner: Well I think there has been at least in the last day a great deal of hang-up about a few things. Viruses like RSV and RLV cannot be found in the sarcomas and chickens generally or in the mouse leukemias. We have never found RLV in any mouse and we have studied all the strains of mice in the last 5 years. So I think these artificial viruses are something that do not relate too much to what happens naturally. It has been possible to study a great many myxoviruses of which you know that the genome is there, by the presence of the antigens – the gs in the beginning and later on the specific antibodies to the virus particles. Now this kind of evidence for virus being present and doing something in what is related to tumors, seems to me much greater than the evidence for these molecular mechanisms that have been discovered recently. If the polymerase – certainly a very important entity – is integrating viral genome into the cell genome, it would appear right now from many of the data that were presented at this meeting, that the polymerase did it maybe 300 million years ago or much earlier. What one is studying now are regressive phenomena, which reflect changes brought about through inbreeding. The geneticists here have pointed out many different ways of bringing out this expression. Those persons working in *in vitro* systems, primarily in the mammalian system, but also in the chicken system, have demonstrated that virus that comes out of the cell through long term culture or by rescuing in reverse as Dr. Hanafusa does or by induction with chemicals, is still an RNA tumor virus. This virus has genes that can be activated in cells as can be demonstrated in many different ways and I think that if the virus has a polymerase then it becomes important.

H.M. Temin: I would just say that perhaps one difference is that where Dr. Huebner likes to simplify things, I have always liked to complicate things and secondly to say that it is good that he still likes this theory because I think it is important to like different theories so people will try to work hard and to develop experimental evidence to disprove other people's theories. But I think it will be a little more difficult than we might think at the present time and I again want to reiterate that the gs antigen may be as much as, or rather, only 3% of the virus genome. Thus when we find the gs antigen — when that is clearly demonstrated by immunologic means — we don't know what else is present there. I just think that at the present time we have to keep in mind the kinds of possibilities: one, that the rest of the information is also present, and is not expressed but is activated, or this other idea that perhaps the rest of the information does not exist at a given time but is created subsequently.

H.S. Kaplan: If I may interject two quick comments. One is that somebody has once said that all people may be divided into two categories: the lumpers and the splitters, and it would appear that this pertains here. The other generalization that seems to be valid is that all those people who propose theories can be relied upon to be among the foremost proponents of their own theories, and this is perhaps understandable.

P. Bentvelzen: The finding of the RNA-dependent DNA polymerase in virions of the RNA oncogenic viruses has complicated the situation very much. Several authors believe that this finding legalizes ideas as presented by Dr. Huebner or me on the genetic transmission of RNA oncogenic viruses. I am glad that they accept our ideas at the moment, but they do this for the wrong reason. If a provirus *sensu* Temin would exist — and the finding of the polymerase makes this very likely — then it has nothing to do with the provirus I have postulated for vertical transmission and the oncogene of Dr. Huebner. If the enzyme would have anything to do with vertical transmission it must then be very easy to change one virus for another with regard to transmission by the gametes. In my studies on MTV which have taken eight years I have never observed such a thing. Only that virus strain will be transmitted genetically in a given mouse strain which is indigenous to that mouse strain. Introduction of another virus strain leads only to milkborne transmission of that strain. I am working in the mouse leukemia field for only a few years. So far I did not observe a genetic transmission of artificially introduced virus strains. I have screened the literature extensively for this but there is no indication whatsoever that a change in vertical transmission would occur. There seems to be a very stable relationship between host genome and indigenous virus with regard to vertical transmission. This we have explained by the presence of a provirus in the host genome. It is obvious that no RNA-dependent, but only a DNA-dependent DNA polymerase is needed for the continuity of the relationship between host genome and virus.

In our publications on provirus for vertical transmission we emphasized that it had to be transcribed (free viral RNA has to be present) before a tumor would develop. We also stated that the released viral RNA has to be replicated before neoplastic conversion could take place. Rather hypocritically I wrote that for our provirus it was not important whether the viral RNA was replicated via a DNA or an RNA intermediate. But we hoped that it would be an RNA one because otherwise things would become so complicated. It is rather ironical that the finding of the RNA-DNA polymerase has convinced many sceptics of the correctness of my provirus hypothesis.

For me the big question is whether our provirus hypothesis is really compatible with the Temin provirus idea. We say that a provirus is already present in the host genome. Why would it be necessary that a new one be established to get neoplastic conversion? If refined molecular biological studies would demonstrate that both our provirus hypothesis for vertical transmission and Temin's hypothesis for replication and neoplastic transformation are correct, a lot of thinking has to be done to reconcile both ideas. I think it to be correct to state once more that the finding of the RNA-dependent DNA polymerase has more complicated our ideas on the RNA oncogenic viruses than that it has resolved many problems.

H.M. Temin: Some people thought that it at least cleared up a few things, so let us not throw away everything.

H.S. Kaplan: I think it would be useful if Dr. Temin and Dr. Huebner would try to stipulate as clearly and quickly as possible for us exactly what differences they perceive between the protovirus hypothesis and the oncogene hypothesis.

H.M. Temin: As I understand the oncogene theory, a DNA copy of the whole viral RNA would exist in the germ line. This DNA is activated to make and stabilize the RNA and so forth. I think that the oncogene theory perhaps should be modified so that we don't have to think of this DNA as linked to the virus genes; it is easier to work with. In the protovirus idea we would only have a little bit of DNA homologous to virus present, which may be making RNA, and their action would be the creation of new DNA sequences in development and so ultimately there would be the same end product as visualized by the oncogene theory, but from a very different starting position. Now unfortunately Dr. Spiegelman keeps telling me that one cannot do molecular hybridization with mammalian cells and so perhaps we'll have to wait until someone develops good genetic tests to resolve these two models.

R.J. Huebner: The big difference at the present time is in relation to cancer as it occurs naturally — and Dr. Temin talked about what he found in a model system. What I am saying is that we have a great deal of evidence that there is a great deal of association with the viral genome or oncogenic gene and the tumor activity under natural and induced circumstances where we did not put in a virus which we created.

H.M. Temin: May I clarify that again. In the case of the model system, such as transformation by RSV, we start with the whole RNA presumably and that infects the cell and then creates the DNA directly. What we were talking about in these other systems is a completely different mechanism.

R.J. Huebner: I want to admit that I don't know much about the mechanisms but we did not know anything about the mechanism by which influenza virus works either, but we do know enough to do a lot with it.

Part II. Invited participants: P. Bentvelzen, F. Jacob, G. Klein and S. Spiegelman

H.S. Kaplan: An important approach to problems discussed at this conference is by the technique of somatic cell hybridization. Doctors Klein and Jacob have some comments on this question.

G. Klein gave a summary of the work of E.M. Fenyö, G. Gruendner, G. Klein, E. Klein and H. Harris (Expt. Cell Res., in press) dealing with the antigen expression and C-type virus release of hybrid cells prcduced by the fusion of the two Moloney lymphoma sublines, YAC and YACIR, with the L-cell derived mouse fibroblast strain, A9. YAC and YACIR are sublines of the same original Moloney lymphoma, differing in the expression of MLV-determined surface antigens (Fenyö, Klein, Klein and Swiech: *J. Natl. Cancer Inst.* 40 (1968) 69-89), and Moloney virus release (Fenyö, Biberfeld, Klein E., *J. Natl. Cancer Inst.* 42 (1969) 837-856). The YACIR subline was selected by passage in Moloney-virus immunized mice *in vivo,* interrupted by cytotoxic exposure to anti-Moloney sera *in vitro,* in the presence of complement. Its MLV-induced surface antigen concentration is reduced approximately tenfold, compared to the original YAC tumor, and it releases little or no infectious virus. Virus can be recovered by co-cultivation with sensitive JLSV-9 cells, but 10^4 times more cells are needed for successful recovery than with the original YAC line. The A9 partner cell also releases C-type virus, the "L-cell virion" and it also expresses the MLV-induced surface antigen. The hybrid lines YAC/A9 and YACIR/A9 were established by Sendai virus induced fusion. The presence of the A9-genome was demonstrated by the metacentric chromosome markers characteristic for this line, and by the L-type surface antigen. Presence of the YAC and YACIR genome, respectively, was demonstrated by typing sera with anti-H-2[d] specificity.

Both hybrid lines showed full expression of the MLV-induced surface antigen, entirely comparable in concentration to the antigen present on the YAC line. This means that the surface antigen suppression, characteristic for the YACIR line, was released in the YACIR/A9 hybrid.

The YAC/A9 hybrid showed a high degree of C-type virus release, as judged by immunogenicity and infectivity of culture supernatants. In contrast, there was no detectable virus release from the YACIR/A9 hybrid.

This means that the suppression of virus release, characteristic of the YACIR line, was imposed upon the A9 partner, restricting the production of the C-type virus produced by this line. Taken together, the results demonstrate that the production of C-type virus and the expression of virus-controlled surface antigen are under at least partially independent control. This confirms previous indirect postulates, based on the independent variation of surface antigenicity and virus production in a series of Moloney virus induced lymphoma lines (Klein, Klein and Haughton, *J. Natl. Cancer Inst.* (1966) 36 607-621). An interesting phenomenon is that the hybrids show the fibroblastic growth pattern instead of the lymphoid one, characteristic for the YAC and YACIR lines. In some of the hybrids the lymphoid pattern gradually reappeared, which is associated with the loss of several A9 chromosomes.

Furthermore the hybrids are not malignant or only very weakly tumorigenic. Reappearance of malignancy was also associated with the loss of A9 chromosomes.

F. Jacob: We happened also to produce some hybrids between highly malignant cells, but for completely different reasons. We are trying to analyze the properties of some myeloma cells which are highly malignant and which produce antibodies. We wanted to see whether the hybrids would produce the antibodies or not. In most of these hybridizations with either high or low malignant partners, we found that some of the clones had the property of contact inhibition and turned out to be very low-malignant hybrids even when the two parents were highly malignant. Exactly the same type of phenomenon was observed by Dr. Klein.

Now to come back to the question of our chairman, the hybridization procedure is a very high potent tool, but I think one has to be a little careful in the interpretation that can be given to the results. In many cases people are using two different types of cells, generally of completely different origin, let us say mouse and man. Each of these produces a particular specialized product, say X and Y. They then ask the question whether the hybrid will or will not produce X and Y, thinking that from that they will be able to derive a conclusion whether it is a negative or a positive system of regulation which is coming into the picture. Most generally the hybrids do not produce either X or Y. Now I think that one has to be cautious in talking about these results in terms of negative or positive phenomena of regulation, repression or other things like that. In most cell cultures in which the expression of a particular product is examined, it turns out that one does not look at the regulation itself which produces the programming of the cells, but just at that expression or non-expression of a program of the cell.

We have been working for a year with David Schubert on the properties of neuroblastoma cells. Now this cell can be grown in suspension in a round form under certain conditions; under other conditions they attach to the plastic dish and they produce clones which differentiate into things which look like neurons. Now it turns out that when one examines this more closely, everything which affects the differentiated state has something to do with the membrane. And very likely what happens there, is that the genetic program, whatever it is in the cell, can be either non-expressed or expressed depending on the state of the membrane.

It has also been shown recently that when two cells are fused, the surface antigens immediately distribute around the hybrids. It seems as if the proteins are in some kind of liquid phase around the membrane and are completely reassorting all around the membrane. And therefore it is extremely likely that the state of the membrane in the hybrid is completely different from the state of the membrane in each of the parents. And therefore the expression of whatever product one looks at in the hybrid may just be the consequence of the state of the membrane and not of some event that would occur on the genome.

So it seems to me that hybridization is an extremely potent tool but that its results have to be interpreted very carefully, and probably have to be applied, at least in the beginning, to a relatively simple case, where the two parents differ by one or very few characteristics only.

J.B. Sheffield: There has been a lot of discussion here about the role of viruses and the role of the cell genome in neoplastic transformation. And the question I would like to address to the entire panel is: if, as so many people have been showing these last few days, there is transmission of genetic information for neoplasm in the genome of the cell, what is the virus doing? Why, in biological terms, does the cell go through all this trouble of making viruses, which are very handy for the researchers?

H.S. Kaplan: Who would like to answer the question? I think, Bentvelzen, it is a good one for you.

P. Bentvelzen: It has not been completely proven yet that somatic cells contain the genetic information for whole tumor virus, but let us assume it is true. I always made the point that what you need for neoplastic transformation is free virus. If you have just a proviral genome and no transcription which means that no virus is produced, neoplastic conversion will not occur. I have quite some evidence that replication of the viral genome is needed for transformation. There is a very good correlation between virion production and the rate of neoplastic transformation in the mouse mammary tumor system. Also G. Pasternak has published several years ago a similar relationship for the mouse leukemia virus, and recently T. Graff told me that he had indications for the same thing in the RSV system. The underlying reason I do not know; maybe many viral genes must be present or virions formed (annexing much of the cell machinery involved in normal behavior) for transformation to occur. Of course the provirus theory of Temin for neoplastic transformation is very attractive but far from proven. I do not know whether indeed integration of the DNA copy must occur. I think there are models feasible in which a limited number of DNA copies are being replicated at a certain pace controlled by the host genome. These copies may not actually be inserted into one of the chromosomes. There are also examples in bacteria where phage DNA is replicated together with the host genome but not in an integrated state.

The other question is of course: what is the purpose anyway of this genetic information for virus being present in an organism. You know the very bold theory of Huebner who says that C-type particles are being switched on at least partially in the embryo and have some role in embryogenesis. I have never ventured such thoughts publicly, but we have of course discussed these things at length, especially with Dr. Daams. He always brought up that there must be some function for that information. We have now good evidence that all mice carry an MTV, or at least have information for some MTV traits. Well, I am flirting with the idea that this information is involved in the post-puberal development of the mammary gland. This resembles Huebner's postulate for embryogenesis, but it takes into account that the main development of the mammary gland takes place postnatally. Some support for this idea can be derived from the work of Ben-David and Dr. Heston, who have shown that the mouse mammary tumor virus can promote development of the mammary gland after hormonal stimulation. I am unable to explain why mature virions are produced in several mouse strains, but after all this is a teleological question.

G. Klein: As I understand the question, it is: Cancer is an evolutionary disadvantage for both the virus and the host, since they die. What is the sense of this? – is this the question?

J.B. Sheffield: More or less.

G. Klein: I think we are suffering from a conceptional astigmatism which is introduced by the use of the *in vitro* systems with high efficiency transforming viruses like SV40. First of all, many of these viruses do not transform the natural hosts. And SV40-hamster and SV40-mouse are highly artificial systems. If we concentrate on the naturally occurring viruses, like MTV or the C-type virus, transformation is an extremely rare event. It is really so rare that it is probably quite negligible from the evolutionary point of view, since it occurs mainly at a very late age. I think it is very important to keep in mind that there is distinct competence in viral transformation. Viruses really transform very few, very specialized cells under very peculiar conditions. There are revertants now, as described for the DNA tumor virus system, and also for the Rous system, where you still have the viral genome present, but revertant morphologies. In cell hybrids you can see the maintenance of viral genome in the presence of an ordinary cellular genome, but this is certainly not enough to have the cell behaving in a malignant way. So I do not really think that there is necessarily a detrimental effect of the virus-host association in all situations.

H.S. Kaplan: I would like to follow up the same line and say that there has been perhaps an overemphasis on a somewhat mechanistic relationship between the presence of this information in the cell and the necessary expression as a cancer of some kind. I think we should be cautious first of all — it has already been brought up very clearly today and in previous days — that one of the more remarkable phenomena which goes beyond the genetic specificity is the further, quite fantastic specificity exhibited by these viruses with regard to the type of cell and the state of differentiation of the cell which they transform. This has not been dealt with in any great detail, but it is a remarkable phenomenon and I think it is the next level on which we have to analyze the system, because it indicates that the cell itself is imposing certain environmental, if you like, pictures on the expression of the viral information. And the further related comment is that we have to be cautious about falling into the implied assumption that a carcinogen is required in all cases to get a cancer. We really do not know that, and the fact that many people have now got spontaneous transformation *in vitro*, in cell systems which are released from many of the normal growth restraints in the body, may possibly not require the presence of some latent virus as the explanation. We have just heard that cells can lose chromosomal material from the hybrids. It is also possible that cells that are dividing rapidly and which are diploid, may also lose genetic material in such a way as to lose the material for switching off the undifferentiated state. And if so, they will replicate in perpetuity and for all practical purposes they are cancer cells. I do not know of any evidence which would refute that idea, and I think we should not make the assumption that we need carcinogens, either viral or non-viral, to make cancers. It is quite possible that they are simply a more efficient agent for doing this, but the cancerous process is something that can happen by mechanisms that do not require the mediation of an external or an internal abnormal agent of this kind.

G. Barski: I have a question for Dr. Spiegelman and a comment on Dr. Klein's report. Dr. Spiegelman, have you had the opportunity to check for reverse transcriptase in virus mutants which are non-transforming and which are now available for Rauscher and Gros leukemia and Rous sarcoma viruses? Now about Dr. Klein's very interesting data; I will only add that in homologous mouse hybrids we obtained, we always found a tendency to chromosomal loss *in vitro* and *in vivo*. It was difficult to establish a systematic relationship between this chromosomal loss and appearance or disappearance of malignancy. In other words we have a display of clones in some homologous mouse hybrids in which the chromosomal loss, which is systematic, is not related in a clear way with appearance or disappearance of malignancy. In other species, especially Chinese hamster, we find that mostly malignancy and chromosomal loss go together. This chromosomal loss is sometimes quite dramatic. However, in some cases we have a near complete preservation of both chromosomal sets and still malignant properties.

S. Spiegelman: Actually the one case I know is the one by Hanafusa, who looked at a non-transforming variety he had of the Rous agent and he did not find the polymerase. The other non-transforming variants should be looked at.

J. Svoboda: I would like to mention briefly experiments which are very similar to those Prof. Kaplan already mentioned, and in this case we studied the expression of RSV in mammalian hybrids of the ascitic rat cells, which produce chicken sarcoma virus B77, and A9 cells derived from the mouse strain which is non-permissive for the chicken sarcoma virus. The aim was to study whether it was possible to obtain a progeny of hybrid cells which would be at least either poor virus producers or which would be able to replicate the genome without expression of the whole virion function. We studied ten hybrid clones and in most we found a great repression of virus production; one clone behaved as a virogenic one. So, using this method properly, we can analyze the problem of expression of the viral genome, not having the background of homologous virus genomes present in the chicken cells.

Just a very short comment on the statement of Dr. Bentvelzen that virus formation is probably necessary for transformation. I would like remind him that there are a number of lines which are perfectly transformed with virus and which have all the properties of transformation but the full virions are not formed.

P. Bentvelzen: I did not say full virion, I only said replication of viral RNA.

K. Scherer: Dr. Klein's comment brought back into focus that transformation is a very rare event and the corrolary of this is also trivial, this is that viruses replicate happily everywhere in the animal world. Therefore, I think we should bring into focus that what the virus has to do in order to accomplish its task is to fit into the mechanism of the cell *per se*. Now for those familiar, not so much with viruses and cancer as with the molecular biology of the animals, it is not difficult to understand how the virus would replicate its genome.

However, what is much more difficult to understand is how the virus would be able to express its information in terms of messenger RNA. Unfortunately we do not know very much about messenger RNA information in the animal cells, but one thing is clear: that this is a fantastically complicated process and much more complicated than the replication of macromolecules. And therefore I think we should keep in mind that the essential thing for the virus to do is to fit into this assembly line, and it is not excluded from this point of view that, for example, the reverse transcriptase has to accomplish the task of bringing back into the machinery of the cell the information that the virus needs. It means that integration, maybe of only part of the genome, is necessary for the expression of the information that the virus wants to have expressed.

F. Jacob: I think that the two cases of the MTV and RSV are quite different, and also the problem of the expression and of the insertion has probably to be considered differently. Now in the case of the MTV, if I understand correctly, the idea is that DNA of the virus is within the genome anyway, and then that in order for a tumor to occur you will have to have replication and this is based mainly on the number of particles, which perhaps is not a very strong proof but is a finding anyway. And in the case of the RSV the situation is different and I think the suggestion of Scherer may probably be a very interesting one: that in order for the Rous virus to be able to express and to replicate it should first go to the genome where the necessary punctuation for transcription is put in. RSV behaves different from, let us say polio. Whereas the polio RNA appears to function as a messenger, probably the RSV as such, when it comes in, does not function as messenger. When messenger is asked to be made from DNA, it may be that it is necessary first to insert the RSV as DNA into the host cell DNA in order to provide in this system punctuation for transcription. I think this is a very interesting idea.

R.A. Weiss: I think it is not right to talk about a genome expression in cell hybrids, particularly in the light of Dr. Jacob's comment. When you get a switch-off of particle production it may well be that something is operating at the cell membrane. The budding of the virus particles maybe has nothing to do with the genome expression inside the cell. And I think one could argue the same for the antigen, so I think one should just talk about the expression of details and to be careful in talking about genome activation and so on.

The other thing about cell hybridization, especially when people talk about contact inhibition and degrees of malignancy, is that when you fuse together two malignant cells of the same type (homokaryon) they very often lose a lot of the expression of malignancy. I am thinking further of the very fine work of Bob Pollack where in cultures of SV40 or polyoma transformed cells, hybrid cells or giant cells start to behave as flat revertants. They have the same quality of information but there is a different dosage of chromosomes. They show extreme contact inhibition, and in fact they revert to the malignant state when they begin to lose chromosomes again, and become more like the diploid state. And here there is nothing about fusing two different kinds of cells and this is a very common phenomenon in any transformed cell line. The giant cells which naturally arise tend to be less malignant in this way. And one more point, when I started using Sendai virus, not for inducing cell fusion but just helping viruses to get in, I started using the same stock as H. Harris uses. I found that UV inactivated Sendai virus preparations contain live leukosis virus, in large quantities, because after all it is grown in eggs. Molecular biologists do not care whether eggs contain RIF and even if the latter do not, it is beginning to seem likely that when you passage myxo-viruses through eggs which contain helper factors that you will release the helper viruses. So any studies on the biochemical level looking at changes in RNA synthesis patterns must take into account that most people are using Sendai virus which contains live leukosis virus.

G. Klein: As to the homokaryons, and also to the hybrids between two sarcoma cells — we have done such experiments, but I had no time to mention it — they remain highly malignant. So, in other words, there is something specific about the lymphoma-sarcoma type of complementation that cannot be reproduced by sarcoma hybrids. On the second point, of course, I completely agree with what you say about the *in vitro* behavior, but I think, and this is why I have been stressing this all the time, the only criterion of malignant behavior is the *in vivo* growth and that is what we are trying to use.

N.J. Duker: Before Dr. Temin left he quoted Dr. Spiegelman as saying that DNA hybridization of mammalian DNA is impossible, could Dr. Spiegelman comment on this?

S. Spiegelman: I did not say it was impossible, but it is difficult. Let me point out something. The nature of the hypotheses we have been listening to today from Temin and also from Huebner, are distinguishable experimentally quite clearly because they make two rather sharp distinctions. The Huebner hypothesis predicts that there exists in the genome of the cell the information contained in the virus. You should therefore be able to find it by molecular hybridization. It essentially should all be there. The Temin hypothesis says that initially all the information is not there. It gets put there by gene amplification involving the use of the reverse transcriptase. We are taking RNA message, make a DNA copy and it goes back again, and so you extend the message that way. So Temin would predict two things. According to his hypothesis, in the non-cancer cell you should find less information than corresponds to the information you find in the virus, and furthermore he makes the prediction that normal cells must contain reverse transcriptase. This is not an enzyme, according to his hypothesis, which is unique to the oncogenic RNA viruses. Thus those are, in principle, testable hypotheses.

Now, the use of molecular hybridization to get an answer to this problem is not a trivial one. We developed a method of RNA-DNA hybridization with bacteria and bacterial viruses, and we were dealing with organisms of a genome size of the order of about 10^9 daltons, or lower in the case of the T phages. Now as soon as you go to things like mammals you increase the amount of genetic information per genome by 3 orders of magnitude. And I mean an experiment where, in the case of bacteria, one can find a gene by molecular hybridization in an annealing reaction which takes say twelve hours. Since in a mammal each gene which is represented only once is present in 1/1000 the molar concentration per gamma of DNA, what took us twelve hours to do will take 12,000 hours to do.

And you cannot carry out those experiments under the usual conditions. That is one thing. So the methods have to be modified, have to be made more sensitive, and you could have predicted with the very simplest calculation that anybody who finds hybridization in mammalian material in experiments which follow the bacterial protocol must be looking at multiple copies. Those are the only ones you would find. And those are the only ones which have been found. In order to find the other ones you will have to devise new tricks. And those tricks really have not as yet been devised to my knowledge. You'll find that most of the published experiments with mammalian hybridization are full of flaws which are perfectly obvious to those who have experience with the technique. For example you very rarely see saturation curves with mammalian material and the reason is very simple: they do not exist. As you keep on pushing your RNA in, you find that you can put more and more RNA in. You can take, for example, the message of the hemoglobin as isolated and try to do a saturation curve with mammalian DNA, and you come to the surprising and unbelievable answer that 4% of the genome is concerned with the synthesis of hemoglobin. Well, clearly there is something wrong. Now what is wrong? In part, it is not simply that the genome is more complicated, and therefore each gene is present in a smaller amount. There is something else going on there. And that is: you apparently can get non-specific pairing which is resistant to ribonuclease. If you do something as simple as this, take the ribosomal RNA, try to do a saturation curve, you get a very complicated thing. It looks as if it is starting to go into a plateau and then it just goes right out. If you make an inverse plot of the data that you get in such experiments, it is perfectly clear that you are looking at two different things. One is a specific pairing and the other is a non-specific pairing. Now the non-specific pairing, curiously enough, and the one which occurs with higher frequency, only occurs at higher inputs of RNA. Now this does not make sense, immediately. But if you look at what has been going on in Manford Eigen's laboratory on the study of the hybridization process as a reaction, you see that they have shown very elegantly by their fast reaction kinetic methods that hybridization is a two-step process. One is a nucleation phenomenon which requires the formation of a perfectly paired triplet and then the thing goes very fast. But the first step, the pairing of the first three bases, is the slow reaction. Now when you are doing perfect pairing there is no problem. But look what happens supposing an RNA molecule is trying to pair imperfectly. It has to get over that first step, because if it makes a triplet and then the next base is unpaired it will fall off again. But if you keep on pushing it, it will bypass some mistakes after a while and zip up later on in the game. But now you have there an imperfectly paired structure. And a lot of what we have been put into the game in the last year and a half, is to find out how to avoid such imperfect pairing. How do you really get good saturation curves which are reliable and how do you get good competition curves which are reliable? In most of the papers which have been published on mammalian systems you will notice very strange competition phenomena. Even in homologous competition you will find somebody putting in, say one gamma labeled RNA and then he chases with a hundred times as much cold homologous RNA, and he only chases out 60% of the counts. Well, there is something wrong. And this is what is wrong. And so one has to devise a procedure which avoids this second plateau and these procedures involve forming the hybridization at the limit of hybridizability, so that only perfectly paired regions can form. This means that the hybridizing you would like to do at high temperature is out of the question because you cannot carry out a long-term hybridization at high temperatures. And the best things to use for this are things like formamide at the proper concentration, and so you can achieve what look like reasonable saturation and competition curves. They are not yet perfect but this is a direction that methods really have to take, and only when these are perfected will it be possible to use the molecular hybridization approach to try to make a decision between the kinds of hypotheses we have been hearing today.

H.S. Kaplan: Thank you very much. I think that it is obvious that we could go on all day and probably the next week but there has to be a time for stopping and this is probably it. I would like to thank the audience and the panelists, including those who had to leave us early, and I would also like, on behalf of all of the foreign participants, once again to thank the Organizing Committee for this invitation to us. Finally, I sincerely hope that Professor Mühlbock has enjoyed, as much as all of us have, this splendid conference in his honor.